T0263867

Don't Forget Your Online Access to ExpertConsult.com

Mobile. Searchable. Expandable.

ACCESS it on any Internet-ready device

SEARCH all Expert Consult titles you own

LINK to PubMed abstracts

ALREADY REGISTERED?

1. Log in at expertconsult.com
2. Scratch off your Activation Code below
3. Enter it into the "Add a Title" box
4. Click "Activate Now"
5. Click the title under "My Titles"

FIRST-TIME USER?

1. *REGISTER*
   - Click "Register Now" at expertconsult.com
   - Fill in your user information and click "Continue"
2. *ACTIVATE YOUR BOOK*
   - Scratch off your Activation Code below
   - Enter it into the "Enter Activation Code" box
   - Click "Activate Now"
   - Click the title under "My Titles"

For technical assistance:
email online.help@elsevier.com
call 800-401-9962 (inside the US)
call +1-314-995-3200 (outside the US)

Activation Code

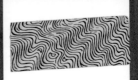

ExpertConsult.com

Echocardiography in Congenital Heart Disease

PRACTICAL ECHOCARDIOGRAPHY SERIES

Look for these other titles in Catherine M. Otto's Practical Echocardiography Series

Donald C. Oxorn
Intraoperative Echocardiography

Linda D. Gillam & Catherine M. Otto
Advanced Approaches in Echocardiography

Martin St. John Sutton & Susan E. Wiegers
Echocardiography in Heart Failure

Echocardiography in Congenital Heart Disease

PRACTICAL ECHOCARDIOGRAPHY SERIES

Mark B. Lewin, MD
Professor and Chief
Division of Pediatric Cardiology
University of Washington School of Medicine
Heart Center Co-Director and Director of Pediatric Echocardiography
Seattle Children's Hospital
Seattle, Washington

Karen Stout, MD
Director, Adult Congenital Heart Disease Program
Associate Professor, Departments of Medicine and Pediatrics
University of Washington School of Medicine
Attending Cardiologist
University of Washington Medical Center and Seattle Children's Hospital
Seattle, Washington

ELSEVIER
SAUNDERS

1600 John F. Kennedy Blvd.
Ste 1800
Philadelphia, PA 19103-2899

ECHOCARDIOGRAPHY IN CONGENITAL HEART DISEASE   ISBN: 978-1-4377-2696-1
Copyright © 2012 by Saunders, an imprint of Elsevier Inc.

No part of this publication may be reproduced or transmitted in any form or by any means, electronic or mechanical, including photocopying, recording, or any information storage and retrieval system, without permission in writing from the publisher. Details on how to seek permission, further information about the Publisher's permissions policies and our arrangements with organizations such as the Copyright Clearance Center and the Copyright Licensing Agency, can be found at our website: www.elsevier.com/permissions.

This book and the individual contributions contained in it are protected under copyright by the Publisher (other than as may be noted herein).

Notices

Knowledge and best practice in this field are constantly changing. As new research and experience broaden our understanding, changes in research methods, professional practices, or medical treatment may become necessary.

Practitioners and researchers must always rely on their own experience and knowledge in evaluating and using any information, methods, compounds, or experiments described herein. In using such information or methods they should be mindful of their own safety and the safety of others, including parties for whom they have a professional responsibility.

With respect to any drug or pharmaceutical products identified, readers are advised to check the most current information provided (i) on procedures featured or (ii) by the manufacturer of each product to be administered, to verify the recommended dose or formula, the method and duration of administration, and contraindications. It is the responsibility of practitioners, relying on their own experience and knowledge of their patients, to make diagnoses, to determine dosages and the best treatment for each individual patient, and to take all appropriate safety precautions.

To the fullest extent of the law, neither the Publisher nor the authors, contributors, or editors, assume any liability for any injury and/or damage to persons or property as a matter of products liability, negligence or otherwise, or from any use or operation of any methods, products, instructions, or ideas contained in the material herein.

Library of Congress Cataloging-in-Publication Data
Echocardiography in congenital heart disease/[edited by] Mark B. Lewin, Karen Stout.
     p. ; cm.—(Practical echocardiography series)
  Includes bibliographical references and index.
  ISBN 978-1-4377-2696-1 (hardcover : alk. paper)
  I. Lewin, Mark B.   II. Stout, Karen.   III. Series: Practical echocardiography series.
  [DNLM: 1. Echocardiography—methods—Handbooks.   2. Heart Defects, Congenital—
ultrasonography—Handbooks. WG 39]
  LC classification not assigned
  618.92'1207543—dc23

                                                                    2011036498

Senior Acquisitions Editor: Dolores Meloni
Editorial Assistant: Brad McIlwain
Publishing Services Manager: Pat Joiner-Myers
Project Manager: Marlene Weeks
Designer: Steven Stave

Working together to grow
libraries in developing countries

www.elsevier.com | www.bookaid.org | www.sabre.org

ELSEVIER   BOOK AID International   Sabre Foundation

Contributors

Peter J. Cawley, MD, FACC
Acting Assistant Professor of Medicine, University of Washington School of Medicine; Attending Cardiologist, University of Washington Medical Center, Seattle, Washington
Thromboembolic Phenomena and Vegetations

Nadine F. Choueiter, MD
Pediatric Cardiology Fellow, University of Washington School of Medicine; Seattle Children's Hospital, Seattle, Washington
Echocardiographic Imaging of Single-Ventricle Lesions

Raylene M. Choy, RDCS
Cardiac Sonographer, Heart Center, Seattle Children's Hospital, Seattle, Washington
Echocardiographic Imaging of Single-Ventricle Lesions

Jeffrey A. Conwell, MD
Associate Professor of Pediatrics, Division of Pediatric Cardiology, University of Washington School of Medicine; Attending Cardiologist, Seattle Children's Hospital, Seattle, Washington
Atrioventricular Septal Defect: Echocardiographic Assessment
Kawasaki Disease: Echocardiographic Assessment

Brandy Hattendorf, MD
Assistant Professor of Pediatrics, University of Washington School of Medicine; Attending Cardiologist, Seattle Children's Hospital, Seattle, Washington
Shunting Lesions
Implications of Pediatric Renal, Endocrine, and Oncologic Disease

Denise Joffe, MD
Associate Professor of Anesthesiology, Department of Anesthesiology, University of Washington School of Medicine; Seattle Children's Hospital, Seattle, Washington
Intraoperative Transesophageal Echocardiography

Troy Johnston, MD
Associate Professor of Pediatrics, University of Washington School of Medicine; Attending Cardiologist, Seattle Children's Hospital, Seattle, Washington
Echocardiography in the Cardiac Catheterization Laboratory

Mariska Kemna, MD
Assistant Professor of Pediatrics, University of Washington School of Medicine; Attending Cardiologist, Seattle Children's Hospital, Seattle, Washington
Myocardial Pathology
Echocardiographic Assessment After Heart Transplantation

Joel Lester, RDCS
Echocardiography Laboratory Supervisor, Heart Center, Seattle Children's Hospital, Seattle, Washington
The Pediatric Transthoracic Echocardiogram

Mark B. Lewin, MD
Professor and Chief, Division of Pediatric Cardiology, University of Washington School of Medicine; Heart Center Co-Director and Director of Pediatric Echocardiography, Seattle Children's Hospital, Seattle, Washington
The Pediatric Transthoracic Echocardiogram
Right Heart Anomalies

Maggie L. Likes, MD

Assistant Professor of Pediatrics, University of Washington School of Medicine; Attending Cardiologist, Seattle Children's Hospital, Seattle, Washington
Right Heart Anomalies

David S. Owens, MD

Acting Assistant Professor of Medicine, University of Washington School of Medicine; Attending Cardiologist, University of Washington Medical Center, Seattle, Washington
Left Heart Anomalies
Myocardial Pathology

Amy H. Schultz, MD

Assistant Professor of Pediatrics, University of Washington School of Medicine; Attending Cardiologist, Seattle Children's Hospital, Seattle, Washington
Conotruncal Lesions
Transposition of the Great Arteries

Brian D. Soriano, MD

Assistant Professor of Pediatrics, University of Washington School of Medicine; Attending Cardiologist, Seattle Children's Hospital, Seattle, Washington
Venous Anomalies
Left Heart Anomalies
Thromboembolic Phenomena and Vegetations

Karen Stout, MD

Director, Adult Congenital Heart Disease Program, Associate Professor, Departments of Medicine and Pediatrics, University of Washington School of Medicine; Attending Cardiologist, University of Washington Medical Center and Seattle Children's Hospital, Seattle, Washington

Margaret M. Vernon, MD

Assistant Professor of Pediatrics, University of Washington School of Medicine; Attending Cardiologist, Seattle Children's Hospital, Seattle, Washington
The Fetal Echocardiogram

Foreword

Echocardiography is a core component of every aspect of clinical cardiology and now plays an essential role in daily decision making. Both echocardiographers and clinicians face unique challenges in interpretation of imaging and Doppler data and in integration of these data with other clinical information. However, with the absorption of echocardiography into daily patient care, there are several unmet needs in our collective knowledge base. First, clinicians caring for patients need to understand the value, strengths, and limitations of echocardiography relevant to their specific scope of practice. Second, echocardiographers need a more in-depth understanding of the clinical context of the imaging study. Finally, there often are unique aspects of data acquisition and analysis in different clinical situations, all of which are essential for accurate echocardiographic diagnosis. The books in the *Practical Echocardiography Series* are aimed at filling these knowledge gaps, with each book focusing on a specific clinical situation in which echocardiographic data are key for optimal patient care.

In addition to *Echocardiography in Congenital Heart Disease*, edited by Mark B. Lewin, MD, and Karen Stout, MD, other books in the series are *Intraoperative Echocardiography*, edited by Donald C. Oxorn, MD; *Echocardiography in Heart Failure*, edited by Martin St. John Sutton, MD, and Susan E. Wiegers, MD; and *Advanced Approaches in Echocardiography*, edited by Linda D. Gillam, MD, and myself. Information is presented as concise bulleted text accompanied by numerous illustrations and tables, providing a practical approach to data acquisition and analysis, including technical details, pitfalls, and clinical interpretation, supplemented by web-based video case examples. Each volume in this series expands on the basic principles presented in the *Textbook of Clinical Echocardiography, fourth edition*, and can be used as a supplement to that text or can be used by physicians interested in a focused introduction to echocardiography in their area of clinical practice.

Patients with congenital heart disease are increasingly encountered in clinical practice due to the success of surgical and medical treatment of these conditions, allowing survival into adulthood. At the same time, each of us may see only a few cases of each type of congenital heart disease because of the wide range of congenital lesions and the variety of surgical repair techniques. Thus, easily accessible and concise information is needed when these patients are seen to ensure that the echocardiographic study is performed and interpreted correctly.

The editors of *Echocardiography in Congenital Heart Disease*, Mark B. Lewin and Karen Stout, are recognized experts with robust clinical experience that includes pediatric, adolescent, and adult patients with congenital heart disease. In this book the editors provide a comprehensive discussion of echocardiography in the patient with congenital heart disease, spanning the entire age range from birth to old age. This book is aimed at all clinicians who care for patients with congenital heart disease, whether in the pediatric or adult setting, including cardiologists, cardiology fellows, cardiac sonographers, anesthesiologists, and cardiac surgeons.

The wealth of information provided in this book is truly awesome. Every clinician who sees patients with congenital heart disease and every echocardiography laboratory will want a copy close at hand.

Catherine M. Otto, MD

Preface

This text is one of four in the *Practical Echocardiography Series*, which covers the range of echocardiographic topics. The topics in the other three volumes in this set include *Intraoperative Echocardiography, Echocardiography in Heart Failure*, and *Advanced Approaches in Echocardiography*. This volume provides a resource for those interested in pediatric and adult congenital echocardiography. The chapters are designed to review basic principles, provide details of image acquisition and interpretation, and describe how echocardiography is used to develop management strategies.

This book will be of interest to cardiology and sonographer trainees, as well as practicing cardiologists and sonographers, as an overview of pediatric and congenital echocardiography. The chapters cover general pediatric echo imaging protocols, individual congenital cardiac diagnoses, cardiomyopathies, and other pediatric organ system disorders in which cardiac structural or functional assessment is necessary. There are also chapters devoted to congenital transesophageal echo as well as echo imaging in the cardiac catheterization laboratory.

Each chapter includes a *step-by-step approach to patient examination*, bulleted points of *major principles*, and lists of *key points*. Those areas where echo can serve as a resource for accurately working through a differential diagnosis are also pointed out. Methods regarding quantitative data analysis and calculations are also included. Numerous echo images and illustrations with detailed figure legends demonstrate important principles. This book does not replace formal training in pediatric and congenital echocardiography but rather serves as a supplement to this training. Accredited training is the only method of obtaining all the tools needed to obtain accurate echocardiographic data, and we fully endorse this process.

Mark B. Lewin, MD
Karen Stout, MD

Acknowledgments

We could never have completed this work if not for the dedication and skills of our authors. The cardiac sonographers at Seattle Children's Hospital and the University of Washington deserve recognition for their commitment to superb imaging and the dedication they show to patients, families, and their colleagues. From Seattle Children's these include Heidi Borchers, RDCS; Colleen Cailes, RDCS; Raylene Choy, RDCS; Mikki Clouse, RDCS; Judy Devine, RDCS; Alison Freeberg, RDCS; Laura Huntley, RDCS; Mary Jordan, RDCS; Joel Lester, RDCS; Danielle Saliba, RDCS; Pauline Suon, RDCS; Shelby Thomas-Irish, RDCS; and Erin Trent, RDCS. From the University of Washington these include Caryn D'Jang, RDCS; Michelle Fujioka, RDCS; Yelena Kovalenko, RDCS; Amy Loscher, RDCS; Todd Zwink, RDCS; Pamela Clark, RDCS; Sarah Curtis, RDCS; Jennifer Gregov, RDCS; Carol Kraft, RDCS; Chris McKenzie, RDCS; Joannalyn Sangco, RDCS; and Rebecca G. Schwaegler, RDCS. Special thanks to Catherine Otto, MD, for her careful attention to detail and dedication to this project. We also wish to acknowledge Natasha Andjelkovic, Bradley McIlwain, and Marla Sussman at Elsevier, who kept us on track and on time.

Of course, finally (and most importantly) the unwavering support of our families cannot be overlooked. Deb, Johanne, Julien, and Cal are always in our hearts!

Mark B. Lewin, MD
Karen Stout, MD

Contents

Glossary

2C two-chamber view
4C four-chamber view
5C five-chamber view
2D two-dimensional
3D three-dimensional
A4C apical four-chamber view
AA aortic arch
AAO aortic arch obstruction
ACC American College of Cardiology
AHA American Heart Association
AI aortic insufficiency
ALCAPA anomalous origin of the left coronary artery from the pulmonary artery
Ao aorta
APB absent pulmonary valve
AR aortic regurgitation
aRV atrialized right ventricle
AS aortic stenosis; atrial septum
ASD atrial septal defect
ASO arterial switch operation
AV atrioventricular; aortic valve
AVC atrioventricular canal; aortic valve closure
AVR aortic valve replacement
AVS atrioventricular septum
AVSD atrioventricular septal defect
AVV atrioventricular valve
AVVR atrioventricular valve regurgitation
bpm beats per minute
BSA body surface area
BT Blalock-Taussig
BVF bulboventricular foramen
cc-TGA congenitally corrected transposition of the great arteries
CFD color flow Doppler
CHD congenital heart disease
CI confidence interval
CM cardiomyopathy
CMR cardiac magnetic resonance imaging
CoA coarctation of the aorta
CPB cardiopulmonary bypass
CS coronary sinus
CT computed tomography
CW continuous wave
Cx circumflex coronary artery

DA ductus arteriosus
DAo descending aorta
DCM dilated cardiomyopathy
DCRV double-chamber right ventricle
DILV double-inlet left ventricle
DKS Damus-Kaye-Stansel (procedure)
DORV double-outlet right ventricle
dP/dt rate of change in pressure over time
DSE dobutamine stress echocardiography
dT/dt rate of increase in temperature
d-TGA dextro-transposition of the great arteries
E early diastolic peak velocity
E' early diastolic tissue Doppler velocity
ECG electrocardiogram
echo echocardiography
EF ejection fraction
EFE endocardial fibroelastastosis
ET ejection time
FAC fractional area change
FO foramen ovale
FS fractional shortening
GOS Great Ormond Street
GV great vessel
HCM hypertrophic cardiomyopathy
HIV human immunodeficiency virus
HLHS hypoplastic left heart syndrome
HR heart rate
IAS interatrial septum
ICE intracardiac echocardiography
ILB inferior limbic bands
IVA isovolumic acceleration
IVC inferior vena cava; isovolumic contraction
IVCT isovolumic contraction time
IVRT isovolumic relaxation time
IVS interventricular septum; intact ventricular system
IVSD inlet ventricular septal defect
LA left atrium
LAA left atrial appendage
LAD left descending artery
LAE left atrial enlargement
LAX long axis view
LCA left coronary artery
LCC left coronary cusp

LLPV left lower pulmonary vein
LM left mural leaflet
LMCA left main coronary artery
LPA left pulmonary artery
LRV lower reference value
LSVC left superior vena cava
L-TGA levo-TGA
LUPV left upper pulmonary vein
LV left ventricle
LVE left ventricular enlargement
LVED left ventricular end-diastolic dimension
LVH left ventricular hypertrophy
LVM left ventricular mass
LVN left ventricular noncompaction
LVO left ventricular outflow
LVOT left ventricular outflow tract
LVOTO left ventricular outflow tract obstruction
LVP left ventricular pressure
LVPW left ventricular posterior wall
MAPCA major aortopulmonary collateral artery
m-BT modified Blalock-Taussig
ME midesophageal
MIPG maximal instantaneous pressure gradient
M-mode motion display (depth versus time)
MPA main pulmonary artery
MPI myocardial performance index
MPR mulitplanar reconstruction
MR mitral regurgitation
MRI magnetic resonance imaging
MS mitral stenosis
MV mitral valve
MVI myocardial videointensity
NBTE nonbacterial thrombotic endocarditis
NCC noncoronary cusp
PA pulmonary artery; pulmonary atresia
PA/IVS pulmonary atresia with intact ventricular septum
PAP pulmonary artery pressure
PAPVC partial anomalous pulmonary venous connection
PAPVD partial anomalous pulmonary venous drainage
PASP pulmonary artery systolic pressure
PBF pulmonary blood flow
PBL posterior bridging leaflet
PDA patent ductus arteriosus; posterior descending artery
PE pericardial effusion
PFO patent foramen ovale
PHTN pulmonary hypertension
PI pulmonary insufficiency
PIPG peak instantaneous pressure gradient
PISA proximal isovelocity surface area
PLAX parasternal long axis view
PPV positive pressure ventilation
PR pulmonary regurgitation
PS pulmonary stenosis
PSAX parasternal short axis view

pulmV pulmonary valve
PV pulmonary vein
PVR pulmonary vascular resistance
PW pulsed wave
Q_p pulmonary volume flow rate
Q_s systemic volume flow rate
RA right atrium
RAA right atrial appendage
RAE right atrial enlargement
RAP right atrial pressure
RCA right coronary artery
RCC right coronary cusp
RCM restrictive cardiomyopathy
RI right inferior leaflet
RLPV right lower pulmonary vein
ROA regurgitant orifice area
RPA right pulmonary artery
RUPV right upper pulmonary vein
RV right ventricle
RVD right ventricle diameter
RVDCC right ventricle–dependent coronary circulation
RVE right ventricule enlargement
RVEDV right ventricular end-diastolic volume
RVH right ventricular hypertrophy
RVO right ventricular outflow
RVOT right ventricular outflow tract
RVOTO right ventricular outflow tract obstruction
RVP right ventricular pressure
RWMA regional wall motion abnormality
s second
SAM systolic anterior motion
SAX short axis view
SBF systemic blood flow
SC subcostal
SCD sudden cardiac death
SCLAX subcostal long axis view
SCSAX subcostal short axis view
SD standard deviation
SLB superior limbic band
SLE systemic lupus erythematosus
SR strain rate
SSFP single-state free-precession
SSN suprasternal notch
SV single ventricle; stroke volume
SVC superior vena cava
TA tricuspid atresia
TAPSE tricuspid annular plane systolic excursion
TAPVC total anomalous pulmonary venous connection
TAPVD total anomalous pulmonary venous drainage
TDI tissue Doppler imaging
TEE transesophageal echocardiography
TG transgastric
TGA transposition of the great arteries

TOF tetralogy of Fallot
TR tricuspid regurgitation
TS tricuspid stenosis
TTE transthoracic echocardiography
TV tricuspid valve

UE upper esophageal
URV upper reference value
VS ventricular septum
VSD ventricular septal defect
VVI velocity vector imaging

I

PEDIATRIC AND CONGENITAL IMAGING PRINCIPLES AND TECHNIQUES

The Pediatric Transthoracic Echocardiogram

1

Joel Lester and Mark B. Lewin

Imaging Planes

KEY POINTS

- Imaging planes may be unique to each individual patient; for example, in the setting of a newborn with a diaphragmatic hernia, the typical views may be obtained from nonstandard locations on the chest because the heart is displaced significantly within the thoracic cavity.
- Best practice is to obtain two-dimensional (2D) imaging before spectral or color flow Doppler. This allows for an anatomic frame of reference before the addition of physiologic data.
- Before acquisition of Doppler data, an anatomic 2D image should be recorded to document the curser position.
- Ergonomics should be considered at all times (Figs. 1-1 and 1-2). Make yourself comfortable. Based on patient age, location where study is being performed, and other environmental conditions (i.e., patient instrumentation, patient body position restrictions, lighting conditions), accommodations may be required to optimize image acquisition. This can make the difference between an exam that shows the pathology at a quality level, which allows for an accurate diagnosis, and a study that is incomplete, requiring subsequent imaging or resulting in incorrect management decisions.
- Standard adult imaging planes and views apply. However, variations of these views are required to optimally image atypical anatomy and cardiac position.
- Nonstandard views are frequently used to assess complex anatomy and track the route of extracardiac anatomic structures and vessels that cannot be seen in a single view. For example, a right ventricle (RV)-to-pulmonary

Continued

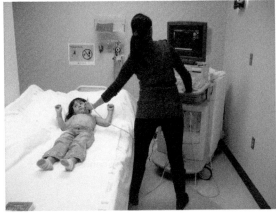

Figure 1-1. This image shows poor ergonomics including the patient is positioned too far from the sonographer, there is no arm support, the patient bed is too low, the sonographer is standing, and the echocardiography (echo) machine is too far away from the patient. All these factors result in poor sonographer posture that drastically increases the likelihood of injury to the back, neck, and shoulders. It also makes it difficult to sustain this position for any length of time, which may be required if the anatomy is difficult to sort out.

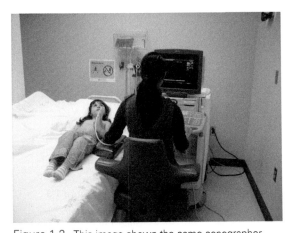

Figure 1-2. This image shows the same sonographer and patient with a drastic improvement in ergonomics. The patient has been moved closer to the sonographer, the bed has been raise, the sonographer is seated, and the echo machine is pulled closer to the patient, reducing the amount of reaching the sonographer has to withstand. Note the ergonomic "tools" used: the specialized chair and arm support cushion. The result is a more comfortable sonographer, which will reduce the risk of injury and increase the ability to scan for longer periods of time.

artery (PA) conduit may require evaluation in three separate imaging planes to obtain a complete assessment: parasternal to visualize the mid-conduit, apical to image the conduit origin, and subcostal to image the distal end at the pulmonary branch bifurcation.

- With the use of nonstandard views, it is critical to acquire confirmatory points of reference,

to obtain longer clips, and to demonstrate anatomic relationships via sweeps from one plane to the next. This will allow the interpreting physician the opportunity to render the most accurate diagnosis.

- Use annotation on the clip to communicate findings and relay information as to the intent of clip acquisition (Table 1-1, Figs. 1-3 to 1-10).

TABLE 1-1 IMAGING PLANES

Window	View	Basic Anatomy Viewed
Left parasternal	LV long axis Slice 2 in Figure 1-3	LV Ventricular septum MV (and supporting structures) AV LA CS Proximal aortic root
	RV inflow Slice 1 in Figure 1-3	RV TV (and supporting structures) RA
	RV outflow Slice 3 in Figure 1-3	RVOT Pulmonary valve Proximal main PA
	Short axis Slices 1, 2, and 3 in Figure 1-4	LV MV (and papillary muscles) AV Ventricular septum Coronary artery origins RVOT Pulmonary valve Main PA and branches TV AS PVs LPA/ductal
Apical	4C Figure 1-5	LV, RV VS AS AVVs Cardiac crux LA, RA RV moderator band Pulmonary venous flow/connection
	Slice 3 in Figure 1-3	CS
	"Five" chamber Slice 1 in Figure 1-5	LVOT
	Further anterior angulation	RVOT, pulmonary valve
	3C Figure 1-6	All structures noted in parasternal long axis views
Subcostal	4C Figure 1-7	LV, RV VS AS Left and right ventricular AVVs LVOT, RVOT

TABLE 1-1   IMAGING PLANES—cont'd

Window	View	Basic Anatomy Viewed
Subcostal—cont'd	Short axis Figure 1-8	VS RVOT AS IVC SVC
Right parasternal	Long axis	SVC Azygous vein Superior aspect of AS Ascending aorta RPA RCA
	Short axis	Ascending aorta RPA PPV
Suprasternal notch	Long axis Figure 1-9	Aortic arch Head and neck vessel branching Innominate vein RPA
	Short axis Figure 1-10	Ascending aorta Arch sidedness PV crab view Additional branch PA views

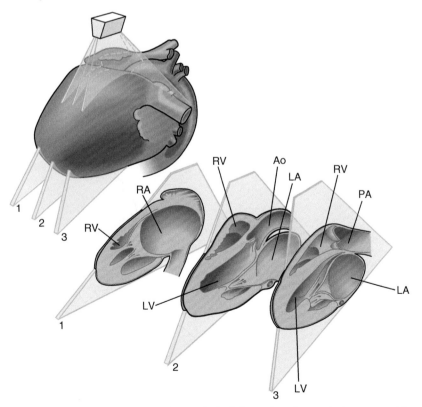

Figure 1-3. Parasternal long axis view: plane 1, right ventricular inflow; plane 2, standard parasternal long axis view through the left ventricle (LV); plane 3, right ventricular outflow. *(Adapted from Snider RA, Serwer GA, Ritter SB. Echocardiography in Pediatric Heart Disease. St. Louis: Mosby; 1980.)*

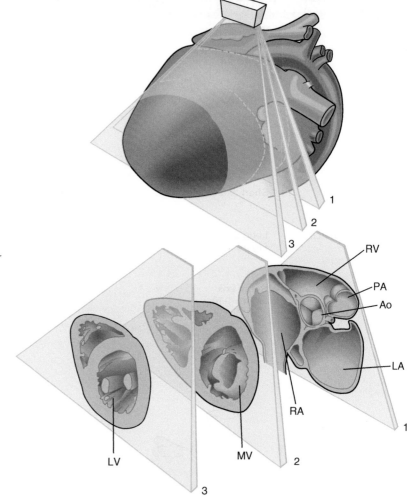

Figure 1-4. Parasternal short axis view: plane 1 at the base of the heart, plane 2 at the level of the mitral valve (MV), plane 3 is through the apical segment. *(Adapted from Snider RA, Serwer GA, Ritter SB.* Echocardiography in Pediatric Heart Disease. *St. Louis: Mosby; 1980.)*

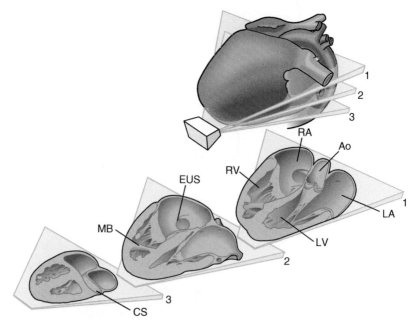
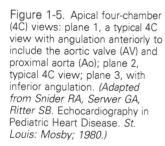

Figure 1-5. Apical four-chamber (4C) views: plane 1, a typical 4C view with angulation anteriorly to include the aortic valve (AV) and proximal aorta (Ao); plane 2, typical 4C view; plane 3, with inferior angulation. *(Adapted from Snider RA, Serwer GA, Ritter SB.* Echocardiography in Pediatric Heart Disease. *St. Louis: Mosby; 1980.)*

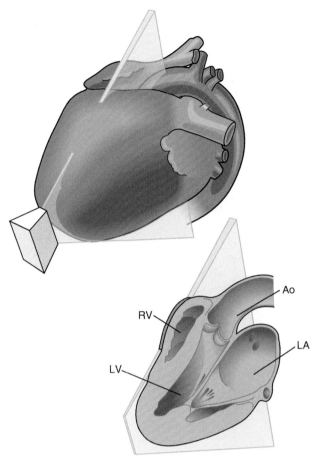

Figure 1-6. Apical three-chamber (3C) view, 90-degree counterclockwise rotation from the apical 4C view. *(Adapted from Snider RA, Serwer GA, Ritter SB. Echocardiography in Pediatric Heart Disease. St. Louis: Mosby; 1980.)*

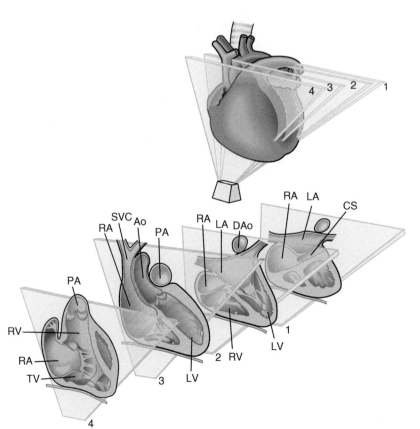

Figure 1-7. Subcostal 4C views. Plane 1 is with inferior angulation, plane 2 is a typical 4C view, plane 3 is with slight anterior angulation, and plane 4 has further angulation to include the right ventricular outflow tract (RVOT). *(Adapted from Snider RA, Serwer GA, Ritter SB. Echocardiography in Pediatric Heart Disease. St. Louis: Mosby; 1980.)*

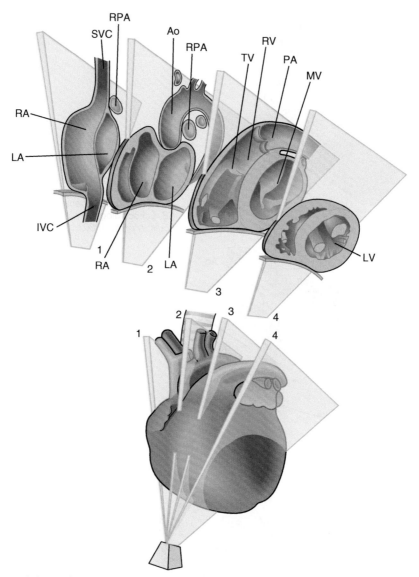

Figure 1-8. Subcostal short axis view, 90-degree clockwise rotation from the subcostal 4C view. Plane 1 is the bicaval view, plane 2 includes more of the atrial septal and aortic arch, plane 3 shows excellent visualization of the RVOT, and plane 4 is through the ventricular apex. *(Adapted from Snider RA, Serwer GA, Ritter SB. Echocardiography in Pediatric Heart Disease. St. Louis: Mosby; 1980.)*

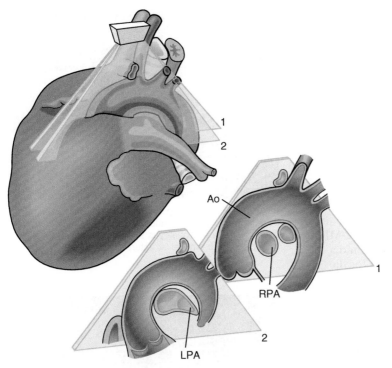

Figure 1-9. Suprasternal notch: long axis view. *(Adapted from Snider RA, Serwer GA, Ritter SB. Echocardiography in Pediatric Heart Disease. St. Louis: Mosby; 1980.)*

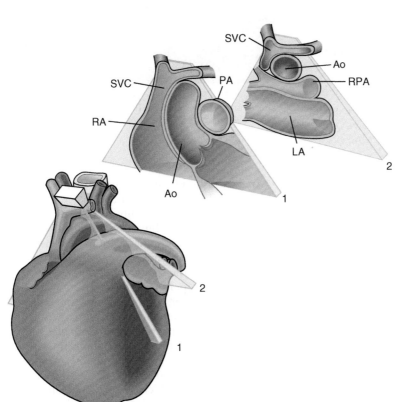

Figure 1-10. Suprasternal notch: short axis view. *(Adapted from Snider RA, Serwer GA, Ritter SB. Echocardiography in Pediatric Heart Disease. St. Louis: Mosby; 1980.)*

Transducers

- Whenever possible, the highest frequency transducer should be used. A higher frequency can provide better resolution, thus increasing accuracy in identifying smaller or more closely spaced structures.
- When performing pediatric echocardiography (echo), it is vital to have access to multiple transducers. Patient size and body habitus can vary widely, from the extremely premature infant weighing as little as 500 g to the adolescent weighing more than 100 kg. For each of these patients, numerous transducers may be required during the performance of a single study. It is typical for a 10- to 12-MHz transducer to be used for newborns, and a 1- to 3-MHz transducer to be used for the largest of patients.
- The same machine gain settings for image optimization apply as in all aspects of echo. However, adjustment in the Nyquist limit settings is common. For turbulent pathologic lesions (high cardiac output states, valve stenosis or regurgitation, a shunting lesion), the Nyquist limit is adjusted upward to avoid background noise. On the other hand, when assessing low-velocity flow (e.g., flow through pulmonary veins [PVs] or coronary arteries), the Nyquist limit settings are adjusted downward to enhance the opportunity to identify flow in these structures.
- New technologies continue to improve transducer quality, allowing for more versatility. A single transducer can now image in a wide array of imaging frequencies that can be changed easily on the machine's control panel.
- When appropriate, a lower frequency can be used to improve both color and spectral Doppler sensitivity. Keep in mind that this can result in degradation in 2D image quality. As a general rule, lower frequencies have better Doppler signals.
- New imaging modalities such as tissue Doppler imaging, harmonic imaging, and velocity vector imaging can also determine transducer selection. These features are being incorporated more and more as research is confirming their usefulness (Figs. 1-11 and 1-12).

Protocols

- Exam protocols should be followed to ensure that all structures are demonstrated and no important detail is overlooked.

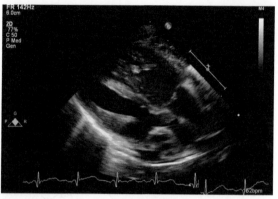

Figure 1-11. This image shows appropriate transducer selection with a high-frequency transducer on a newborn patient. The image quality is smooth with more detail and better suited to smaller structures.

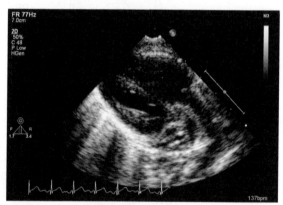

Figure 1-12. This image shows the same patient with an inappropriate transducer. The image quality is poor, and small structures are not nearly as well defined. The transducer frequency is too low.

- An established baseline protocol for any echo lab is of the utmost importance.
- A protocol should not only include the sequence of views but also include all expected measurement locations and methods of obtaining those measurements.
- In some labs, the sonographer will create a preliminary report, and this can be a part of the overall lab protocol. This postprocedure component of the lab protocol serves to further refine expectations and enhances the sonographer-physician relationship.
- Guidelines set by accrediting bodies can be a good place to start. This will establish a framework from which to develop a lab protocol most appropriate to the individual lab. Such a starting point will ensure that all necessary study and reporting components are included.

- There must be room for variation to further investigate pathology, take additional measurements, or account for patient movement or activity. Once straying from the protocol, it is important to return to the protocol to ensure that all views and information are comprehensively covered.

Sample Pediatric Protocol for a New Patient (Derived from Seattle Children's Hospital Protocol)

This document is meant to be a guideline. The echocardiographic procedure may be modified at the sonographer's discretion.

- Remember that a narrow sector creates better resolution, with both 2D and color. Be careful not to lose your frame of reference when using a narrow sector in 2D. All structures should be assessed by 2D imaging first; do not be too quick to put the color on!
- When acquiring any type of Doppler information, it is important to be as parallel as possible to flow to measure maximal velocity. It is important, especially with pathology, to perform Doppler imaging from multiple windows to ensure measurement of the maximal velocity. Always acquire a clip demonstrating your cursor placement before displaying spectral Doppler or M-mode tracings.

Acquiring Clips
- Use 3-second clips if the heart rate (HR) is more than 100 beats per minute (bpm) or there is an irregular rhythm (or at any time); three-beat clips may be used if the HR is less than 100 bpm and it is in sinus rhythm.

Parasternal Long Axis View
- 2D left ventricular long axis view. Demonstrate valve and ventricular function. Examine the coronary sinus (CS) for dilation. Focus on the mitral valve (MV) and aortic valve (AV) (separately); use zoom function if appropriate. Measure aortic annulus, sinus, and sinotubular junction in systole.
- Color Doppler of the MV and AV (separately, without zoom). Be sure to clip sweeps of the valves to evaluate for any anatomic abnormalities or eccentric regurgitation.
- Use color Doppler to evaluate the interventricular septum for any defects. Be sure to sweep all the way posterior and anterior. This may require multiple clips and may also require adjusting the Nyquist limit and gain.

- 2D image of the right ventricular inflow: evaluate tricuspid valve (TV) and right ventricular function.
- Color Doppler across the TV, evaluating for stenosis and regurgitation. Pulsed wave (PW) Doppler/continuous wave (CW) Doppler ultrasound of tricuspid regurgitation (TR) if angle is appropriate.
- 2D image of the right ventricular outflow tract (RVOT)/PA: evaluate pulmonary valve leaflets.
- Color Doppler across the pulmonary valve. PW Doppler RVOT and pulmonary valve. (A patent ductus arteriosus [PDA] may be seen from this view.)

Parasternal Short Axis View
- Obtain 2D clip with cursor demonstrating where the M-mode will be obtained.
- Obtain M-mode of the aortic root/left atrium (LA) (measure dimensions at end systole).
- Obtain M-mode of the right ventricular wall/RV/interventricular septum/left ventricle (LV)/left ventricular posterior wall (measure right ventricular wall and RV at end-diastole; interventricular septum/LV/left ventricular posterior wall measurements done in diastole and systole). M-mode should be performed at the MV leaflet tips (between the tip of the papillary muscle and the leaflet tips; M-mode will show just a little bit of the leaflet). Record image of M-mode with measurements to show where measurements were made.
- Zoom up on the aortic valve. 2D imaging to evaluate number and function of leaflets. Evaluate coronary artery origins by 2D and color Doppler (will need to turn Nyquist limit down to 30s or even 20s; keep color box small). Screen for an abnormal coronary vessel coursing between the aorta and PA.
- 2D sweep from the AV to the left ventricular apex. Be sure to have a good look at the MV structure (evaluate for cleft and papillary muscle structure).
- Color Doppler: Clip with color on the AV and a separate clip of color on the MV. Color sweep along both sides of the interventricular septum, from the AV to the left ventricular apex (may have to slide down an interspace to image the apical aspect). This may take multiple clips to view the entire septum.
- 2D of the right ventricular inflow.
- Color Doppler imaging across the tricuspid valve. PW Doppler/CW Doppler ultrasound of TR, if applicable.
- 2D imaging of the RVOT/pulmonary valve/main pulmonary artery/pulmonary artery branches. Zoom in on the pulmonary valve and measure the annulus.

- Color Doppler imaging from the RVOT through the branches (use a long, narrow sector). PW Doppler ultrasound of the RVOT, pulmonary valve, main pulmonary artery (if applicable), and right and left pulmonary branches. CW Doppler ultrasound across the pulmonary valve/main pulmonary artery. Evaluate for a PDA.
- Evaluate PVs with 2D and color Doppler imaging. May need to turn the Nyquist limit down and/or the gain up. Evaluate the atrial septum (AS) with 2D and color Doppler.

High Left Parasternal View
- This is a good view with which to evaluate for a PDA.
- From the parasternal short axis view, slide up an interspace or two and rotate counterclockwise.
- Visualize the right PA, left PA, and descending aorta. If a duct is present, you should be able to see a third "finger" or "prong."
- Further rotation may align with the long axis view of the ductus and show its insertion into the descending aorta.
- Add color Doppler and look for ductal flow.
- Be careful not to miss a pure right-to-left shunt.
- If a PDA is present, measure the diameter and also document flow with PW Doppler and CW Doppler ultrasound.

Four-Chamber Apical View
- 2D clip to evaluate function. Clip showing sweeps all the way anterior and all the way posterior to evaluate the CS (may need to do two separate clips).
- 2D zoom on the TV and MV. Make annular measurements.
- Color Doppler on the TV (be sure to sweep through the entire valve). PW Doppler to evaluate TV inflow. CW Doppler to detect any TR, and measure peak velocity.
- Color Doppler on left heart (right PV, left lower PV, and MV). Evaluate PW Doppler pattern in the right PV. PW Doppler the MV inflow, measure the time interval from MV closure to MV opening for use in Tei index calculation. CW Doppler regurgitation if applicable.
- Tissue Doppler imaging of the septal and lateral MV annulus. Measure peak systolic velocity, peak E′ (early diastolic tissue Doppler velocity), and peak A′ (diastolic tissue Doppler velocity with atrial contraction). Tissue Doppler imaging of the lateral tricuspid annulus.
- Obtain a 2D five-chamber view of aortic outflow by angling anteriorly. Demonstrate

color across the left ventricular outflow tract (LVOT) and AV. PW Doppler of the AV; measure the ejection time and the velocity time integral. The velocity time integral should be measured above the AV.
- Color sweeps of the ventricular septum, particularly the apex, to rule out muscular ventricular septal defects.

Apical Three-Chamber or Long Axis View
- 2D imaging to evaluate function. Demonstrate color across the MV and AV.

Subcostal Images
Abdominal Views (Uninverted)
- 2D clip demonstrating abdominal situs. Identify the inferior vena cava (IVC) (within liver) and aorta in cross section. Ensure that there is no dilated azygous vein (posterior to the liver and adjacent to the vertebral body).
- 2D sweep demonstrating cardiac position and IVC connection to the right atrium (RA). If clinically of concern, evaluate hemidiaphragm motion.
- 2D and color clips of the IVC/hepatics. PW Doppler of the IVC (if angle is poor for IVC, you can perform Doppler imaging of the hepatic vein).
- 2D and color clips of the abdominal aorta. Pulsed wave (PW) Doppler imaging of the abdominal aorta, evaluating for diastolic runoff and flow reversal. Optimize the angle for Doppler imaging as much as possible.

Subcostal Long or Four-Chamber View (Inverted Imaging)
- 2D clips demonstrating all four chambers. This should include sweeps that go from the diaphragm through the RVOT.
- Rotate slightly clockwise to evaluate the interatrial septum (IAS). Acquire 2D images of the septum. Perform CF Doppler across the AS to evaluate for an atrial shunt. Be sure to sweep all the way posterior and anterior and include the entire length of the AS.
- Color Doppler across the atrioventricular valves (AVVs) and the semilunar valves.
- Color Doppler on the interventricular septum, evaluating for a defect. Be sure to extend all the way anterior and posterior.

Subcostal Short Axis View
- Acquire 2D images, sweeping from the bicaval view to the apex. A true short axis view of the ventricle can be obtained by rotating clockwise. This is particularly important when evaluating a common AVV.
- Color Doppler of the bicaval view, evaluating the AS and systemic venous return. This is a

good view to evaluate for any atrial septal defects (ASDs), and it is particularly important to rule out a sinus venosus defect of the superior vena cava (SVC) or IVC type.

- Color Doppler sweeps from the bicaval view all the way to the apex, including the ventricular septum and outflow tracts. The right upper PV can be seen slightly rightward of the SVC. The ventricular septum should be evaluated for any defects.

Subcostal Right Ventricular Inflow/Outflow View

- Rotate counterclockwise from the four-chamber (4C) view and angle anteriorly and toward the right shoulder to obtain a RVOT view.
- Acquire a 2D and color flow image.
- This is an excellent view to evaluate for right ventricular muscle bundles or anterior malalignment of the infundibular septum.
- Perform PW Doppler and CW Doppler through the RVOT and pulmonary valve, if applicable.

Suprasternal Notch View

- 2D long axis view of the aortic arch (want to see all three head and neck vessels if at all possible). Color Doppler of the aortic arch. PW Doppler proximal and distal to the isthmus, and CW Doppler through the descending aorta.
- 2D sweep over to the SVC (demonstrating innominate vein connection, if possible). Color and PW Doppler of the SVC, either from this view or from the short axis view.
- Color sweep to the left to make sure that there is not a left SVC or left vertical vein (may need to turn Nyquist limit down and/or gain up).
- 2D short axis sweep demonstrating arch sidedness. Starting position should show aorta in cross section, innominate vein. Sweep superiorly to identify the first branch of the aorta, then follow the first branch to determine whether it branches.
- Color Doppler sweep demonstrating branching pattern and vessel pulsatility, starting from the short axis view. Because you

are visualizing the innominate artery branching into a subclavian and common carotid artery all in a short axis, turn down the Nyquist limit so that these vessels will fill. CF Doppler and PW Doppler of the SVC if not done from the long axis view.

- 2D still image demonstrating PA branches, with measurements.
- 2D "crab view" demonstrating PVs entering LA, if possible.
- Color Doppler on "crab view" demonstrating pulmonary venous return (may need to lower color scale and/or increase gain). To optimize frame rate, in larger patients, you may need to evaluate right and left PVs separately.
- These views can be used to evaluate for any central lines.

Right Parasternal

- These views should be used if subcostal views are suboptimal, particularly if you are unable to rule out a sinus venosus ASD from a subcostal bicaval view.
- 2D imaging of the SVC entering the RA. Also able to view the IAS and the right upper PV.
- Color Doppler of the SVC entering the RA and the IAS. This is a good window to evaluate for sinus venosus defect and anomalous pulmonary venous return.
- A right parasternal short axis view may also be used to evaluate coronary artery anatomy if left parasternal views are suboptimal.

Suggested Reading

1. Lai WW, Mertens LL, Cohen MS, Geva T, eds. *Echocardiography in Pediatric and Congenital Heart Disease: From Fetus to Adult.* Oxford, UK: Wiley-Blackwell; 2009.
2. Snider AR, Serwer GA, Ritter SB. *Echocardiography in Pediatric Heart Disease.* 2nd ed. Philadelphia: Mosby-Year Book; 1997.
3. Silverman NH. *Pediatric Echocardiography.* Baltimore, MD: Williams & Wilkins; 1993.
4. Seward JB, Tajik AJ, Edwards WD, Hagler DJ. *Two-Dimensional Echocardiographic Atlas. Volume 1: Congenital Heart Disease.* New York: Springer; 1987.
5. Otto C. *The Practice of Clinical Echocardiography.* 3rd ed. Philadelphia: Saunders Elsevier; 2007.
6. Otto C, Schwaegler RG, eds. *Echocardiography Review Guide.* Philadelphia: Saunders/Elsevier; 2008.

The Fetal Echocardiogram

Margaret M. Vernon

2

Background

As recently as the early 1990s, less than 10% of infants undergoing cardiac surgery in the first month of life received a diagnosis before birth. Today, reported rates of prenatal diagnosis frequently approach 50%.

A variety of maternal or fetal disorders may place a fetus at increased risk for congenital heart disease (CHD) (Table 2-1). If present, a fetal echocardiogram is indicated, and timely referral is recommended. Combined, approximately 5% of pregnancies are referred for in utero evaluation. Abnormal or unsatisfactory (the inability to establish normal) cardiac views obtained as part of an obstetric anatomic survey account for more than 20% of all referrals for in utero evaluation and lead to more than half of all prenatal diagnoses. The anatomic survey, a nearly universal mid-pregnancy ultrasound scan, includes a four-chamber (4C) view of the heart and, if possible, views of both outflow tracts. A positive family history accounts for another nearly 20% of all referrals. However, these are the source of less than 5% of all prenatal diagnoses.

Cardiac Embryology and In Utero Physiology

Cardiac Embryology
- The heart begins as a straight tube oriented in a caudocranial direction.
- Complex looping and septation follow; abnormal looping patterns and incomplete septation form the basis for many forms of CHD.
- By the eighth week post-conception, cardiogenesis is complete.
- By the 10th week post-conception, ventricular contraction can be detected. Transvaginal ultrasound can then detect ventricular contraction (the fetal heart beat).
- By 18 weeks post-conception, transabdominal ultrasound can be used to identify many congenital lesions with a high degree of accuracy and precision.

Fetal Circulation
The fetal circulation differs from the postnatal circulation in several ways. Three shunts exist prenatally: the ductus venosus, foramen ovale (FO), and ductus arteriosus.

In the fetus, oxygenated blood returns to the body through the umbilical vein having just taken up oxygen in the placenta. As the blood within the umbilical vein approaches the liver, the majority flows through the ductus venosus directly into the inferior vena cava (IVC) before entering the right atrium (RA) where preferential streaming occurs.

Blood originally from the ductus venosus flows across the FO into the left atrium (LA) and left ventricle (LV), whereas blood from the abdominal IVC joins that from the superior vena cava (SVC) and flows preferentially through the tricuspid valve (TV) into the right ventricle (RV).

The blood entering the LV is then pumped out of the ascending aorta, where it supplies the coronary, carotid, and subclavian arteries (and hence the heart, brain, and upper body) with relatively richly oxygenated blood.

Blood entering the RV is pumped out of the pulmonary artery (PA). Because the lungs are fluid filled and offer high resistance to flow, most of the blood passes, not to the lungs, but through the ductus arteriosus and into the low-resistance descending aorta. Here it mixes with blood from the ascending aorta before ultimately returning to the placenta for oxygen uptake by way of the two umbilical arteries.

Overview

Echocardiography is the main diagnostic modality used to evaluate the fetal heart. The optimal timing for performance of a comprehensive transabdominal fetal echocardiogram is 18 to 20 weeks' gestation. In select cases, late first trimester evaluation may be possible. Evaluation late in gestation is often complicated by a more "fixed" fetal position, which may limit the available acoustic windows.

A complete fetal echocardiogram includes two-dimensional (2D) evaluation of cardiac anatomy,

TABLE 2-1	INDICATIONS FOR FETAL ECHOCARDIOGRAPHY

Maternal Indications	Fetal Indications
Family history of CHD including prior child or pregnancy with CHD	Abnormal obstetric screening ultrasound
Metabolic disorders (e.g., diabetes)	Extracardiac abnormality
Exposure to teratogens	Chromosomal abnormality
Exposure to prostaglandin synthetase inhibitors (ibuprofen)	Arrhythmia
Infection (rubella, coxsackie virus, parvovirus B19)	Hydrops
Autoimmune dx (e.g., Sjögren syndrome, SLE)	Increased first trimester nuchal translucency
Familial inherited disorder (Marfan, Noonan syndromes)	Multiple gestation and suspicion for twin-twin transfusion syndrome
In vitro fertilization	

TABLE 2-2	COMPONENTS OF THE FETAL ECHOCARDIOGRAM

Overview	Fetal number and position Stomach position and abdominal situs Cardiac position
Biometric examination	Cardiothoracic ratio Biparietal diameter and head circumference Femur length Abdominal circumference
Cardiac imaging	4C view LVOT RVOT Great arteries Three vessel view Bicaval view Ductal arch Aortic arch
Doppler examination	IVC and SVC PVs Ductus venosus FO AVVs Semilunar valves Ductus arteriosus Transverse aortic arch Umbilical artery Umbilical vein
Measurement data	AVV diameter Semilunar valve diameter Main PA Ascending aorta Branch PAs Transverse aortic arch Ventricular length Ventricular short-axis dimensions
Examination of rate and rhythm	M-mode of atrial and ventricular wall motion Doppler examination of atrial and ventricular flow patterns

spectral and color Doppler interrogation, and an assessment of cardiac function and rhythm. The components of a comprehensive evaluation are listed in Table 2-2, although not all may be visualized in every fetus at every examination. Similar to transthoracic imaging, fetal echocardiography depends on the ability to obtain standard views and evaluate structures in orthogonal views. The fetus may be very active, and the examiner may need to piece together many partial images to form a composite picture, particularly in the presence of complex CHD.

Study Protocol

2D Images
Fetal Position
Single sweep from the uterine fundus to the cervix to establish fetal position (vertex, breech, or transverse).

Abdominal and Cardiac Situs
Although uncommon as a whole, CHD and abnormalities of laterality (heterotaxy syndrome) are commonly found together. It is essential to establish abdominal and cardiac situs:
- Doublecheck that the "P" is to the right of the screen (this should never change).
- Rotate/move the transducer on the maternal abdomen as necessary to orient the fetus such that the fetal head is to the right of the screen (Fig. 2-1).

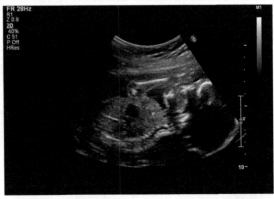

Figure 2-1. Fetus oriented with the head to the screen right (as the sonographer faces it) for cardiac and abdominal situs determination.

- Rotate the transducer 90 degrees clockwise into a transverse cut; the fetus is now oriented with the head into the screen (this is the same orientation as a computed tomography (CT) or magnetic resonance imaging (MRI) scan. Right and left are then established, depending on the position of the fetal spine (up or down), and a reviewer can reliably interpret fetal right from left, utilizing a standard practice approach.

- Find the stomach and the heart and establish cardiac (levo, dextro, or mesocardia) position and abdominal situs.

The Four-Chamber View

The 4C view is the most important in a comprehensive examination of the fetal heart (Fig. 2-2A). The image is obtained in a transverse scanning plane (cross section). Once an acceptable image

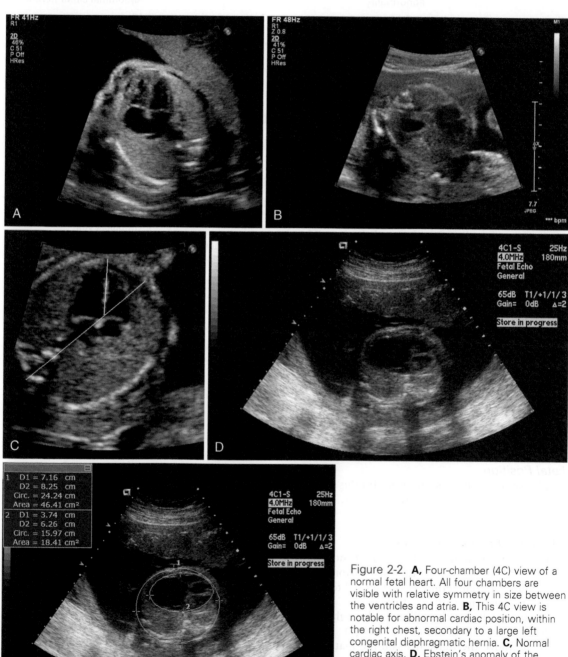

Figure 2-2. **A,** Four-chamber (4C) view of a normal fetal heart. All four chambers are visible with relative symmetry in size between the ventricles and atria. **B,** This 4C view is notable for abnormal cardiac position, within the right chest, secondary to a large left congenital diaphragmatic hernia. **C,** Normal cardiac axis. **D,** Ebstein's anomaly of the tricuspid valve leading to massive cardiomegaly. **E,** Abnormal cardiothoracic ratio confirms visually apparent cardiomegaly.

KEY POINTS

- Attention to alignment cannot be over-emphasized. Anatomic relationships can easily be visually manipulated.
- Comprehensive cardiac evaluation should include sweeps rather than solely a series of still frame captures. Sweeps allow for mental reconstruction and are essential to understanding complex cardiac lesions.

is obtained, cardiac position, axis, and size are assessed. Cardiac position can be influenced by the presence of extracardiac abnormalities that displace the heart within the thorax. Examples include congenital cystic adenomatoid malformations, diaphragmatic hernia (see Fig. 2-2B), and intrathoracic pulmonary sequestration. Normal cardiac axis can be confirmed by visually drawing a line from the spine to the sternum. The interventricular septum intersects that line at an approximately 45-degree angle (see Fig. 2-2C). Axis deviation can be seen in a variety of congenital heart lesions such as Ebstein's anomaly of the TV (see Fig. 2-2D). Normally the fetal heart occupies about one third of the thorax. If there is any doubt on visual inspection, the circumference of each can be measured and compared (the cardiac-to-thoracic ratio). A normal cardiac-to-thoracic ratio is 0.55 ± 0.05 (see Fig. 2-2E).

KEY POINTS

- The 4C view is the most informative of all views.
- It is essential to be able to obtain this view quickly and to be thoroughly familiar with the features that denote normality.

Take time to assess all components of the 4C view. This view is abnormal in at least 50% of complex congenital heart disease.

- Symmetry in size of the RA and LA and RV and LV: Late in gestation, the RV may be slightly larger than the LV.
- Determination of left versus right ventricular morphology: The RV, in its normal position, is posterior to the sternum and identified by the presence of the moderator band (Fig. 2-3A). Postnatally, the trabeculation pattern may be quite distinct between the RV and LV; prenatally, this may be less conspicuous. Notice the slightly more apical location of the tricuspid annulus (see Fig. 2-3B) in comparison with the mitral valve.

- Valve morphology and function: The valve leaflets should open fully and appear thin. Leaflets should show complete coaptation.
- Intracardiac shunts: The presence of the foramenal flap in the LA as well as the coronary sinus. Evaluation for myocardial dropout suggestive of a ventricular septal defect. Pertinent to evaluate in a short axis view perpendicular to the interventricular septum, the thin membranous septum is subject to dropout artifact when imaged solely parallel to the septum. Color Doppler may be helpful. Atrial septal defects (ASDs), in particular secundum defects, can be quite difficult, if not impossible, to detect because of the normal patency of the FO.
- Pulmonary venous return: The pulmonary veins (PVs) are often best evaluated in the 4C view (see Fig. 2-3C and D).
- Pericardial effusion (PE).

The Outflow Tracts

Combined with the 4C view, visualization of both the right ventricular outflow tract (RVOT) and left ventricular outflow tract (LVOT) identifies well more than one half of all congenital heart lesions.

- Establishing the origin of the main PA from the RV and the aorta from the LV is mandatory.
- The LVOT can be obtained by rotating the transducer from the 4C view and angling very slightly toward the fetal right shoulder, similar to the transition by transthoracic imaging in a pediatric patient. Once the LVOT is opened up, rocking the transducer slightly anteriorly (and cranially) will allow visualization of the main PA arising from the RV in normally related great arteries.
- The main PA and ascending aorta should crisscross.
- In transposed great arteries, the aorta and PA are oriented parallel to each other as the PA arises from the LV and courses posteriorly before bifurcating.
- If the great arteries are not clearly seen crossing, the possibility of a conotruncal malformation, specifically transposition of the great arteries, should be investigated.
- The outflow tracts can also be evaluated in a short axis image similar to the pediatric parasternal short axis. In this image, the PA is seen wrapping around the aorta, which is visible en face.

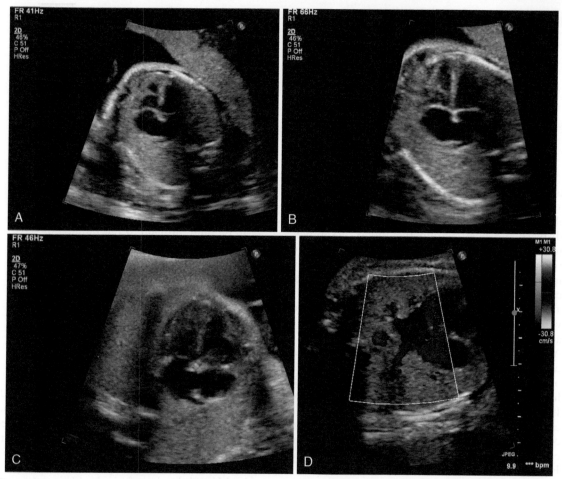

Figure 2-3. **A,** The right ventricle is identified by the presence of the moderator band and increased myocardial trabeculations compared with the LV. The descending aorta is seen directly behind the left atrium (LA). **B,** Note the slight apical offset of the tricuspid annulus in comparison with the mitral valve. **C,** Pulmonary veins are well seen entering the LA from the right and left lung fields. **D,** Color Doppler confirms two-dimensional imaging of the pulmonary veins.

KEY POINT
• Identifying two semilunar valves is only half of the task. One must identify the branching of the PAs and the brachiocephalic arteries to be confident that the great arteries are normally related.

Aortic and Ductal Arches

The aortic and ductal arches can be assessed in either the long axis (LAX) view or by sweeping cranially from the 4C view.

- In the long axis view, the aortic arch takes a tight curve as it courses from ascending to descending, often described as a "candy cane" appearance (Fig. 2-4).
- The ductal arch stretches from the anterior chest all the way back to its entry into the

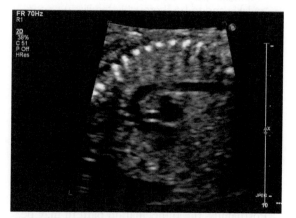

Figure 2-4. In the long axis view, the aortic arch follows a tight curve, resembling a "candy cane." In this image, the brachiocephalic vessels are identified along the transverse arch, confirming the great artery is the aorta.

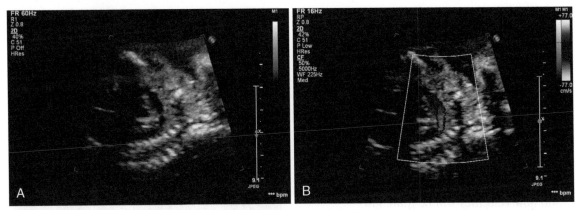

Figure 2-5. **A,** In the long axis view, the ductal arch follows a distinctly different course from that of the aorta; its course is more angular as it connects the pulmonary artery (PA) with the descending aorta. **B,** Color Doppler evaluation of the ductal arch.

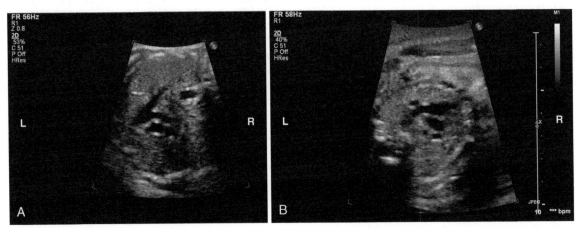

Figure 2-6. **A,** The normal three-vessel view. From anterior to posterior and left to right in decreasing size are the main pulmonary artery (PA), the ascending Ao, and the right SVC. **B,** The three-vessel view in the presence of a persistent left SVC (LSVC). Note the presence of a fourth vessel to the left of the main PA.

descending aorta, commonly referred to as having a "hockey stick" appearance (Fig. 2-5A and B).

- Alternatively, starting from the three-vessel view (described later), one can follow the course of the aorta from the rightward ascending to the leftward descending aorta. Additionally, the continuation of the main PA as the ductus arteriosus, which then joins the leftward descending aorta, is obtained.

Systemic and Pulmonary Venous Return

- The entry of the superior vena cava (SVC) and IVC into the RA is documented in an image identical to that of the transthoracic bicaval view.
- In addition, the three-vessel view (Fig. 2-6A) is obtained to evaluate for the presence of a persistent left-sided SVC (see Fig. 2-6B). This

view also confirms the normal relationship of the great arteries. It is obtained by sweeping cranially from the 4C view to the level of the superior mediastinum. From anterior to posterior and in decreasing size from left to right, the main PA, ascending aorta, and SVC are seen.

- The PVs are often best evaluated in the 4C view. By 2D imaging, PVs can be seen entering the LA; this can be confirmed by color Doppler.

Doppler Evaluation
Color Doppler

- In addition to obtaining clear 2D images of each structure, flow is evaluated with color Doppler and pulsed-wave (PW) Doppler.
- Careful 2D images are arguably more important to the successful detection of pathology.

- Color Doppler can often quickly confirm normal flow patterns. The sample volume is set as narrow as possible.
- Color Doppler evaluation of the aortic and ductal arches showing normal antegrade flow is essential because flow reversal is consistent with severe CHD such as semilunar valve hypoplasia or atresia.
- Color Doppler is often helpful in evaluating the ventricular septum, but one must remember that due to the in utero parallel circulation, the pressure is essentially the same between the right and left ventrides and flow velocities will be quite low.
- Valve regurgitation and/or stenosis can be detected similar to transthoracic imaging.

PW Doppler

- Compared with postnatal imaging, the velocity settings are much lower. PW Doppler values change with advancing gestation and normal valves have been established.
- The highest velocity of flow is in the ductus arteriosus, which may reach 2 m/s when the fetus is near term gestational age.
- Similar to transthoracic imaging, color Doppler is often used to help position the PW Doppler sample volume.
- Important to use a small sample volume.
- Transducer manipulated on the maternal abdomen to maximize the obtained velocity by aligning the sample volume with the direction of blood flow.

Function

- Evaluation of heart size, heart rate (HR), and the presence or absence of hydrops can provide clues to cardiac function.
- Systolic function is both qualitatively estimated and can be quantified by calculating shortening fraction from either 2D images or M-mode tracings. The left and right ventricular shortening fractions are both in the range of 34 ± 3% from 17 weeks' gestation until term.
- Diastolic function can be evaluated by analyzing PW Doppler tracings of ventricular inflow, ductus venosus, and umbilical vein flow patterns.

Measurements

Although not all structures require measurement, especially if visually there are no concerns based on 2D images, structures can be measured and compared with established normals for varying gestation ages.

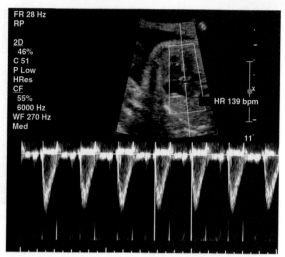

Figure 2-7. The fetal HR is calculated by measuring the time from the onset of aortic flow in successive beats.

Rate and Rhythm Assessment

Once a comprehensive assessment of the cardiac anatomy is complete, the HR and rhythm are documented.

- The rate and rhythm of the fetal heart are evaluated by mechanical surrogate events, specifically, the movement of the atria and ventricles or blood flow across valves.
- The HR is typically obtained using a Doppler tracing obtained with the sample volume just distal to the aortic valve (Fig. 2-7). The time from onset of flow from one beat to the next is obtained and then using the following conversion a rate in beats per minute (bpm) is calculated.
- Average HR is 140 bpm at 20 weeks' gestation, decreasing to 130 bpm by term gestation.
- Fetal bradycardia is defined as a persistent HR of less than 80 bpm.
- It is important to differentiate between HRs out of the normal range but occurring as a physiologic response (sinus bradycardia and sinus tachycardia) from those that arise because of a disturbance in the rhythm-generating mechanism within the heart.
- Rhythm disturbances are fairly common; the majority are benign and self-limiting. Most arrhythmias will be immediately obvious on the 4C view (too fast, too slow, or irregular); however, the M-mode and PW Doppler provide additional information.
- The majority of both benign and serious arrhythmias occur in structurally normal hearts.
- Normal fetal rhythm is regular with a 1:1 atrial to ventricular relationship.

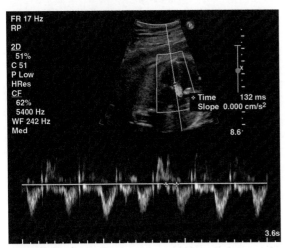

FR 17 Hz
RP

2D
51%
C 51
P Low
HRes
CF
62%
5400 Hz
WF 242 Hz
Med

Time   132 ms
Slope 0.000 cm/s²

8.6·

3.6s

Figure 2-8. Normal sinus rhythm is established by documenting an atrial contraction before each aortic Doppler profile and then measuring the time from atrial contraction to aortic outflow, the mechanical PR, a surrogate for the electrocardiographic PR interval.

- Sinus rhythm is established by measuring the time from the beginning of the mitral A wave corresponding to atrial contraction to the beginning of aortic outflow. This is defined as the mechanical PR interval (Fig. 2-8) and is the mechanical equivalent of the electro-cardiographic PR interval.
- A mechanical PR interval of greater than 200 m is considered prolonged.

Suggested Reading
Background
1. Friedberg M, Silverman N, Hornberger L, et al. Prenatal detection of congenital heart disease. *J Pediatr.* 2009;155: 26-31.
   Recent multicenter prospective evaluation of the frequency of and factors influencing the prenatal detection of CHD.
2. Wimalasundera RC, Gardiner HM. Congenital heart disease and aneuploidy. *Prenat Diagn.* 2004;24:1116-1122.
   In as many as one third of fetuses with a prenatal diagnosis of CHD, an associated chromosomal abnormality is identified. In addition, the majority of fetuses with CHD and aneuploidy have extracardiac anomalies. This is a recent review of the frequency

and types of aneuploidy associated with commonly diagnosed CHD.
3. Pajkrt E, Chitty LS. Fetal cardiac anomalies and genetic syndromes. *Prenat Diagn.* 2004;24:1104-1115.
   In addition to an increased incidence of cardiac anomalies among fetuses with aneuploidy, there is an increased association with genetic syndromes. This article reviews genetic syndromes commonly associated with CHD.

Fetal Circulation and Neonatal Transition
1. Rychik J. Fetal cardiovascular physiology. *Pediatr Cardiol.* 2004;25:201-209.
   Review of fetal cardiovascular physiology and the unique elements that distinguish the fetal cardiovascular system from the postnatal cardiovascular system. Includes a discussion of the response to in utero stress.

The Fetal Echocardiogram
1. Yagel S, Cohen SM, Achiron R. Examination of the fetal heart by five short-axis views: a proposed screening method for comprehensive cardiac evaluation. *Ultrasound Obstet Gynecol.* 2001;17:367-369.
2. Allan LD, Paladini D. Prenatal measurement of cardiothoracic ratio in evaluation of heart disease. *Arch Dis Child.* 1990;65:20-23.
   Retrospective evaluation of the normal cardiothoracic ratio and the impact of CHD or hydrops on the cardiothoracic ratio.
3. Schneider C, McCrindle BW, Carvalho JS, Hornberger LK, et al. Development of Z-scores for fetal cardiac dimensions from echocardiography. *Ultrasound Obstet Gynecol.* 2005;26:599-605.
   Establishes Z scores for a set of measurements routinely obtained during a comprehensive fetal echocardiographic study. Allows for comparison with gestational age as well as femur length or biparietal diameter acknowledging variability in fetal size.
4. Al-Ghazali W, Chapman MG, Allan JG. Doppler assessment of the cardiac and uteroplacental circulations in normal and abnormal fetuses. *Br J Obstet Gynaecol.* 1988;95:575-580.
5. Api O, Carvalho J. Fetal dysrhythmias. *Best Pract Res Clin Obstet Gynaecol.* 2008;22:31-48.
   Recent review of fetal dysrhythmias and their management.
6. Pasquini L, Gardiner HM. PR Interval: A comparison of electrical and mechanical methods in the fetus. *Early Hum Dev.* 2007;83:231-237.
   Prospective comparison of the mechanical PR interval with a signal-averaged electrocardiogram obtained on the maternal abdomen. Discussion of the limitations of the mechanical PR interval, a surrogate for fetal cardiac electrical activity.
7. Huhta J. Fetal congestive heart failure. *Semin Fetal Neonatal Med.* 2005;10:542-552.
   Reviews fetal heart failure and introduces a novel scoring system for serial evaluation, the Cardiovascular Profile Score.

Echocardiography in the Cardiac Catheterization Laboratory

3

Troy Johnston

Background

Interventional catheter techniques are now well established for the treatment of congenital heart disease (CHD). Echocardiography is an essential adjunct to fluoroscopy during certain interventional catheterization techniques. The improved imaging resulting from the addition of echocardiography may lead to increased procedure success with improved safety and decreased fluoroscopic time. Procedures include transcatheter closure of atrial septal defects (ASDs), patent foramen ovale (PFO), and ventricular septal defects (VSDs), balloon atrial septostomy, balloon mitral valvuloplasty, and percutaneous aortic valve replacement. Echocardiography is used to assess the anatomy, guide the procedure, and assess the immediate result. The techniques used include transthoracic echocardiography (TTE), transesophageal echocardiography (TEE), and intracardiac echocardiography (ICE).

Cooperation and clear communication between the proceduralist and the echocardiographer are essential. All team members need to understand the procedural and imaging requirements for technical success.

Echocardiographic Techniques

Multiple echocardiographic techniques are used during interventional procedures. The choice of technique is determined by technical issues associated with the modality, experience with the technique, and the use of general anesthesia.

The simplest technique is TTE. The supine position of the patient and the fluoroscopic imaging equipment may increase the complexity of image acquisition. Careful attention is required in order not to contaminate the sterile field. Despite these limitations, this technique is capable of providing good-quality imaging.

TEE provides excellent imaging and is the standard technique for most centers. This technique usually requires general anesthesia.

ICE uses an ultrasound catheter that is steerable and deflectable. The most commonly used catheter (AcuNav catheter; Biosense Webster, Diamond Bar, CA) comes in 8- and 10-French sizes. It has a 64-element vector phased-array transducer (5.5–10 MHz) at the tip of the catheter. It produces a two-dimensional (2D) sector of 90 degrees with color Doppler imaging. ICE can be performed by the interventionalist without the need for an echocardiographer. The greatest limitation of this technique is the catheter cost.

Real-time three-dimensional (3D) echocardiography is a more recently developed technique that can be used to image the anatomy, catheters, and devices. It allows for improved understanding of the relationships between the device and cardiac structures. The image quality and resolution are inferior to those of the other 2D techniques (Table 3-1).

Transcatheter Closure of Atrial Septal Defects/Patent Foramen Ovale

Technique

TEE is most often used. It provides excellent image quality. ICE provides comparable image quality without the need for general anesthesia.

Step-by-Step Approach

1. **Assess Anatomy.** Secundum ASDs and PFO are amenable to transcatheter closure.
2. **Dynamic Sizing.** A sizing balloon is often used to measure the stretched diameter of the ASD.
3. **Device Placement.** Live imaging during device placement is required to assess the relationship of the device to cardiac structures.
4. **After Device Release.** Complete assessment of the device is performed after device release.

TABLE 3-1   ADVANTAGES AND LIMITATIONS OF EACH TECHNIQUE

Technique	Advantages	Limitations	Use
Transthoracic	Ease of use Good image quality 3D real time	Access to patient difficult Interference with sterile field	Balloon atrial septostomy Pericardiocentesis
Transesophageal	High-quality imaging Does not interfere with the sterile field 3D real time	Invasive Often requires general anesthesia and intubation	Any procedure
Intracardiac	High-quality imaging No need for general anesthesia	Far-field imaging Invasive Vascular complications (rare) Operator learning curve Increased cost	ASD/PFO closure Balloon mitral valvuloplasty Transcatheter aortic valve implantation

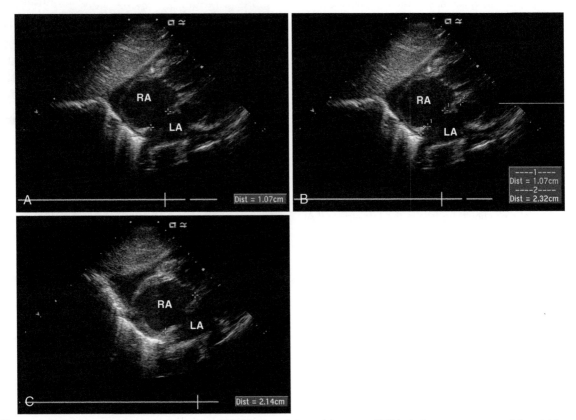

Figure 3-1. Transesophageal echocardiographic evaluation of the atrial septum (AS) includes measurement of the atrial septal defect (ASD) diameter (**A**), septal rims (**B**), and the total septal length (**C**).

KEY POINTS

- Before closure attempt, the anatomy of the atrial septum (AS) is assessed. Morphology, maximum diameter, defect number, total septal length, adequacy of the rims, and distance of the defect from the surrounding structures must be determined (Fig. 3-1).
- The assessment for a PFO should include the length of the tunnel and the assessment of an associated atrial septal aneurysm. An intravenous injection of agitated saline solution bubbles is performed to identify the presence of a right-to-left shunt.
- The Eustachian valve should be assessed. A large Eustachian valve or Chiari network does not preclude the ability to place a device.
- Color Doppler should be performed to assess for additional defects and the presence of fenestrations.

KEY POINTS—cont'd

- The devices that are currently available are indicated for secundum ASDs and PFO. The exact location of the defect needs to be determined.
- The pulmonary veins (PVs) should be assessed. The presence of partial anomalous pulmonary venous return may indicate surgical referral to address both anomalies.

- The entire rim needs to be assessed. The presence of a circumferential rim of at least 5 mm is ideal for closure. The exception is the retroaortic rim. Deficiency of the retroaortic rim does not preclude device placement.

KEY POINTS

- Color Doppler assessment is performed during balloon inflation. Careful attention is paid to the point at which any left-to-right flow is eliminated. The diameter of the balloon is measured at this stop-flow diameter. The narrowest diameter, or waist, in the balloon is measured (Fig. 3-2).
- This diameter is used for device sizing. Different devices have different sizing guidelines.

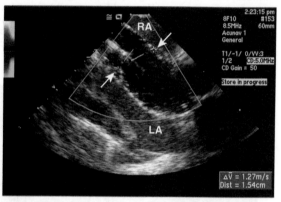

Figure 3-2. Intracardiac echocardiography (ICE) image of a sizing balloon straddling the AS. The waist of the balloon (*arrows*) is measured at the point where the left-to-right atrial shunt ceases. Note that the color box is larger than the balloon at the level of the AS.

Transcatheter Closure of Muscular Ventricular Septal Defects

Technique
TEE generally provides the best imaging for percutaneous closure of muscular VSDs.

Step-by-Step Approach
1. **Assess Anatomy.** Percutaneous closure is possible for select muscular VSDs.

KEY POINTS

- The left atrial disk of the device is deployed first. A view with good visualization of the mitral valve (MV) and AS is required. The left atrial disk should be free in the left atrium (LA) during extrusion from the sheath. It should not be opened in the PVs, left atrial appendage, or MV.
- After the device has been fully deployed, echocardiography should determine whether all the rims have been captured. Often the interventional cardiologist will need to "wiggle" the device to help visualize the rims within the space between the right and left disks.
- The relationship of the deployed device to the MV, pulmonary venous return, and superior vena cava (SVC) is important before final release of the device (Fig. 3-3). Any interference with these cardiac structures most often is an indication for device removal.

KEY POINTS

- The location of the defect and size must be determined. The presence of additional defects and their relationship to each other is important. Due to the right ventricular trabeculations, any individual defect may have multiple channels on the right side of the septum (Fig. 3-4).
- The distance from the defect to the atrioventricular and semilunar valves should be measured.

KEY POINTS

- The presence of residual shunt is assessed after release.
- The relationship of the device to intracardiac structures should be carefully assessed before deployment.
- Assess for complications.

2. **Device Placement.** The device can be positioned with echocardiographic and fluoroscopic guidance, but only echocardiography can reliably visualize the ventricular septum (VS).

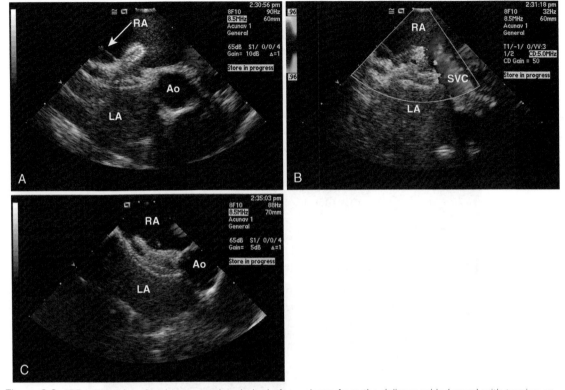

Figure 3-3. ICE image of an Amplatzer septal occluder before release from the delivery cable (*arrow*) with tension on the right atrial disk (**A**). The superior vena caval flow is unobstructed by the Amplatzer septal occluder (**B**). After release of the device, the right atrial disk rests flush against the right side of the AS (**C**).

KEY POINTS

- Echocardiography is helpful to assess whether the desired course across the VS has been accomplished. In the case of multiple channels or defects in the VS, successful device placement often requires placement within a particular channel or defect.
- Usually the left ventricular disk is deployed first. It needs to be visualized during deployment to confirm the location in the left ventricle without entrapment in the MV, including the MV apparatus.
- After the right ventricular disk has been deployed, the device is assessed to ensure adequate location of the device with the septum captured between the disks. The device size should also be assessed. The device size should be large enough so that the disks are larger than the diameter of the VSDs.
- It is important, particularly with high muscular defects, to ensure that the device does not interfere with the function of the aortic valve.

3. **After Device Release.** Echocardiography is key to assess the immediate results of device placement.

KEY POINTS

- Device location is assessed in addition to residual shunt.
- The presence and size of additional defects are assessed. Large enough additional defects may necessitate the placement of additional devices.
- Assessment for complications should complete the examination.

Balloon Atrial Septostomy

Balloon atrial septostomy is often performed to improve mixing in patients with transposition of the great arteries. In this setting it can be done at the bedside with TTE guidance. A septostomy may also be required for palliation of other congenital lesions. Echocardiographic imaging can be used to assess the adequacy of the procedure.

Technique
TTE is usually adequate. On the rare occasion when atrial septostomy is performed in adult patients, TEE or ICE may be required.

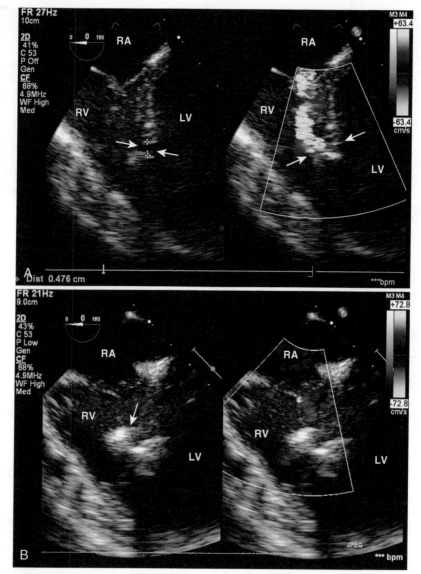

Figure 3-4. Transesophageal four-chamber (4C) view of the ventricular septum (VS) can be used to identify the presence and location of muscular ventricular septal defects (VSDs) (*arrows*) (**A**). After device placement, the relationship of the right atrial disk (*arrow*) to the tricuspid valve (TV) is demonstrated (**B**). Color interrogation of the TV is performed to assess the presence and degree of regurgitation.

Step-by-Step Approach

1. **Assess Anatomy.** The presence of inadequate atrial level communication is confirmed by echo.

> **KEY POINT**
>
> • The atrial septal anatomy is assessed to determine the location and size of the atrial level shunt.

2. **Balloon Atrial Septostomy.** Echocardiographic guidance is more than adequate to perform balloon atrial septostomy safely.

> **KEY POINT**
>
> • Imaging of the AS is required during catheter manipulation. A transthoracic four-chamber view provides adequate visualization so that the catheter tip can be placed in the LA. The balloon should be visualized during inflation. The relationship of the balloon to the MV, left atrial appendage, and PVs must be determined to minimize complications. Correct placement of the balloon in the LA must be verified before pulling the balloon through the AS (Fig. 3-5).

3. **After Balloon Atrial Septostomy.** Echocardiography confirms an increase in the size of the atrial communication.

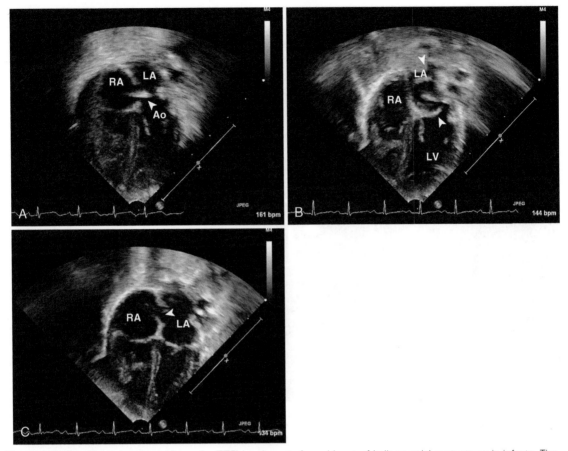

Figure 3-5. Transthoracic echocardiography (TTE) is adequate for guidance of balloon atrial septostomy in infants. The apical 4C view provides good visualization of both atria, the AS, and the mitral valve (MV). The balloon catheter tip (*arrow*) is seen before (**A**) and after (**B**) inflation. Confirmation of correct balloon position in the left atrium (LA) is crucial before pulling the balloon catheter. The ASD (*arrow*) is visualized after each septostomy to assess adequacy (**C**).

> **KEY POINT**
>
> • The adequacy of the septostomy is assessed after each left-to-right pull. 2D and Doppler color assessment should be performed to determine the size of the enlarged atrial septal communication.

Balloon Mitral Valvuloplasty

Balloon mitral valvuloplasty is a much more common procedure in older patients with rheumatic MV disease. However, it may be useful for select patients with congenital MV stenosis.

Technique

TEE with general anesthesia provides the highest quality imaging. TTE can be used, but the quality of imaging is inferior to that of TEE. Fluoroscopy cannot be performed simultaneously with TTE without inadvertent radiation exposure to the sonographer. ICE can be used, but the image quality is inferior. Adequate images can be obtained if the catheter tip is positioned in the right ventricle.

Step-by-Step Approach

1. **Initial Assessment.** The primary use of echocardiography is to assess the efficacy of the procedure; and it allows early identification of complications.

> **KEY POINTS**
>
> • The anatomy of the MV and mechanism of stenosis should be confirmed. Any mitral insufficiency should be quantified. The MV area can be measured (Fig. 3-6).
> • The ideal candidate has stenosis at the level of the valve leaflets. The efficacy of balloon mitral valvuloplasty is less in the presence of a hypoplastic annulus or a double-orifice MV.
> • Although rare, the presence of a left atrial thrombus should be excluded.

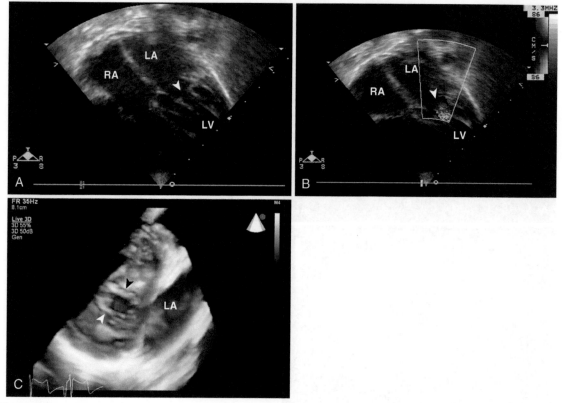

Figure 3-6. In children, TTE is often adequate to assess the MV during mitral valvuloplasty. Assessment should include two-dimensional (**A**) and color interrogation (**B**) of the MV (*arrow*). Three-dimensional echo (**C**) may provide more information about the MV leaflets (*arrows*) and mechanisms of stenosis or insufficiency.

2. **Balloon Dilation.** Echocardiographic visualization of the balloon during inflation is often helpful.

KEY POINTS

- Echo can be used to monitor balloon positioning and visualize balloon inflation.
- The balloon should be positioned through the main orifice of the valve and not through the MV chordal attachments.

---

3. **After Balloon Dilation.** Echocardiography is used to assess the success of the procedure.

KEY POINTS

- After each balloon dilation, the degree of mitral insufficiency should be quantified.
- The MV opening should be examined closely to assess commissural splitting.
- A comparison of valve area is often helpful.
- Hemodynamic data are very difficult to interpret because the MV gradient is dependent on preload and cardiac output.

---

4. **Detection of Complications.** Echocardiography is used to identify complications.

KEY POINTS

- Hemopericardium can be secondary to transseptal atrial catheterization or wire puncture. Echocardiographic guidance can be used to perform pericardiocentesis.
- Severe mitral regurgitation (MR) is identified by echocardiography.

Transcatheter Aortic Valve Implantation

Transcatheter aortic valve implantation is an investigational technique.

Technique

TEE is the most common technique used for transcatheter aortic valve placement. TTE can be used if there is a contraindication to general anesthesia.

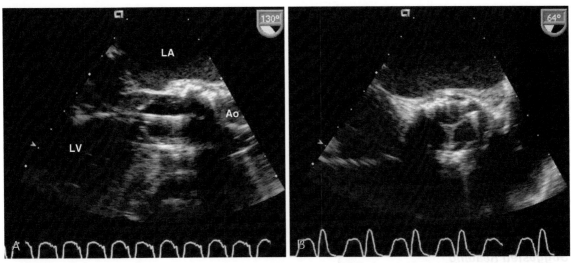

Figure 3-7. **A,** Long axis view by transesophageal echocardiography (TEE) of deployment of percutaneous aortic valve replacement. The delivery balloon is inflated in the left ventricular outflow tract across the stenotic aortic valve. Note the rapid heart rate reflecting rapid ventricular pacing needed to deploy the valve in a stable position. **B,** TEE short axis of the deployed aortic valve. The valve leaflets are closed, and the stent is seen across the aortic annulus.

Step-by-Step Approach

1. **Assess Anatomy.** Accurate assessment of aortic valve anatomy is dependent on echo.

KEY POINTS

- The aortic valve annulus should be measured. Accurate measurement of the annulus is a crucial component of valve sizing.
- The aortic valve anatomy (tricuspid) should be assessed and any calcifications identified.
- The aortic root dimensions should be measured.
- Left ventricular size and function should be assessed.
- The MV anatomy should be determined and any insufficiency quantified.
- If an apical approach is used, echocardiography can identify the left ventricular apex for determining the surgical incision site.

2. **During the Procedure.** Echocardiography can be used to confirm correct wire placement and balloon position during dilation (Fig. 3-7A).
3. **After Deployment.** Echocardiography is crucial to the assessment of the valve after deployment (see Fig. 3-7B).

KEY POINTS

- Echocardiography is important during wire placement. The wire course should be carefully visualized. The relationship of the wire to the MV apparatus is important. The wire course should be free of the MV apparatus.
- Echocardiography can be used for balloon positioning during the aortic valvuloplasty and then to assess the presence and extent of aortic insufficiency.
- Valve placement can be assessed to ensure correct location of the device during deployment.

KEY POINTS

- The position of the valve in relation to the aortic annulus is identified.
- Valve function is assessed for stenosis or insufficiency.
- Aortic valve insufficiency can be assessed to quantify the extent and determine the location of the regurgitant jet. There is often a small amount of regurgitation associated with the wire. Assessment should be performed both before and after wire removal.
- The presence and extent of paravalvular leaks should be identified. The device should be evaluated for incomplete expansion or malposition (Box 3-1).

BOX 3-1   Role of Echo in Interventional Catheterization

1. Echo is a crucial adjunct to fluoroscopy for many complex interventional catheterization procedures.
2. High-quality imaging is important.
3. The echocardiographer needs good knowledge of the procedure.
4. A team approach is required with good communication between the echocardiographer and the interventional cardiologist.
5. The choice of technique (TTE, TEE, or ICE) depends on the procedure and whether general aesthesia is needed.

Suggested Reading

1. Hellenbrand WA, Fuhey JT, McGowan FX, et al. Transesophageal guidance of transcatheter closure of atrial septal defect. *Am J Cardiol*. 1990;66:207-213.
2. Hijazi ZM, Shivkumar K, Sahn DJ. Intracardiac echocardiography during interventional and electrophysiological cardiac catheterization. *Circulation*. 2009;119:587-596.
3. Kim S, Hijazi ZM, Lang R, et al. The use of intracardiac echocardiography and other intracardiac imaging tools to guide non-coronary cardiac interventions. *J Am Coll Cardiol*. 2009;53:2117-2128.
4. Moss RG, Ivens E, Pasupati S, et al. Role of echocardiography in percutaneous aortic valve implantation. *J Am Coll Cardiol Imaging*. 2008;1:15-24.
5. Mullen MJ, Dias BF, Walker F, et al. Intracardiac echocardiography guided device closure of atrial septal defects. *J Am Coll Cardiol*. 2003;41:285-292.
6. Perk G, Lang RM, Garcia-Fernandez MA, et al. Use of real time three-dimensional transesophageal echocardiography in intracardiac catheter based interventions. *J Am Soc Echocardiogr*. 2009;22:865-882.
7. Silvestry FE, Kerber RE, Brook MM, et al. Echocardiography-guided interventions. *J Am Soc Echocardiogr*. 2009;22:213-229.

Intraoperative Transesophageal Echocardiography

4

Denise Joffe

KEY POINTS

- There is a vast spectrum of abnormalities in patients with congenital heart disease (CHD), and there are usually several appropriate surgical options for repair. The echocardiographer must have an excellent understanding of the surgical repair to interpret intraoperative findings.
- The intraoperative presurgical transesophageal echocardiography (TEE) is used to confirm the diagnosis and help guide the hemodynamic management before cardiopulmonary bypass (CPB), if needed. Because of the unique views and excellent resolution of TEE, new abnormalities are occasionally diagnosed prerepair that call for a revision of the surgical plan.
- With the less than ideal conditions of the operating room with respect to lighting, time constraints, and labile hemodynamic conditions, examinations are more directed and less detailed than a comprehensive transthoracic study.
- The hemodynamic condition of the patient under anesthesia may differ from baseline and may alter findings. For example, the severity of valve regurgitation may be less under anesthesia. The decision to repair or replace a valve is best made based on preoperative imaging. At the conclusion of a bypass, satisfactory hemodynamic conditions should be present for assessment of TEE.
- Postprocedure TEE is used to evaluate the repair and to guide postbypass hemodynamic management. There are circumstances when residual abnormalities are left because of surgical limitations or patient considerations. For example, these compromises are frequently made in the case of valvular heart disease in very young patients.
- TEE has significant limitations in the direct assessment of the aortic arch and descending aorta because the trachea interferes with adequate imaging. Doppler techniques may demonstrate indirect evidence of flow but are often suboptimal. Consequently, TEE is rarely used in the repair of isolated coarctations or interruptions of the aorta.

Practical Considerations

- Ensure an adequate level of anesthesia before probe placement, especially in patients at risk of complications from sympathetic stimulation, e.g., patients with tetralogy of Fallot (TOF), other forms of dynamic outflow tract obstruction, pulmonary hypertension (PHTN).
- The TEE probe may cause hemodynamic or respiratory changes in young patients because of its proximity to the left atrium (LA), pulmonary veins (PVs), and airway. When there is doubt about the cause of a serious hemodynamic or airway problem, it is best to remove the probe.
- To avoid damping of an arterial waveform by the TEE probe, place a left radial or lower extremity arterial line in patients with aberrant right subclavian arteries.

Atrial Septal Defects (Table 4-1)

- Secundum atrial septal defect (ASD)
- Primum ASD
- Sinus venosus ASD
- Coronary sinus (CS) ASD

KEY POINTS

All Atrial Septal Defects
- Left-to-right (L→R) shunt results in right heart enlargement.
- Associated lesions include left superior vena cava (LSVC), mitral regurgitation (MR), pulmonary stenosis (PS), partial anomalous pulmonary venous drainage (PAPVD).
- Significant tricuspid regurgitation (TR) may occasionally result from right ventricle (RV) enlargement or PHTN.

TABLE 4-1   BASIC ECHO PRINCIPLES WHEN IMAGING ASDs

Defect	Best TEE Views*	What to Look for on 2D Imaging	CFD and Spectral Doppler
All ASDs		• Measure size of ASD in multiple planes. • Examine IAS for multiple defects. • Examine MV/TV structure/function, especially for prolapse/clefts. Measure MV/TV annulus. • Examine pulmV. Look for restricted motion, doming leaflets, commissural fusion. • Examine PV drainage. • Identify RAE/RVE. • Assess biventricular function. • PHTN/RVH/R→L shunt/systolic flattening of IVS in systole may indicate Eisenmenger syndrome. • Look for an LSVC between the LUPV and the LAA (ME 2C, 4C view).	• PW/CFD to identify size/direction of flow (L→R in uncomplicated ASD). • Grade MR, TR. • PW of PV may show higher baseline velocities secondary to high PBF, but pulsatility is preserved and peak/mean velocities are not significantly elevated. • If TR is present: CW is used to measure $RVP = PAP = 4V_{TR}^2 + RAP$. • CFD/CW to assess for PS. Velocities up to 2.5 m/s at the pulmV may result from ASD flow alone (deep TG LAX, ME ascending aortic SAX views).
Secundum ASD	ME four chamber ME AV SAX ME RV inflow-outflow ME bicaval Deep TG bicaval equivalent	• Defect in area of FO (ME 4C, ME bicaval; ME RV inflow-outflow, deep TG LAX with 90-degree rotation so that SVC and IVC are seen (deep TG bicaval equivalent). • Examine MV for prolapse.	
Primum ASD	ME four chamber ME LAX ME modified 5C ME AV LAX TG basal SAX TG LAX Deep TG LAX	• Defect in posterior/inferior IAS at crux of heart, above AVV (ME 4C view). • Both AVVs originate at same level. • Examine MV structure/function, especially for cleft, obstructing chords. Measure MV annulus (ME 4C, TG basal SAX view). • Look for LVOTO (ME LAX, ME AV LAX, deep TG LAX, ME modified 5C view).	• Assess MV/note all regurgitant jets/grade MR. • CFD/CW/PW to assess LVOTO (deep TG LAX, TG LAX views).
Sinus venosus ASD	ME four chamber ME two chamber ME bicaval Deep TG bicaval equivalent	• Superior defect located above FO near SVC (ME bicaval, ME 4C views, deep TG LAX bicaval view equivalent). • Inferior defect located in inferior part of IAS below FO near IVC. • Locate anomalous PV drainage.	• CFD/PW/2D to assess drainage of all PVs: • R PV (ME bicaval with rightward rotation, ME 4C views). • L PV (ME 4C, ME 2C views). • Examine SVC/IVC for evidence of aliasing/high normal velocity flow suggestive of anomalous PV drainage (advance and withdraw probe to locate upper and lower veins).
Coronary sinus ASD	ME four chamber ME two chamber ME LAX ME bicaval	• Defect anywhere along course of CS (ME 4C view scanning inferiorly/posteriorly near IVC, ME 2C views, CS in AV groove, ME bicaval view adjacent to entrance of IVC). • Measure CS size. • Use contrast saline solution injection into L hand to determine if LSVC is present: with LSVC and CS ASD→immediate opacification of LA prior to RA. With CS ASD but without LSVC→bubbles first enter RA (via innominate and right SVC).	

*See the Appendix on page 57 for schematics of these views. CFD, color flow Doppler; FO, fossa ovalis; IAS, interatrial septum; LAA, left atrial appendage; LUPV, left upper pulmonary vein; PAP, pulmonary artery pressure; PBF, pulmonary blood flow; pulmV, pulmonary valve; PW, pulsed wave Doppler; RAE, right atrial enlargement; RAP, right atrial pressure; RVE, right ventricle enlargement; RVH, right ventricle hypertrophy; RVP, right ventricular pressure.

Secundum Atrial Septal Defects (Fig. 4-1)

- May have multiple defects.
- If left untreated, Eisenmenger syndrome develops in about 5% (irreversible pulmonary vascular disease).

Primum Atrial Septal Defects (also called Partial Atrioventricular [AV] Canal, Defect)

- Almost always associated with a cleft mitral valve (MV) (Fig. 4-2).
- Left ventricular outflow tract obstruction (LVOTO) can develop from:
  - Long tunnel-like obstruction of the left ventricular outflow tract (LVOT) ("goose-neck" deformity).
- The development of a discrete membrane in the LVOT.
- Aberrant chords inserting into the interventricular septum (IVS) and obstructing left ventricle (LV) outflow.
- Membranes and tunnel-like obstruction tend to occur years after a primary repair.

Sinus Venosus Atrial Septal Defects

- Superior defects are most common; inferior defects are very rare.
- Sinus venosus ASDs are associated with PAPVD, especially right PVs that drain into the superior vena cava (SVC) or right atrium (RA).
- TEE has superior ability to visualize the anatomy of sinus venosus ASDs and drainage of PVs compared with TTE.

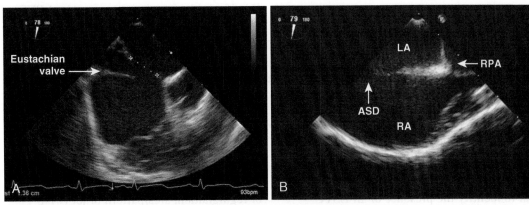

Figure 4-1. **A**, Midesophageal (ME) right ventricular inflow-outflow view demonstrating a 1.4-cm secundum atrial septal defect (ASD). **B**, ME bicaval view showing a secundum defect in the area of the fossa ovalis. The full extent is not visible in this view. Note that there is right pulmonary artery (PA) enlargement.

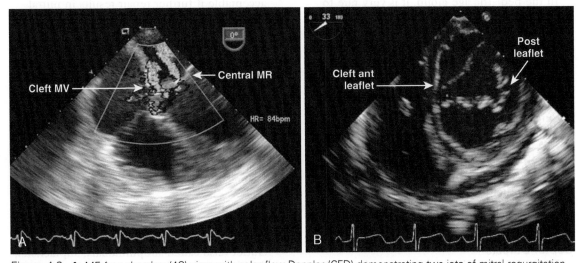

Figure 4-2. **A**, ME four chamber (4C) view with color flow Doppler (CFD) demonstrating two jets of mitral regurgitation (MR). One originates from the medial area of the cleft, and a second from a more central jet of MR was from a coaptation defect as a result of annular dilation (not well seen in this frame) and not from the cleft. This patient had closure of her primum ASD and cleft mitral valve (MV). The acute reduction in left ventricular volume decreased the central MR to trace to mild. Note also that both atrioventricular valves (AVVs) originate at the same level of the center (crux) of the heart. **B**, Transgastric basal short axis (SAX) view of a cleft MV. The cleft is clearly seen in the anterior mitral leaflet.

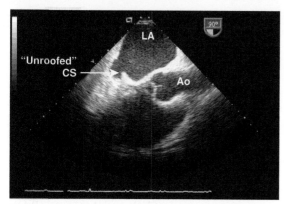

Figure 4-3. Two-dimensional (2D) modified ME two-chamber view showing the unroofed coronary sinus (CS) in the atrioventricular (AV) groove. The shunt goes from the left atrium to the coronary sinus to the right atrium.

Coronary Sinus Atrial Septal Defects (also called Unroofed Coronary Sinus)

- Results in shunting between the LA and the RA via the missing "roof" of the CS. The amount of unroofing is variable (defect may be partial or complete) (Fig. 4-3).
- Associated defect very common: LSVC, PAPVD, other complex CHD such as heterotaxy syndrome.
- The CS may appear large even without an LSVC because of flow from the shunt. It is crucial to identify the presence of an LSVC because it alters the surgical repair.

Principles of Surgical Management

- In the pediatric age group, it is very rare to have to perform a concomitant tricuspid valve (TV) repair, but it may be necessary in older patients with moderate to severe TR.

Secundum Atrial Septal Defects

- Device closure in catheterization lab or surgical closure.
- Surgical closure is a stitch closure or closure with a pericardial patch.

Primum Atrial Septal Defects

- Surgical patch closure is necessary.
- Even without MR, the cleft is often closed to avoid the late development of MR.

Sinus Venosus Sinus Atrial Septal Defects

- Patch closure of defect with anomalous PV baffled to the LA.
- The SVC-RA junction may be augmented with a pericardial patch to avoid SVC obstruction: two-patch technique may be

necessary, one to baffle the PV and one to augment the SVC.
- When PVs drain into the high SVC or there is difficulty making an unobstructed baffle, a Warden procedure may need to be performed in which the SVC is disconnected and reattached to the right atrial appendage. The PV "stump" (the cardiac end of the SVC containing the anomalous PV) is baffle closed to the LA.

Coronary Sinus Atrial Septal Defects

- Without an LSVC, simple patch closure of the CS orifice. The CS drains into the LA, resulting in minimal cyanosis (right-to-left shunt).
- With an LSVC, the CS is covered in the LA and the ostium is allowed to drain into the RA. If a bridging vein is present, the LSVC can be ligated and the CS orifice closed. If an LSVC is not recognized, a simple patch closure will result in unacceptable cyanosis.

Postoperative TEE Assessment

- Verify ASD closure. A bubble contrast study is often a helpful adjunct to visualize shunts.
- Assess MV function. After a primum repair, MR can be eccentric and composed of multiple jets. Grading can be difficult. Use the vena contracta width (<3–5 mm is ideal), density of spectral jet, duration of regurgitation, area/pattern of jet (wrap around ventricle), and effect on PV flow pattern. Less than mild MR is best for a durable repair, but moderate MR may be acceptable if further repair results in mitral inflow obstruction.
- Sinus venosus ASD: Confirm appropriate drainage of PVs into the LA without narrowing of PV, SVC, SVC baffle, or SVC-RA appendage anastomosis. SVC and PV flow should be laminar, low velocity, and phasic.
- After device closure it is important to verify the absence of pulmonary venous obstruction.

Ventricular Septal Defects (Table 4-2)

- Perimembranous (also called infracristal, subaortic, paramembranous, conoventricular)
- Inlet (also called AV canal [AVC] type)
- Outlet (also called subpulmonary, supracristal, doubly committed, subarterial, infundibular, conal)
- Muscular
- Malalignment type (with anterior or posterior deviated outlet septum)

TABLE 4-2 BASIC ECHO PRINCIPLES WHEN IMAGING VSDs

Defect	Best TEE Views*	What to Look for on 2D Imaging	CFD and Spectral Doppler
All VSDs		• Measure size of VSD. Size can be compared to size of aortic valve (small, <25%; moderate, 25–75%; large, >75%; or roughly small, 1–2 mm; moderate, 3–5 mm; large, >5mm). • Look for multiple VSDs. • Assess LAE/LVE. • Assess TV, RAE. Measure annulus if dilated. • Assess biventricular function. • PHTN/RVH/R→L shunt/systolic flattening of IVS in systole may indicate Eisenmenger syndrome. • Look for subpulmonary/subaortic obstruction. • Look for associated lesions.	• CFD/CW to classify size/ direction of shunt. (Flow is L→R during systole with a small reversal during the early part of diastole in an uncomplicated VSD.) • CW to measure RVP = PAP = SysBP − $4V_{vsd}^2$, or RVP = $4V_{TR}^2$ + RAP. In the absence of RVOTO, RVP = PAP. With RVOTO, PAP = RVP − RVOT gradient. • CFD/CW/PW to assess AI. Use vena contracta, width of jet compared to LVOT, flow reversal in descending Ao, AI deceleration slope/ deceleration time. • CFD/CW to assess TR.
Peri-membranous VSD	ME four chamber ME LAX ME modified 5C ME AV SAX ME RV inflow- outflow ME AV LAX Deep TG LAX	• From RV: defect adjacent to septal leaflet of TV. • From LV: defect adjacent to RCC and NCC (ME 4C, ME AV SAX, ME RV inflow-outflow, modified 5C views, obtained by withdrawing/ flexing the probe slightly from ME 4C view). • Septal TV leaflet tissue can completely/partially close defect. • Examine AV cusps for structure/ function especially thickness, prolapse (RCC/NCC) (Fig. 4-4A).	
Inlet VSD	ME four chamber ME LAX ME RV inflow- outflow ME AV LAX TG basal SAX TG :LAX Deep TG LAX	• Located inferiorly/posteriorly in inlet septum adjacent to AVV (ME 4C view or leftward rotation from ME RV inflow-outflow view or rightward rotation from ME LAX view absent/scooped out appearance of inlet septum seen). • Often associated with an AVC defect (see below). • Examine valve for override (>50% opens into the opposite ventricle) or for straddling chords that cross the IVS and insert in the opposite ventricle (Fig. 4-5) (ME 4C view). • Examine LVOT for chords, membranes, tunnel-like LVOTO.	• CFD/CW to assess AVV stenosis/regurgitation. • CFD/CW to assess for LVOTO (deep TG LAX, TG LAX views).
Outlet VSD	ME LAX ME modified 5C ME AV SAX ME RV inflow- outflow ME AV LAX Deep TG LAX Deep TG RVOT	• From RV: defect anterior/adjacent to pulmV in RVOT (ME AV SAX, deep TG LAX, ME RV inflow-outflow views). • From LV: defect between LCC/RCC (ME AV LAX view with rightward rotation). • Examine AV cusp for structure/ function, especially thickness, prolapse (RCC) (Fig. 4-4B) (ME RV inflow-outflow, ME AV LAX views with rightward rotation).	• CFD/CW/PW to assess AR.

Continued

TABLE 4-2   BASIC ECHO PRINCIPLES WHEN IMAGING VSDs—cont'd

Defect	Best TEE Views*	What to Look for on 2D Imaging	CFD and Spectral Doppler
Muscular	ME four chamber ME LAX ME AV LAX TG mid SAX Deep TG LAX Deep TG RVOT	• Defect in muscular inlet/outlet/mid-ventricular/apical septum. • Perform careful sweep of entire IVS because multiple defects are common.	
Malalignment type	ME LAX ME AV SAX ME AV LAX Deep TG LAX	• Anterior deviation typical of TOF and is associated with RVOTO. Look for other components of TOF (see TOF). • Posterior deviation typical of interrupted aortic arch/coarctation and results in subaortic stenosis. Assess mechanism/severity of LVOTO. It may be possible to see evidence of coarctation/interruption/hypoplastic Ao (scanning up and down from descending aortic LAX). • Look for PDA (UE aortic arch SAX, ME ascending aortic SAX).	• CFD/CW to assess RVOTO/LVOTO (in presence of a PDA, the gradient may not be present). • CFD/PW to assess for coarctation. Look for aliasing and persistent antegrade flow in diastole. • CFD/CW to assess for a PDA and direction of flow (UE aortic arch SAX, ME ascending aortic SAX).

*See the Appendix on page 57 for schematics of these views.

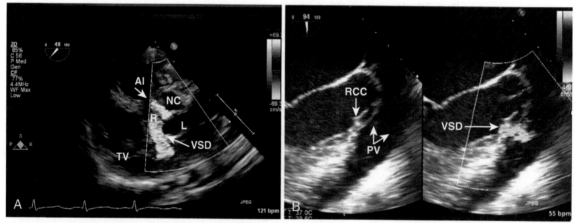

Figure 4-4. A, 2D and CFD ME RV inflow-outflow view demonstrating the proximity of the defect to the TV and the AV. There is mild-moderate AI that was seen to originate from a prolapse of the RCC. **B**, 2D and CFD ME AV LAX view demonstrating an outlet defect that is adjacent to the RCC in the left ventricle (LV) and entering the right ventricle (RV) underneath the pulmonary valve.

KEY POINTS

All Ventricular Septal Defects
• Left-to-right (L→R) shunt at the ventricular level results in left heart enlargement.
• Associated lesions include aortic regurgitation (AR), ASD, double-chamber right ventricle (DCRV), coarctation/other complex CHD.
• Significant TR may occasionally result from PHTN.

Perimembranous/Outlet Defects
• Due to Venturi effect from ventricular septal defect (VSD) flow, right coronary cusp (RCC) and noncoronary cusp (NCC) at risk of prolapse with the development of AR.

Inlet Defects
• Often part of an AVC defect or a component of heterotaxy syndrome.
• Abnormalities of the AVV and LVOT are common.

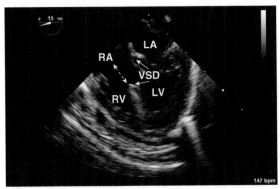

Figure 4-5. 2D ME 4C view demonstrating an inlet VSD in a patient with an overriding tricuspid valve (TV) with straddling chords. The straddling chords are not well seen. The *stippled line* represents where the crest of the interventricular septum would join the AV annulus. More than 50% of the TV opens into the LV, consistent with the definition of an overriding valve.

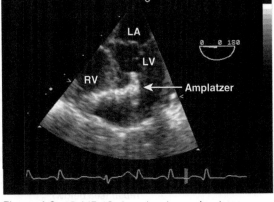

Figure 4-6. 2D ME 4C view showing an Amplatzer device that was placed through a muscular VSD using a right ventriculotomy (hybrid approach). This picture was taken immediately before release of the device.

Muscular Defects
- May be difficult to locate, especially if there are multiple defects in the trabeculated RV apex.
- Defect may partially/completely close with surrounding muscle.

Malalignment Type
- Outlet (infundibular) septum is deviated anteriorly or posteriorly and fails to join the interventricular septum (IVS) resulting in a VSD and outflow tract obstruction.
- Anterior deviation results in a VSD and right ventricular outflow tract obstruction (RVOTO) (TOF).
- Posterior deviation is typical of interrupted aortic arch/coarctation complexes and results in a VSD and LVOTO.

Principles of Surgical Management
- In the presence of a large VSD, PHTN, evidence of Eisenmenger syndrome, or R→L flow through the VSD, cardiac catheterization may be required to assess pulmonary vascular resistance (PVR) before closure of a VSD.
- At this time, devices are not yet approved for routine closure of VSDs, although devices for closure of muscular/perimembranous defects are available. A hybrid approach with catheter access through a right ventriculotomy with TEE guidance is useful in some cases (Fig. 4-6).
- Surgical closure is with a synthetic patch via RA/RV/infundibular (transpulmonary)/transaortic/rarely LV approach.

- Approach to some defects may require take-down of tricuspid valve for adequate exposure.
- TV repair/annuloplasty ring may rarely be necessary if RV hypertension has caused severe TR.
- Surgical management in patients with subaortic obstruction from a posterior malaligned VSD is complex and may involve LVOT enlargement (Konno procedure) or may have to follow a single ventricle (SV) pathway.

Postoperative TEE Assessment
- Verify VSD closure and look for residual/additional VSDs. Residual acceptable VSD flow should be high velocity (restrictive). About 40% of patients have a residual VSD on intraoperative TEE. Most are small or moderate. Long-term follow-up shows that the majority close. Additional parameters to quantitate size are Q_p/Q_s (pulmonary/systemic blood flow) determined by intraoperative blood gas analysis (<1.5, small; 1.5–2, moderate; >2, large) or right ventricular pressure/left ventricular pressure (RVP/LVP) (<0.5, small; 0.5–0.75, moderate; >0.75, large).
- Measure RVP/PAP using TR or VSD jet velocity.
- Verify that ASD/PFO is closed.
- Examine TV/AV. Look for prolapse/perforation of a cusp or poor resuspension of the TV around annulus. Confirm that there is no significant TR or AR.
- Examine biventricular function. New or worsening ventricular dysfunction can be secondary to bypass and cross clamp CPB, a ventriculotomy, or injury to a coronary artery.

TABLE 4-3   BASIC ECHO PRINCIPLES WHEN IMAGING AVC DEFECTS

Best TEE Views*	What to Look for on 2D Imaging	CFD and Spectral Doppler
ME four chamber ME LAX TG basal SAX TG mid SAX TG LAX Deep TG LAX	• Examine IAS for primum defect/secundum ASD/PFO. • Examine the configuration of the AVV. Look for straddling/aberrant chords/AVV override, MV cleft, leaflet prolapse (ME 4C, ME LAX, TG basal SAX deep TG LAX views). • Assess the inlet VSD. • Evaluate size/function of ventricles and whether the defect is balanced (ME 4C, TG mid-SAX views). • Look for LSVC; *it alters surgical repair* (see below).	• CFD/PW to assess ASD size/direction of flow (should be L→R in uncomplicated AVC). • CFD/CW to assess VSD size/direction of flow (should be L→R in uncomplicated AVC). • Grade AVV stenosis/regurgitation. • Identify possible LVOTO with CFD and measure gradient (deep TG LAX, TG LAX, ME LAX views). • Measure RVP/PAP with TR/VSD jet.

*See the Appendix on page 57 for schematics of these views.

Atrioventricular Canal Defects (also called Atrioventricular Septal Defects or Endocardial Cushion Defects) (Table 4-3)

- Partial AVC
- Transitional AVC
- Complete AVC

Partial AVC
- Consists of a primum ASD, cleft MV (see Primum ASD)

Transitional AVC
- Consists of a primum ASD, cleft MV, restrictive VSD

Complete AVC
- Consists of a primum ASD, inlet VSD, and common AVV.
- Single AVV with multiple leaflets, usually an anterior (superior) and posterior (inferior) leaflet that bridges the IVS and several lateral leaflets (Fig. 4-7).
- AVV regurgitation is often multifactorial.
- Straddling chords that insert in the opposite ventricle may prohibit the creation of two competent AVVs and necessitate a SV repair.
- Often the RV appears small compared with the LV because of the large VSD. Concerning is a small LV (unbalanced AVC), which may indicate the need for a SV repair.
- Repair before 4 to 6 months of age is ideal to avoid pulmonary vascular disease.
- Associated lesions: TOF.
- Late development of LVOTO in about 5% of patients (see Primum ASD for etiology of LVOTO).

Principles of Surgical Management
- A one- or two-patch technique or the so-called Australian technique (stitch closure of VSD with patch closure of ASD) is used to close the ASDs/VSDs and bridge the anterior/posterior leaflets.
- The atrial patch is usually placed so that the CS drains into the LA. An LSVC draining to the CS would preclude that.
- Residual MV cleft is usually closed unless significant valve distortion would result in mitral stenosis (MS)/MR.
- May have to accept even moderate residual regurgitation to avoid early valve replacement.

Postoperative TEE Assessment
- Verify closure of ASDs/VSDs.
- AVV without stenosis/prolapse/flail. Minimal/acceptable degree of regurgitation. Regurgitant jets may be multiple/complex and difficult to grade.
- Measure PAP if TR is present.
- Assess biventricular function.

Tetralogy of Fallot (Table 4-4)

- TOF with PS
- TOF with pulmonary atresia
- TOF with an AVC
- TOF with an absent pulmonary valve
- Double-outlet RV (DORV)-TOF spectrum

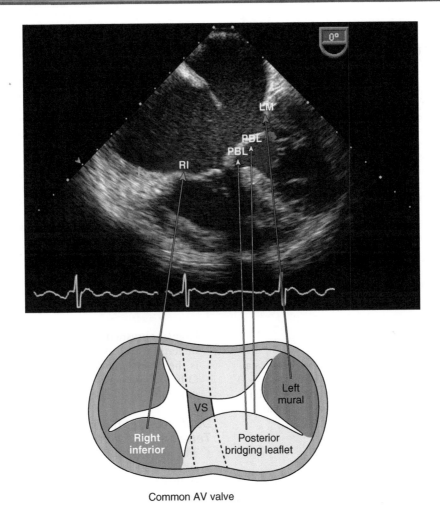

Common AV valve

Figure 4-7. 2D ME 4C view in a patient with a complete AVC defect with an inset of a schematic of the configuration of a common AVV typical of patients with Down syndrome. *Arrows* in the 2D picture indicate corresponding leaflet in the schematic. Lateral leaflets are the left mural (LM) and right inferior (RI), bridging leaflet is the posterior bridging leaflet (PBL). *(Adapted with permission from Joffe D, Oxorn D. Transitional atrioventricular canal. Anesth Analg. 2009; 109[2]:358-360.)*

TABLE 4-4	BASIC ECHO PRINCIPLES WHEN IMAGING TOF	
Best TEE Views*	**What to Look for on 2D Imaging**	**CFD and Spectral Doppler**
ME four chamber ME LAX ME modified 5C ME AV SAX ME RV inflow-outflow ME AV LAX ME bicaval TG mid SAX Deep TG RVOT	• Examine IAS for ASD/PFO. • Assess VSD location(s)/size (ME AV LAX, ME LAX, withdraw from ME 4C, ME RV inflow-outflow, ME AV SAX, deep TG LAX views). • Assess RVH/biventricular function/size (ME 4C, TG mid SAX, ME RV inflow-outflow views). • Examine origin/course of coronary arteries. • Look for abnormalities in course of descending aorta (see above).	• CFD to assess size/direction of atrial/ventricular level shunts. • Direction of ASD/VSD flow may be dynamic depending on RVOTO. • Continuous flow signals (not in the location of) strongly suggestive of MAPCAs.
ME asc aortic SAX ME AV SAX ME RV inflow-outflow Deep TG RVOT UE aortic arch SAX	• Assess morphology/function of pulmV. Look for doming leaflets with commissural fusion. Measure annulus Z score. Z score < −2.5 to −3 generally warrant transannular patch. • Assess level(s) of RVOTO/PA stenosis. Examine RV/RVOT; measure pulmonary annulus/PAs as far distally as possible.	• CFD/CW to identify/measure RVOTO/PA stenosis (ME RV inflow-outflow, ME ascending aortic SAX, deep TG LAX turn leftward/antiflex, UE aortic arch SAX views).

*See the Appendix on page 57 for schematics of these views.

KEY POINTS

All Forms of Tetralogy of Fallot
- Consist of RVOTO, an anterior malaligned VSD, RVH, and an overriding aorta. The VSD is usually large and unrestrictive. Associated defects include PFO, ASD, and additional VSDs.
- RVOTO is secondary to a combination of obstruction at multiple levels: subpulmonary/infundibular narrowing/pulmonary valve annular hypoplasia/PS/main pulmonary artery (PA) or branch PA hypoplasia. RV hypertrophy results from obstruction and worsens over time. Rarely, there is intracavitary obstruction similar to a double-chamber RV.
- There is a 25% incidence of a right aortic arch (the arch goes over the right bronchus, but this is not seen by TEE). However, abnormalities in the course of the descending aorta should increase suspicion because although a left arch can exist with a right descending aorta, it is unusual.
- Coronary artery anomalies are common. In about 3%, the left anterior descending artery comes from the right coronary artery (RCA) and crosses the RVOTO.
- Over time dilation of the ascending aorta can develop in patients with conotruncal abnormalities (TOF, transposition of the great arteries [TGA], truncus arteriosus), which may progress and may become a risk for rupture or dissection. It may also cause AR.

Tetralogy of Fallot with Pulmonary Stenosis
- The most common location of PA hypoplasia is the left PA at the insertion point of the ductus. The left PA is not well seen by TEE.
- Rarely there can be aortopulmonary collateral arteries.

Tetralogy of Fallot with Pulmonary Atresia
- Atresia may be limited to the valve or may involve the subpulmonary infundibulum.
- Variable degrees of hypoplasia of the main or branch PAs. There can be nonconfluent PAs, PAs supplied by a ductus with or without multiple aortopulmonary collateral arteries, and absent PAs. In the latter case, pulmonary blood flow is supplied by multiple aortopulmonary collateral arteries.
- Patients require a preoperative cardiac catheterization to delineate PA anatomy/identify multiple aortopulmonary collateral arteries. Not reliably seen on TTE/TEE.

Tetralogy of Fallot with an Atrioventricular Canal
- Components of both diseases present, but RVOTO results in less PBF and a smaller common AVV orifice than with an isolated AVC, making the repair more difficult.
- The malaligned VSD has inlet extension.

Tetralogy of Fallot with an Absent Pulmonary Valve
- Pulmonary annulus is hypoplastic with no pulmonary valve leaflets, resulting in severe pulmonary valve insufficiency (PI). PAs are large/aneurysmal. Often there is severe RV dilatation. The degree of airway compromise is the overriding determinant of prognosis.
- Other components of TOF present include dynamic RVOTO that causes "tet spells."

Double-Outlet Right Ventricle – Tetralogy of Fallot Spectrum
- The aorta overrides the IVS by more than 50%.
- With a subaortic VSD and subpulmonary obstruction, the physiology resembles TOF. Intracardiac anatomy resembles TOF, although the aorta is more rightward and there is no aortic-MV continuity.

Principles of Surgical Management
(Table 4-5)

Postoperative TEE Assessment
- Immediately post-bypass, there may be acute worsening of right ventricular diastolic and systolic function secondary to multiple factors such as bypass and ischemic cross-clamp times, a ventriculotomy, or, rarely, coronary injury. Additional volume and pressure loads on the RV from PI, AVV regurgitation, residual VSD, or RVOTO can create an intolerable hemodynamic burden. The postoperative course is especially difficult after TOF with AVC if the repair is suboptimal. Interpretation of post-CPB TEE must take these facts into account.
- Visualize the VSD patch and look for a residual VSD. Reexamine the IVS because lower right ventricular pressures may unmask previously unrecognized VSDs.

TABLE 4-5   PRINCIPLES OF SURGICAL MANAGEMENT

Defect	Most Common Surgical Apapproach
All TOF (except TOF-PA)	• Complete repair consists of VSD closure/division/limited resection of RV muscle bundles/pulmonary valvotomy and commissurotomy/transannular patch/PA plasty if indicated. RA/RV approach for VSD, and may need separate infundibular incision for obstructing outlet components. • Atrial fenestration/PFO usually left to preserve cardiac output in the event of diastolic dysfunction of the RV (restrictive right ventricular physiology).
TOF-PS	• Surgical approach/timing varies. Options for cyanotic patients include palliation with systemic-to-pulmonary shunt (rarely ductal stent) versus complete repair.
TOF-PA	• Complex. Often requires staged procedures.
TOF-AVC	• Both lesions are usually repaired simultaneously.
TOF-APV	• May require translocation/plication of PAs or valved RV-PA conduit in addition to TOF repair.
DORV	• The spectrum of repairs varies from a TOF-like repair to an arterial switch procedure and occasionally other options. • In TOF spectrum, VSD closed with a patch so that left ventricular outflow is baffled to the aorta. May also need subaortic conus resection.

- Exception: TOF with pulmonary atresia. It is often necessary to fenestrate the VSD or leave it open completely.
- Locate/measure residual RVOTO. Obstruction with RVP more than two thirds systemic requires revision. The exception is myocardial hypertrophy causing dynamic obstruction, which generally resolves with time and/or altered hemodynamic management (volume loading, decreasing inotropic support, etc.).
- Assess PI/conduit function.
- Examine PFO/atrial shunt and note direction of flow. R→L flow provides a crude indication of right ventricular diastolic dysfunction and provides an explanation for systemic desaturation.
- Assess biventricular function. Postoperative right ventricular systolic function may be preserved even in the presence of significant residual RVOTO, so normal function does *not* rule out RVOTO.

Transposition of the Great Arteries (Table 4-6)

- Dextro transposition of the great arteries (d-TGA)
- DORV-transposition spectrum
- Congenitally corrected TGA

Dextro Transposition of the Great Arteries
- The aorta originates rightward and anteriorly from the RV, the PA originates from the LV.

- A VSD is present in 20%, and 20% of those have PS.
- Must have a source of intracardiac mixing: PDA/PFO/ASD/VSD.
- A small number have an interrupted aortic arch/coarctation.
- Coronary arteries usually arise from aortic sinuses that face the PA: sinus 1 (anterior)/sinus 2 (posterior), but the origin and course are often abnormal.

DORV-TGA Spectrum
- The aorta arises from the RV, and the PA originates from the LV but overrides the RV more than 50%. With a subpulmonary VSD, physiology resembles TGA.

Congenitally Corrected TGA
- Often referred to as L-TGA (levo-TGA).
- There is atrioventricular and ventriculoarterial discordance. Physiologically correct but anatomically inverted. The aorta exits anteriorly and to the left from the right-sided LV.
- The RA connects to the anatomic LV and LA to anatomic RV.
- Associated VSD, PS, Ebstein's anomaly of the left-sided TV are common.

Additional Facts
- Low LV wall thickness/mass in combination with a "banana-shaped" LV may indicate an "unprepared LV" and increase the likelihood of needing mechanical support after an arterial switch operation (ASO) in the rare patient

TABLE 4-6   BASIC ECHOCARDIOGRAPHIC PRINCIPLES WHEN IMAGING d-TGA

Best TEE Views*	What to Look for on 2D Imaging	CFD and Spectral Doppler
ME four chamber ME LAX ME asc aortic SAX ME RV inflow-outflow ME AV LAX ME bicaval TG mid SAX TG LAX Deep TG LAX	• Examine IAS, ASD usually large. • Assess VSD size/location/extension. Confirm it can be closed without compromising RV size or AVV function or causing LVOTO (ME 4C, ME LAX, ME RV inflow-outflow, deep TG LAX views). • Great vessels (GV) are parallel and often seen in the same orientation in transverse/longitudinal views (ME LAX, ME AV LAX, ME RV inflow-outflow with leftward scanning, deep TG LAX, ME ascending aortic SAX views). • TGA: pulmonary valve–mitral valve continuity, subaortic conus, and anterior/posterior GV (Fig. 4-8A). • DORV: bilateral subarterial conus and the GV are usually more side by side than in TGA (Fig. 4-8B). • Examine morphology/function of both outflow tracts and semilunar valves and look for obstruction. • Assess biventricular function/wall thickness/orientation of IVS. • Note origin/course of the coronary arteries. Look for intramural/interarterial course. • Look for a PDA.	• CFD/PW to assess size/direction of ASD flow. • CFD/CW to assess size/direction of VSD flow. • Examine both outflow tracts/measure gradients. • Examine both semilunar valves for stenosis/insufficiency. • Examine coronary flow. • MR jet used to estimate PAP. • Determine predominant direction of flow in PDA and measure aortic to PA gradient (see text).

*See the Appendix on page 57 for schematics of these views.

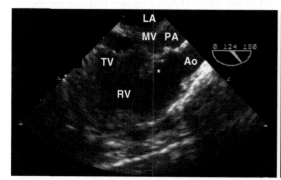 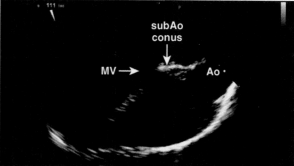

Figure 4-8. Double-outlet RV (DORV) versus transposition of the great arteries (TGA). **A**, 2D ME right ventricular inflow-outflow view in a patient with d-TGA. The aorta (Ao) is anterior to the PA and comes off the RV. There is PA-MV continuity and a subaortic conus (*asterisk*). **B**, ME LAX view in a patient with DORV. The aorta overrides the RV by more than 50%, and there is a subaortic conus resulting in a lack of continuity between the aortic and mitral valves. Note the PA and the aorta are more side by side, so the PA is not visible in this anteroposterior image of the great vessels. There is a large subaortic VSD.

who is older than 2 to 3 months at the time of the ASO.
• If a PDA is present, the predominant direction of flow can provide important information. If high-velocity left-to-right flow (aorta to PA), it suggests low PAP/LV pressure. If right-to-left flow, it suggests PHTN or coarctation/interrupted aortic arch.
• The RCA and left main coronary artery (LMCA) are easiest to identify (≥60%) by TEE. The left anterior descending artery and the left circumflex coronary artery (Cx) are more difficult. More than 95% of patients with d-TGA have a right-dominant system.
• Distinguish structural pulmonary obstruction (LVOTO) from dynamic obstruction secondary to septal bowing into the LV. The former may preclude performing an ASO, whereas the latter resolves after the ASO.

Principles of Surgical Management

- An atrial septostomy is performed before surgical repair if there are no other sources of mixing.
- ASO. The aorta is moved posteriorly, and the main PA is moved anteriorly. A Lecompte maneuver is performed: the right PA is moved anterior to the aortic arch so that the main PA/PA branches are anterior to the aorta. The coronary arteries are translocated to the aorta. Intracardiac shunts are closed.
- With VSD and PS, options include the Rastelli procedure/Nikaidoh procedure (aortic translocation)/ASO with LVOT enlargement/others.
- The Rastelli procedure is the standard treatment. The VSD is closed by baffling LV outflow to the anterior aorta/PA is transected/RV-PA direct anastomosis or via a conduit. However, long-term survival is compromised by
  - LVOTO/RVOTO secondary to the long angulated course of the baffle.
  - The RV-PA conduit needs several replacements during the patient's lifetime and is prone to compression and accidental re-entry during reoperations.
- Nikaidoh procedure: a combination of an ASO, an autograft valve replacement with the coronary arteries moved as buttons or en bloc (Ross component), and a Konno (see section on LVOT abnormalities). An RV-PA direct anastomosis or via a conduit is required, although the conduit is in a more favorable location compared with a Rastelli (Fig. 4-9). A Nikaidoh procedure is an option when the VSD is not in an optimal location for a Rastelli procedure, i.e., an inlet VSD.
- ASO with LVOT enlargement. Given the complexity of these approaches, performing an ASO/LVOT enlargement may be a reasonable option in select patients (predominantly valvular PS with mild to moderate subvalvular PS amenable to enlargement/resection).
- The management of the patient with congenitally corrected TGA is controversial. The three general approaches are:
  - Ignore the abnormal connections and repair associated defects. However, this leaves the RV as the systemic ventricle and results in a high incidence of TR and complete heart block.
  - Perform a double switch (an ASO and atrial switch) after a preliminary PA band if necessary. The ideal timing is before the prepubescent age group. This complex procedure restores the LV to the systemic ventricle but leaves the patient with intra-atrial baffles.
  - Cardiac transplantation.

Postoperative TEE Assessment

- TEE has a limited ability to directly assess coronary flow. Use surrogate indicators of perfusion such as wall motion and MR.
- Verify closure of ASD/VSD.
- Confirm a lack of obstruction at the aortic and pulmonary anastomosis. Measure gradients.
- Assess biventricular function, especially regional wall motion abnormalities.
- MR may be related to poor ventricular function, ischemia, or overly aggressive volume resuscitation.
- If an aortic arch abnormality was repaired, verify patency as much as possible. Look for low velocity laminar flow in the aorta without a diastolic gradient.
- Examine coronary flow using CFD/PW (see earlier discussion). Coronaries are often implanted above the sinuses. PW pattern consists of a late systolic peak and a slower diastolic decrease in velocity (Fig. 4-10). A peak systolic velocity greater than 0.6 cm/s or velocity-time integral greater than 0.14 may be abnormal and should prompt visual inspection of the coronary arteries by the surgeon and a careful evaluation of regional wall motion.
- Congenitally corrected TGA—verify repair of associated defects if physiologic repair was done. If a double switch was performed, see previously described considerations for evaluation post-ASO. In addition, verify atrial baffle patency without obstruction/stenosis.

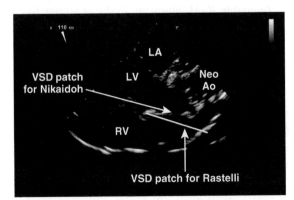

Figure 4-9. 2D ME LAX view in a patient with d-TGA, pulmonary stenosis, and a VSD after a Nikaidoh procedure. Note that the almost vertical VSD patch is baffled to the now posteriorly located aorta. The subaortic area is wide open. There is also a RV-PA conduit that can be identified anteriorly by its increased echogenicity. The *solid line* marks the approximate angle of a VSD patch if a Rastelli procedure had been performed (see text).

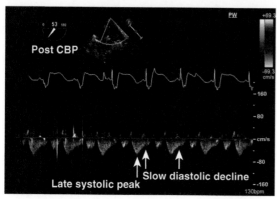

Figure 4-10. Pulsed wave imaging of the implanted left coronary artery after an arterial switch operation demonstrating a late systolic peak with a slower decline in coronary blood flow during diastole.

Total Anomalous Pulmonary Venous Drainage (Table 4-7)

- Supracardiac total anomalous pulmonary venous drainage (TAPVD)
- Cardiac TAPVD
- Infracardiac TAPVD
- Mixed TAPVD

KEY POINTS

All Forms of TAPVD
- All PVs drain to a location other than the LA.
- They usually drain to a horizontal confluence behind the LA, then to a vertical vein, and then a systemic vein (innominate, SVC, azygos, CS, inferior vena cava [IVC], or other veins).
- A PFO is necessary for survival.
- Usually an isolated defect except when associated with heterotaxy syndrome.
- Patients with obstructed TAPVD often present as neonates in extremis.

Supracardiac TAPVD
- Most common type (50% of cases).
- Vertical vein usually anterior to left PA but occasionally between the left PA and left bronchus creating pulmonary venous obstruction. As PAP increases, the "vicelike" compression worsens.

Cardiac TAPVD
- About 25% of cases.
- The PV confluence drains to the CS or RA.
- Can rarely become obstructive or cause mitral inflow obstruction.

Infracardiac TAPVD
- About 20% of cases.
- The PVs drain to vertical confluence behind the LA. The vertical vein descends to the portal vein/ductus venosus/hepatic vein, then to the IVC.
- PV obstruction occurs as the vein descends below the diaphragm.

Mixed TAPVD
- Least common, about 5% of cases.
- No PV confluence—any combination of the previously listed forms is present.

Principles of Surgical Management
- The vertical vein is ligated, and the PV confluence is opened into the LA.
- Sutureless PV repair, a procedure often performed on patients with recurrent PV stenosis, is occasionally performed for primary repairs.
- In the newborn, the PFO is often left open to enable R→L shunting in the postoperative period. If the LA is small, a fenestrated patch is used to close the ASD. The surgery is straightforward, but patients are often severely ill postoperatively with PHTN.

TABLE 4-7   BASIC ECHO PRINCIPLES WHEN IMAGING TAPVD

Best TEE Views*	What to Look for on 2D Imaging	CFD and Spectral Doppler
ME four chamber ME LAX ME mitral commissural ME RV inflow-outflow ME AV LAX ME bicaval TG mid SAX TG two chamber Deep TG LAX UE aortic arch SAX	• PV confluence is easy to identify behind LA (any view of LA). • Assess ASD/PFO. • Assess LA size. • Assess biventricular function. Systolic flattening of septal wall consistent with PHTN. • Massively dilated CS with cardiac TAPVD (any view of LA). • Examine innominate, SVC, CS, IVC; note size.	• Locate PVs with CFD. Look for increased velocity/lack of pulsatility/aliasing. Measure gradient (ME 4C, ME 2C, ME bicaval views). • Atrial shunt is R→L. • Measure $PAP = RVP = 4V_{TR}^2 + RAP$. • If PDA is present, bidirectional or R→L flow suggests elevated PAP. • CFD/PW to examine entry site of PV drainage.

*See the Appendix on page 57 for schematics of these views.

TABLE 4-8   BASIC ECHO PRINCIPLES WHEN IMAGING TRUNCUS ARTERIOSUS

Best TEE Views*	What to Look for on 2D Imaging	CFD and Spectral Doppler
ME four chamber ME LAX ME asc aortic SAX ME AV SAX ME AV LAX ME bicaval TG LAX Deep TG LAX UE aortic arch SAX	• Look for ASD/PFO. • Assess location/size of VSD. • Locate the origin of PAs, usually from posterior left side of truncus or separately off posterior truncus (Fig. 4-11). • Assess PA size (hypoplasia/stenosis rare). • Assess truncal valve: leaflets/thickness/mobility/stenosis/regurgitation. • Assess biventricular size/function. • Examine descending aorta and arch for evidence of abnormality or PDA. • Examine course of the coronary arteries.	• CFD/CW to assess truncal valve regurgitation/stenosis (deep TG LAX, TG LAX, ME LAX, ME AV LAX views). • CFD/CW/PW evaluation of ASD/VSD.

*See the Appendix on page 57 for schematics of these views.

- TAPVD to the CS. The CS is "unroofed" into the LA, and the CS ostium is closed with a patch so that both the CS and anomalous PV drain into the LA.

Postoperative TEE Assessment
- The anastomosis between the PV confluence and LA is usually easy to visualize. Laminar flow should be present, although the PW tracing is often abnormal with flow that does not return to baseline and has a continuous gradient. The tracing can usually be ignored if the anastomosis is widely patent and the patient's clinical status is adequate. Predischarge TTE findings are usually normal. The etiology of the pseudo-obstruction pattern is likely post-CPB changes in LA and LV compliance.
- The direction of the atrial shunt should be noted.
- Measure the PAP if TR is present.
- Assess biventricular function.

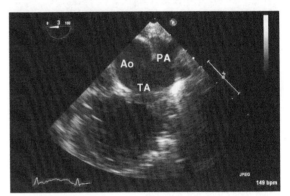

Figure 4-11. 2D ME AV SAX view in a patient with type 1 truncus arteriosus. The main PA originates to the left of the truncal valve.

- Complete early repair with VSD closure and placement of a (valved) RV-to-PA conduit is ideal. An atrial communication is usually left to allow right-to-left shunting.
- The treatment of moderate to severe truncal regurgitation is usually a valve repair, with the expectation that residual regurgitation is likely. Otherwise, a homograft aortic valve replacement is necessary in the neonatal period, although because of the large truncus, a reasonably sized prosthetic valve can be placed earlier than in other forms of CHD (Fig. 4-12).

Postoperative TEE Assessment
- Examine the PFO/atrial fenestration and note the direction of the shunt.
- Verify VSD closure. The size of an acceptable residual defect should be individualized given that the ventriculotomy/residual truncal valve regurgitation/conduit regurgitation (if valveless conduit) may worsen preexisting right ventricular diastolic dysfunction.
- Assess the course of the conduit and assess for stenosis or regurgitation.

KEY POINTS

Truncus Arteriosus (Table 4-8)
- Classified according to the origin of the main PA or, if absent, separate PAs off the truncus (common great vessel [GV] exiting the heart).
- Abnormal truncal valve is very common with more than three leaflets. The valve can be regurgitant, rarely stenotic.
- Associated defects: large subaortic VSD, interrupted aortic arch (10–15%), right aortic arch (25%), aberrant right subclavian artery (5–10%).
- Abnormal coronary anatomy is common.

Principles of Surgical Management
- Low diastolic blood pressure caused by runoff into the PA or ventricle (if truncal regurgitation is present) can result in precarious myocardial perfusion.

- Assess the truncal valve for insufficiency/stenosis.
- Assess biventricular function.
- Evaluate coronary flow if a homograft was required.

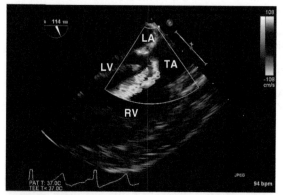

Figure 4-12. CFD ME modified AV LAX view with rightward rotation in a 3-month-old patient with truncus arteriosus. Note the large truncal valve and subaortic VSD. There is prolapse of a left-sided aortic cusp with severe truncal valve regurgitation, mostly into the RV. This patient previously had a modified truncus repair with repair of the truncus and placement of a RV-PA conduit but with the VSD left open. She presented with symptoms of severe right heart failure and had placement of a prosthetic truncal valve, VSD closure, and revision of the RV-PA conduit. The surgeons thought that a truncal valve repair was not possible.

Single Ventricle (Table 4-9)

KEY POINTS

- Includes hypoplastic left heart syndrome, single ventricle (SV) (double-inlet left ventricle [DILV] the most common variant), tricuspid atresia, unbalanced AVC, PA with an intact ventricular septum (PA/IVS), heterotaxy syndrome (Fig. 4-13).
- In DILV, both AVV empty into the LV. A VSD (also referred to by its embryological name, the bulboventricular foramen [BVF]) leads to the outlet chamber. The ventricles and GVs are often transposed. Associated hypoplastic aorta, coarctation, and subaortic obstruction are common. PS/subpulmonary stenosis are also common. In less than 10%, the two coexist.

Principles of Surgical Management

- Usually a three-stage repair leading to a Fontan procedure.
- Stage 1 procedure (see Table 4-10).
- Stage 2: bidirectional cavopulmonary anastomosis (Glenn/Hemi-Fontan procedure).
- Stage 3: Fontan procedure.

TABLE 4-9 BASIC ECHO PRINCIPLES WHEN IMAGING PATIENTS WITH SINGLE VENTRICLES

Best TEE Views*	What to Look for on 2D Imaging	CFD and Spectral Doppler
ME four chamber ME two chamber ME LAX ME mitral commissural ME asc aortic SAX ME RV inflow-outflow ME AV LAX ME bicaval TG basal SAX TG mid SAX TG LAX Deep TG LAX Deep TG RVOT UE aortic arch SAX	• Determine position/size of GV (deep TG LAX, ME LAX, ME LAX, ME RV inflow-outflow, ME ascending aortic SAX views). • Determine morphology/function of semilunar valves/conus (ME LAX, ME RV inflow-outflow views). • Examine biventricular size/function (TG mid-SAX, ME 4C views). • Measure BVF. If less than the size of a normal aortic valve (or <2 cm²/m²), it suggests restrictive flow is likely (ME 4C view). • Examine size/morphology of AVV. Determine Z score (if TV Z < –3 in PA/IVS, SV repair likely). Determine whether valve overrides or has straddling chords (ME 4C, ME LAX views). • Examine venous anatomy. Look for LSVC/anomalous pulmonary venous drainage/unroofed CS. Determine drainage of IVC/hepatic veins. • Examine course of coronary arteries. • Rapid transit of contrast saline solution into pulmonary venous atrium after an intravenous injection suggests pulmonary arteriovenous malformations and may explain cyanosis. Use upper extremity vein injection (Glenn/fenestrated Fontan) or any vein (Kawashima-Glenn or nonfenestrated Fontan procedure).	• Determine size/direction of flow through ASD. • Assess whether BVF restrictive/unrestrictive (<10–20 mm Hg ideal). • CFD/CW to assess LVOT or RVOT (PDA will mask a pressure gradient). • Grade AVVR/stenosis. • CFD/PW to assess for Glenn/PA stenosis. Look for laminar, low-velocity phasic flow in PAs, ME bicaval, ME asc A. SAX, ME RV inflow-outflow. • Look for evidence of coronary sinusoids/fistulae (PA/IVS). • Look for PDA.

*See the Appendix on page 57 for schematics of these views.

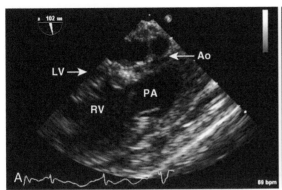
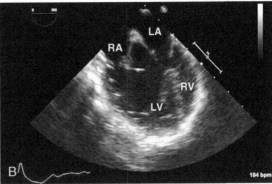

Figure 4-13. **A,** Modified ME AV LAX view in a patient with hypoplastic left heart syndrome. The hypoplastic LV is barely visible in this view. The diminutive aorta is seen posterior to the large PA and RV. **B,** 2D ME 4C view demonstrating a patient with a double-inlet LV. Both AVVs open into the left ventricular cavity. The bulboventricular foramen appears large.

TABLE 4-10	SURGICAL/HYBRID OPTIONS FOR STAGE 1	
Defect	**Surgical Options for Stage 1**	**Additional Points**
HLHS	• Norwood procedure includes arch augmentation/DKS type of anastomosis/atrial septectomy/Sano or BT shunt. • A hybrid procedure with balloon atrial septostomy, PDA stent, and surgically placed bilateral PA bands.	• DKS-PA transected/pulmV and proximal main PA (which is effective systemic outflow vessel) are anastomosed to aorta. • Indications for hybrid procedure not defined. Note that procedure requires bilateral PA band placement. TEE is not typically used.

SV-DILV	• Normal GV: either BT/Sano shunt or PA band usually necessary.
	• With TGA/large BVF: PA band
	• With TGA/restrictive BVF:
	  • Norwood/DKS
	  • PA band/arch/coarctation repair/ +- enlargement of BVF.
		• Size of BVF critical for type/timing of repair. With TGA, systemic flow must cross BVF to reach aorta.
		• Even *potential* for restriction important as obstruction at any time adversely affects ventricular function.
		• PA band is placed on main PA.

Tricuspid atresia	• Same considerations as DILV.	
Unbalanced AVC	• Without PA obstruction-PA band.	
PA/IVS	• SV, $1\frac{1}{2}$, 2 ventricle repair.	• Must not decompress RV in patients with RV-dependent coronary circulation.
Heterotaxy	• Usually SV approach necessary. Procedure(s) depend on associated defects.	• Obstructed TAPVD confers increased risk.

Stage 1
- The principles of long-term management are to preserve systolic and diastolic ventricular function and AVV competence and to keep the PVR as low possible so as to optimize SV physiology.
- During each surgical stage/catheterization, residual or recurrent abnormalities such as arch obstruction or LVOTO, AVV regurgitation, restricted ASD, and aortopulmonary collaterals should be addressed.

Stage 2
- Glenn/Hemi-Fontan procedure: SVC flow is anastomosed to the PAs.

Stage 3
- IVC flow is routed to the PAs via an extracardiac conduit or a lateral tunnel.
- Extracardiac Fontan procedure: The cardiac end of the IVC is suture closed, and the IVC is anastomosed to the PA via a conduit.
- Lateral tunnel Fontan procedure: A tunnel from the IVC to the PA within the

atrium is constructed from prosthetic material.

- A small 3- to 4-mm fenestration may be placed between the conduit/tunnel and the atrium to serve as a "pop off" in the event of high SVC/PAP.
- A Kawashima Glenn procedure is a Glenn procedure performed in a patient with an interrupted IVC and azygos continuation. The Fontan procedure in these patients involves rerouting hepatic venous blood to the PAs via a conduit. This is most commonly necessary in patients with heterotaxy syndrome.

Postoperative TEE Assessment

- Many centers do not perform TEE during isolated Blalock-Taussig (BT) shunt, PA band placement, or Glenn or Fontan procedures because of the limited ability of TEE to visualize the relevant anastomoses.

Stage 1

- BT shunt: flow in PAs/PVs may be visible.
- PA band placement
  - Verify the presence of a large unrestrictive atrial communication.
  - Verify a large unrestrictive BVF in patients with associated TGA and confirm the absence of a VSD gradient after placement of PA band.
  - Measure pressure gradient across the PA band. The band must be sufficiently tight so that favorable conditions (low pulmonary artery pressure) for a SV approach are attained (gradients of about 50 mm Hg). A combination of TEE and clinical data such as systemic saturation, blood pressure, and

direct pressure measurements (RV and PA) can be used. Patients may have to return to the operating room for PA band adjustment.
  - After PA band placement verify the absence of pulmV distortion (in the event that the patient needs a Damus-Kaye-Stansel procedure at a later stage).
- Damus-Kaye-Stansel/Norwood procedure
  - Verify the presence of a large, unrestrictive atrial communication.
  - Examine the proximal end of the Sano shunt for obstruction. Usual velocity is less than 3 m/s.
  - Verify AVV and AV function without regurgitation/stenosis.
  - Verify the absence of arch obstruction. Gradients less than 10 to 20 mm Hg are ideal. Indirect assessment of flow is often necessary. Use CFD/PW to look for aliasing or continuous aortic flow in the descending aorta. A low cardiac output may affect velocity/pressure measurements.
  - Assess ventricular function. Myocardial dysfunction occurs as a result of long CPB and cross-clamp times and primary coronary insufficiency from abnormal coronary anatomy or injury during repair.

Stage 2

- Difficult to visualize the Glenn anastomosis by TEE. Indirect evidence of flow includes low-velocity, laminar flow in SVC/PA and pulmonary venous return to the atrium (Fig. 4-14).

Stage 3

- Verify low-velocity, laminar flow in hepatic veins/IVC after a Fontan procedure.

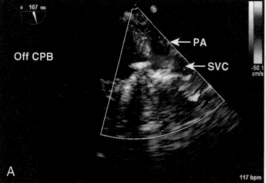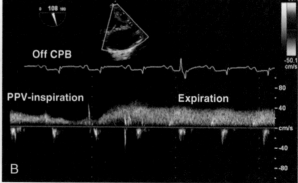

Figure 4-14. **A,** CFD ME bicaval view in a patient after a Glenn procedure. Low-velocity superior vena cava flow is seen to drain into the right PA. **B,** PW imaging of the superior vena cava profile in the same patient. Note the low-velocity, laminar profile and the effect of positive pressure ventilation on decreasing Glenn flow.

- Flow difficult to discern in extracardiac conduit, but ensure that there is no external compression from the conduit.
- Verify patency of fenestration. Intravenous contrast saline solution injection through lower extremity is helpful when Doppler is unclear.

Coronary Artery Abnormalities
(Table 4-11)

- Anomalous origin or course of a coronary artery
- Anomalous origin of the LMCA from the PA
- Intramural course
- Coronary artery fistula

KEY POINTS

Congenital Coronary Anomalies
- The LMCA originates from the left sinus of Valsalva and bifurcates behind the main PA into the anteriorly directed left anterior descending artery and the posteriorly directed Cx.
- The Cx continues laterally and posteriorly in the AV groove. In a left dominant circulation, the Cx becomes the posterior descending coronary artery.
- The RCA originates anteriorly and slightly superior to the origin of the LMCA from the right sinus of Valsalva and courses rightward around the AV groove to the posterior aspect of the heart. In 75% of patients, the RCA becomes the posterior descending artery.
- Both the LMCA/RCA should be similar in size and exit the aortic wall perpendicularly. A large

size discrepancy can occur as a result of aneurysms/coronary fistulae/compensatory enlargement of one coronary artery secondary to increased flow when it is providing collateral circulation.
- Coronary abnormalities often exist in patients with CHD (e.g., TOF, TGA, PA/IVS).
- Isolated congenital coronary abnormalities are revealed in less than 1.5% of angiograms and 0.3% of autopsies.
- High-risk lesions include an abnormal origin of the coronary artery from the aorta with an intramural or interarterial course (especially the LMCA/left anterior descending artery) and anomalous origin of the LMCA from the PA.

TABLE 4-11 BASIC ECHO PRINCIPLES WHEN IMAGING CORONARY ARTERIES

Best TEE View*	What to Look for on 2D Imaging	CFD and Spectral Doppler
ME AV SAX ME RV inflow-outflow ME AV LAX	• Describe origin/course of LMCA/RCA as far as possible. • LMCA (ME AV SAX, ME RV inflow-outflow, occasionally ME AV LAX if viewing left cusp). • RCA (withdraw probe slightly from above views, also seen exiting from right sinus on ME AV LAX view). • If ALCAPA suspected, carefully inspect PA for coronary origin. • If fistulae suspected, right-sided receiving chamber is enlarged.	• May need to decrease velocity scale to image coronary flow. It is important to see flow in vessel as artifacts like transverse sinus can be confused for coronary arteries. • Measure direction/timing of coronary flow. Normal pattern: low-velocity, anterograde flow during diastole. • In ALCAPA look for retrograde flow in the PA. • No coronary flow should be seen between the aorta and PA (interarterial coronary). • Continuous coronary flow signal consistent with coronary fistula. • Abnormal CFD signal into R-sided chamber may represent entry point of coronary fistulae. • CFD/CW to assess MR severity.
ME four chamber ME two chamber ME LAX TG basal SAX TG mid SAX	• Assess biventricular function/ventricle size/RWMAs. Correlate areas of dysfunction with coronary artery distribution (TG mid-SAX, ME 4C, ME LAX, ME 2C views). • Assess MV for evidence of ischemic MR. Measure annulus/check for leaflet prolapse/mobility/evidence of papillary muscle dysfunction (ME 4C, ME LAX, ME 2C views).	

*See the Appendix on page 57 for schematics of these views.

Anomalous Origin of the Coronary Artery from the Aorta

- Origin usually from the opposite aortic sinus of Valsalva.
- Slitlike ostia with stenosis and intramural coronary segments and/or an interarterial course are common (Fig. 4-15).
  - An intramural segment: the coronary artery courses within the wall of the aorta before exiting.
  - An interarterial segment: the coronary artery originates from the opposite aortic sinus and travels between the GVs to supply the appropriate territory.

Anomalous Origin of the LMCA from the Pulmonary Artery

- The LMCA or, very rarely, both coronary arteries arise from the left or right posterior sinus of the PA/posterior main PA or PA branches.
- Early in life when the PVR is increased, there is anterograde flow of deoxygenated blood from the PA.
- As the PVR decreases, reversal of flow in the left coronary system develops with retrograde flow into the PA leading to coronary steal and myocardial ischemia.
- The RCA provides coronary perfusion, including retrograde flow into the PA.
- Patients present as neonates/young infants in congestive heart failure with massive cardiomegaly, severe MR, and cardiogenic shock. Rarely, with enough collateral circulation from the RCA, they can present later in life with symptoms of a L → R shunt (aorta to coronary artery to PA), or symptoms of ischemia, including sudden death.

Coronary Artery Fistula

- The origin from either coronary artery emptying into the right heart (RA, RV, and/or, less commonly, the PA). Usually a solitary fistula.
- Results in enlargement of the involved coronary or aneurysm formation because of increased flow. Can cause steal of flow from the distal segment of coronary. When large, it results in right heart volume overload. Small risk of endocarditis in fistula.

Principles of Surgical/Interventional Management

- Coronary arteries with anomalous origin: Options include unroofing intramural segments/enlarge abnormal ostia/translocation of the coronary artery to the appropriate sinus/translocation of the PA, which can compress the aberrantly located coronary/coronary artery bypass graft.
- Resuspension of the aortic leaflet may be necessary when unroofing a segment that crosses the aortic valve commissure.
- Treatment of anomalous origin of the LMCA from the PA: The coronary artery is translocated to the aorta.
- Most coronary fistulae can be closed using interventional catheter techniques such as coils. Surgical closure is occasionally necessary for very large fistulae.

Postoperative TEE Assessment

- The coronary artery may be difficult to visualize. Use indirect techniques of assessment of perfusion such as regional wall motion abnormalities, and evaluation of MR. However, if there is stunned/hibernating myocardium, improvement may be gradual.

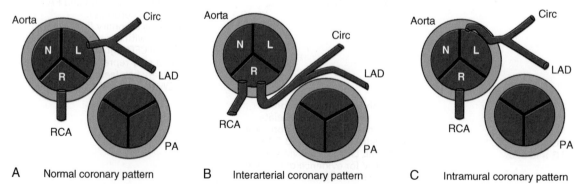

Figure 4-15. A, Normal coronary anatomy. **B,** Interarterial course with the left coronary artery originating aberrantly from the right sinus and coursing between the great vessels. **C,** A left coronary artery with an aberrant origin, ostial stenosis, and an intramural segment. *(Adapted from Eisses M, Verma S, Gurvitz M, Joffe DC. Intramural left coronary artery. Anesth Analg. 2010;111[2]:354–356, Figure 3.)*

MR usually resolves as ventricular remodeling occurs.

- Verify suitable origin/course of repaired coronary. Verify low-velocity anterograde flow from the ostia without obvious stenosis.
- Confirm the absence of prolapse/perforation/other injury to the pulmonary or aortic valves, especially if the aortic leaflet required mobilization and resuspension.
- Assess biventricular function/MR.

Congenital Valvular Heart Disease

KEY POINTS

Tricuspid Valve
Ebstein's Anomaly (Table 4-12)
- Most common isolated congenital abnormality of the TV.
- Abnormal development of the septal and posterior leaflets that are dysplastic and apically displaced create an "atrialized" ventricle.
- There are tethering and shortening of the valve and subvalvar apparatus with a normally positioned annulus.
- There is a variable degree of TR and effective right ventricular hypoplasia. Massive enlargement of the right heart can lead to functional pulmonary atresia and left ventricular dysfunction. Structural pulmonary atresia is rare.
- An atrial-level shunt is usually present and may be necessary for survival,
- Presentation varies from severe cardiac compromise to mild TR.

Principles of Surgical Management
(Table 4-13)
Neonates
- Have more severe disease. May be ductal dependent with severe TR, decreased right ventricular function, and poor anterograde flow from the RV.
- When PVR decreases, anterograde flow generally improves if there is no structural pulmonary atresia.
- If the patient cannot be weaned from prostaglandin or has refractory RV failure, there are a couple of options for this very high risk cohort that are mostly institution dependent:
  - Biventricular repair strategy with TV repair and repair of associated defects.
  - Staged RV approach (Starnes procedure) that ultimately leads to a single ventricle repair.
- Surgical option in the older patients (older than 3 months).
  - May require TV repair or replacement, with/without a Glenn procedure with/without a Fontan procedure.
- Patients with a Glenn procedure and adequate right ventricular function to handle IVC return are left with a $1\frac{1}{2}$ ventricle repair. Patients with inadequate right ventricular output require a Fontan procedure.

Postoperative TEE Assessment
Biventricular Repair Strategy
- Confirm size/direction of flow through atrial/fenestration.

TABLE 4-12 BASIC ECHOCARDIOGRAPHIC FEATURES WHEN IAGING EBSTEIN'S ANOMALY

Best TEE Views*	What to Look for on 2D Imaging	CFD and Spectral Doppler
ME four chamber ME RV inflow-outflow ME bicaval TG mid SAX TG two chamber TG RV inflow Deep TG RVOT UE aortic arch SAX	• Assess TV morphology and mechanism of TR. Evaluate degree of tethering, the subvalvar apparatus, and anterior leaflet size—factors important for repair (ME 4C, ME RV inflow-outflow, TG RV inflow views). • Assess RV function/volume, (ME 4C, ME RV inflow-outflow, TG SAX views). • Examine RVOT for etiology of RVOTO (structural vs. functional) (ME RV inflow-outflow, deep TG LAX, UE aortic arch SAX views). • Evaluate effect of RV size/dysfunction on LV function. • Examine IAS for PFO/ASD.	• CFD/CW/PW to assess TR severity: use area of jet/width of vena contracta/density of spectral Doppler/evidence of systolic flow reversal in hepatic vein. • Enlarged IVC (>20 mm) suggestive of increased RAP. • Assess anterograde flow through RVOT/evaluate RVOTO/assess PI (ME RV inflow-outflow, deep TG LAX, UE aortic arch SAX views). • Measure PAP = RVP (if no RVOTO). With RVOTO: PAP = RVP–RVOT gradient. • CFD/PW to assess ASD. • Check for PDA. Assess size/direction of flow.

*See the Appendix on page 57 for schematies of these views.

TABLE 4-13   SUMMARY OF SURGICAL OPTIONS FOR PATIENTS WITH EBSTEIN'S ANOMALY

Procedure	Key Facts
Valve repair	• Two main types: 1. Anterior leaflet of TV used to form competent valve. 2. "Cone repair." Trileaflet valve is created that originates at true annulus. Both include: • Reduction atrioplasty/fenestrated atrial communication. • Valve repairs may also involve reduction annuloplasty/fenestration of subvalvar apparatus and/or augmentation of anterior leaflet with a pericardial patch. • When necessary, valved pulmonary conduit is placed in order to reduce RV volume load.
RV exclusion or Starnes procedure	• Staged approach: fenestrated patch closure of TV ensuring that CS blood enters the RA. • ASD is enlarged, reduction atrioplasty/aortopulmonary shunt performed. • If there is PI, the PV is oversewn or the main PA disconnected. *RV must be decompressed so that it does not interfere with LV function.*
Glenn procedure	• Must be old enough (about 3 months old minimum). • Usually done in combination with a valve repair.
1½ ventricle repair	• RV can eject IVC return but Glenn procedure needed for SVC flow. • ASD closed.

• Assess biventricular size/function: RCA at risk of injury, especially during these complex valve repairs.
• Confirm adequate TV repair without significant regurgitation/stenosis.
• Verify anterograde pulmonary flow.
• Confirm minimal PI through native PV or RV-PA conduit.
• Measure PAP.

Starnes Procedure
• Confirm large unrestrictive ASD.
• Confirm that the CS empties into the atrium.
• Confirm that the RV is decompressed.
• Confirm adequate fenestration in the pericardial patch.
• Confirm flow in aortopulmonary shunt. Indirect assessment includes flow in PAs/PVs.
• Confirm absence of PI.

KEY POINTS

Pulmonary Valve
• Isolated PS is usually the result of commissural fusion or fusion of the leaflets in a valve with a variable number of cusps. Other than critical PS, it is usually well tolerated. There is often post-stenotic dilation of the PA. When associated with a syndrome such as Alagille, Noonan, and Williams, there is usually annular hypoplasia as well.
• The management of PS is usually interventional except in the case of syndromes in which the success of balloon dilation is limited and patients may require surgical management with placement of a transannular patch.
• Pulmonary insufficiency is often the result of balloon dilation of PS or the use of a transannular patch for TOF repair and may require bioprosthetic valve replacement or RV-PA conduit placement.
• Patients with RV-PA conduits generally require several conduit replacements during their lifetime for stenosis/regurgitation. The introduction of percutaneously placed valves may delay or obviate surgery in appropriate candidates.

KEY POINTS

Mitral Valve (Table 4-14)
• Composed of the mitral annulus, leaflets, chordae, and papillary muscles attached to the anterolateral and posteromedial LV. Abnormalities in any component can result in MV disease.
• Rheumatic disease is the most common cause of MS worldwide. Congenital MS is the most common cause of MS in developing nations.
• Congenital MS consists of a combination of abnormalities of the MV including thick, short, webbed chordae with restricted interchordal spaces (arcade) that produce LV inflow obstruction/MR (Fig. 4-16). The papillary muscles may connect the leaflets directly to the ventricle (papillary commissural fusion). The valve can have a double orifice or be parachute restricting inflow and causing MS.
• Supramitral ring/cor triatriatum are anomalous fibromuscular membranes located in the LA and cause obstructive symptoms that mimic MS. A ring is located below the atrial appendage, and the membrane of cor triatriatum is above the appendage.

TABLE 4-14 BASIC ECHOCARDIOGRAPHIC FEATURES WHEN IMAGING THE MV

Best TEE Views*	What to Look for on 2D Imaging	CFD and Spectral Doppler
ME four chamber ME two chamber ME LAX ME mitral commissural ME AV LAX TG basal SAX TG two chamber Deep TG LAX	• Assess morphology and function of MV/ subvalvar apparatus (Fig. 4-17). Examine leaflets and look for a cleft; examine chordal arrangement, mobility, and the number/location of papillary muscles. Measure Z score diameter and cross-sectional area if; <–3, a SV repair likely (ME 4C, ME 2C, ME LAX, ME AV LAX, ME mitral commissural, TG basal SAX, TG 2C views). • Assess LA, LV size/function. • Examine LA for stasis/thrombus (especially LAA). • Examine morphology, annulus size, and function of TV if evidence of PHTN. • Look for systolic flattening of IVS suggestive of PHTN. • Look for supramitral ring/cor triatriatum.	• CFD: Assess location and quantitate MR/MS. • CW: Mean and peak pressures are flow related but otherwise adequate indicators of MS severity (mean >12–15 severe MS). An atrial level shunt with L→R flow can factitiously decrease the severity of MS as measured by Doppler. Pressure half-time is not reliable in pediatric patients. • If TR is present, measure PAP.

*See the Appendix on page 57 for schematics of these views.

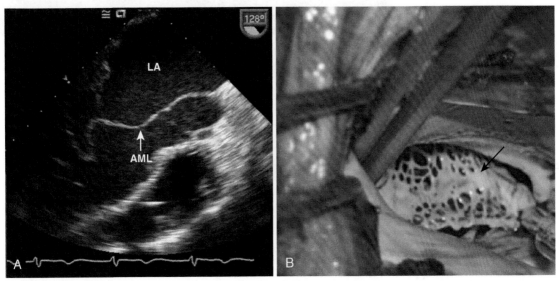

Figure 4-16. **A**, 2D ME aortic valve LAX view in a patient with Shone's anomaly and congenital MV disease. Note the redundant anterior mitral leaflet. This patient also had a parachute MV, although the single papillary muscle is not well seen in this view. She had predominantly MR and not the typical mitral stenosis seen in most of these cases. **B**, An intraoperative picture of the valve seen in **A**. Note the thick, webbed chords with minimal interchordal spaces (*arrow*).

Principles of Surgical Management

• It is preferable to delay valve replacement whenever possible, especially in young patients (younger than 2 years) because of the high morbidity and mortality. The degree of acceptable residual valve dysfunction after a valve repair is greater in infants/young children than in older patients.

• Balloon valvuloplasty may be possible for rheumatic MS and some etiologies of congenital MS, although results are not as long lasting in the latter group. It is only an option in patients with less than mild MR.

• Techniques of valve repair include closure of clefts, chordae lengthening and transfers, triangular resections, commissurotomy, splitting of papillary muscles, fenestrating webbed chords, pericardial patch augmentation of deficient leaflets, and annuloplasty techniques.

• Mechanical prosthetic valves have a lower profile (smaller sewing ring and lower transvalvular gradient) compared to bioprosthetic valves.

• The Cx coronary is at risk of injury during placement, especially in patients with small annulus.

• Supra-annular placement of a mitral prosthesis may be necessary in young children. The atrial appendage is left above the prosthesis. The LA may need augmentation to decrease atrial hypertension.

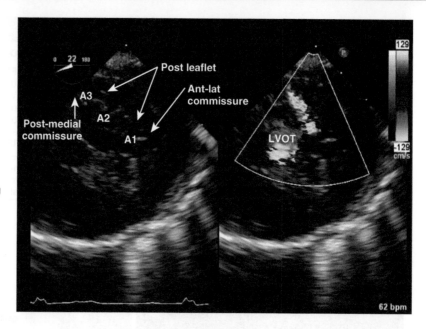

Figure 4-17. 2D and CFD modified transgastric basal SAX view of the MV with the MV scallops labeled (A1, A2, A3). Note that the posterior leaflet has the corresponding nomenclature. Scallops are not well delineated in the very young patient. The CFD image shows the MR jet originates near the anterolateral commissure.

- Rarely the Ross II procedure has been used. The pulmonary autograft is used in the mitral position and a valved conduit in the pulmonary position.
- "Membranes" from supramitral rings/cor triatriatum are resected when obstructive.

Postoperative TEE Assessment

- Ensure an adequately seated valve with complete fixation of the valve to the annulus (unless it was placed in the supra-annular position).
- If supra-annular placement is necessary, the left atrial appendage should be above the valve and should not appear overly distended.

- With a bileaflet valve, both leaflets should be seen to open and close.
- Prosthetic valves: characteristic "signature" regurgitant jets occur at hinge points of the leaflets. Identify and grade pathologic paravalvular/transvalvular jets. Inflow pressure gradients should be within the valve manufacturer's acceptable range.
- Bioprosthetic valves: at most, trace to mild central MR acceptable.
- Assess for LVOTO and aortic valve dysfunction from an oversized valve impinging on the LVOT.
- Measure PAP, although it seldom decreases acutely.

KEY POINTS

Aortic Valve/LVOT Abnormalities
(Table 4-15)

- Bicuspid aortic valve. The most common congenital abnormality with an incidence of 1% to 2%.
- About one third remain asymptomatic, one third develop stenosis, one third develop insufficiency. Symptoms tend to occur after childhood.
- Critical aortic stenosis in the newborn is a result of a deformed valve with one to four cusps.
- Often associated with variable degrees of hypoplastic left-sided structures: MV, LV, LVOT, aorta. May have endocardial fibroelastosis where fibrous tissue replaces myocardium.
- Various grading schemes developed to determine whether one- or two-ventricle repair is best.

- Subaortic membranes are fibromuscular membranes with attachments to the septum and often to the aortic and MV. AR occurs in about 50% of patients from turbulent flow and/or involvement of the valve in the fibromuscular process.
- The combination of left heart obstructive lesions including coarctation/aortic stenosis/subaortic stenosis/supramitral ring or other forms of congenital MS is referred to as Shone's complex.
- The aorta consists of the root (aortic annulus, cusps, sinuses, and sinotubular junction), ascending aorta, proximal and distal transverse arches, isthmus, and descending aorta. The dimensions of the aorta decrease from ascending to descending aorta.
- Each component should be measured and examined to determine the etiology and guide the surgical repair.

TABLE 4-15 BASIC ECHOCARDIOGRAPHIC FEATURES WHEN IMAGING THE AV AND LVOT

Best TEE Views*	What to Look for on 2D Imaging	CFD and Spectral Doppler
ME LAX ME modified 5C ME asc aortic SAX ME AV SAX ME RV inflow-outflow ME AV LAX TG LAX Deep TG LAX	• Assess morphology/function of AV. Thick/doming valve is common. Calcified valve is uncommon. Identify areas of perforation or prolapse for potential repair (ME RV inflow-outflow, ME AV SAX, ME LAX, ME AV LAX, ME ascending aortic SAX, TG LAX, deep TG LAX views). • Bicuspid valves: fusion of L/R cusps or R/NCC, rarely L/NCC. Evaluate in systole. Cusp size is often uneven with eccentric orifice. • Examine LVOT/subvalvular area for obstruction. • Assess LV function/hypertrophy/size/brightness (indication of EFE). • Examine LA for membranes. • Examine MV (see MV exam). • Examine IAS for PFO/ASD. • Measure aortic root/aorta.	• CFD/CW/PW: Identify AI/AS and direction of jet. Measure width of vena contracta/deceleration slope of AI jet/flow reversal in descending aorta. • Measure LVOT gradient (deep TG LAX, TG LAX views). Modified Bernoulli equation may not be applicable with multilevel LVOTO. • CFD/CW to assess MV inflow (see above). • Measure PAP. • Check for persistent gradient in diastole in descending aorta for evidence of obstruction. • Check for PDA; assess size/direction of flow. R→L in critical LVOTO.

*See the Appendix on page 57 for schematics of these views.

Principles of Surgical Management

• Balloon valvuloplasty is the procedure of choice for isolated AS in pediatric patients and is done without TEE guidance. The goal is to provide even mild relief of LVOTO without causing more than mild AR.

• Homograft/autograft valves (Ross procedure) can be used to minimize the hemodynamic effects of sewing rings in very young patients. Both procedures are technically challenging and involve reimplantation of coronary arteries.

• Autograft valves grow with the patient and have a low risk of endocarditis. The procedure can be performed in combination with the Konno procedure to enlarge the LVOT (Ross-Konno procedure).

• A Konno procedure involves enlarging the annulus "into" the IVS using a surgically created VSD. It may be required in patients needing a prosthetic valve replacement and annular enlargement with or without subaortic enlargement. This allows for the placement of a larger prosthetic valve (two or three sizes larger than the native annulus) and reduces LVOTO.

• Simple resection of a subaortic membrane is associated with a high rate of recurrence. Very aggressive resection on all surfaces in combination with a myomectomy may be associated with a decreased rate of recurrence and a lower incidence of AR. A modified Konno procedure (LVOT enlargement without prosthetic valve placement) can be performed if there is more tunnel-like subaortic obstruction or in patients with multiple recurrences of the membrane (Fig. 4-18).

Postoperative TEE Assessment

• Verify the integrity and function of the valve repair/replacement. Acoustic shadowing can make TEE evaluation difficult. Epicardial echo may be helpful.

• Prosthetic valves have characteristic "signature" regurgitant jets. Identify and grade pathologic paravalvular/transvalvular jets (Fig. 4-19).

• Bioprosthetic valves should have less than mild central AR.

• Assure that the valve gradient is within manufacturer's specification.

• Homografts are very fragile and prone to injury during implantation. Accept trace AR for an adequate long-term result.

• Konno/modified Konno procedure: verify that there is no new/residual VSD.

• Subaortic membrane resection. Ensure that the membrane is adequately resected with an acceptable gradient. Mean gradients less than 20 mm Hg are ideal, but varies with the presurgical gradient. Verify that the MV is intact. Assess the aortic valve for injury from the resection as well as improvement in

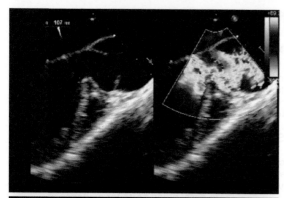

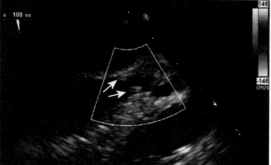

Figure 4-18. 2D and CFD ME LAX in a patient with a subaortic membrane. **A**, Note the discrete membrane that is clearly visible in the left ventricular outflow tract. The aliasing begins at the level of the membrane. **B**, ME LAX view showing recurrent obstruction after a previous discrete membrane resection. There is complex subaortic narrowing *(arrows)* with extension to the MV and the aortic valve. There was a 40 mm Hg mean gradient and moderate AI.

preoperative AR. Verify that there is no new VSD.
- Examine the coronary arteries if a Ross or homograft valve replacement was performed.
- Assess systolic and diastolic ventricular function and regional wall motion.

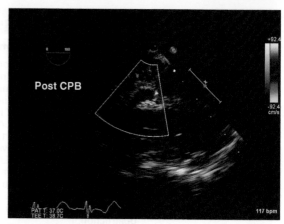

Figure 4-19. 2D and CFD ME AV LAX in a 3-month-old patient with truncus arteriosus after aortic valve repair with bileaflet prosthetic valve. Residual severe hemodynamically significant AR was very difficult to locate because of acoustic shadowing. Epicardial scanning was not helpful. Two attempts at returning to bypass could not locate the leak, although reinforcement sutures were placed between the annulus and valve. Eventually it was determined that one of the leaflets was not closing properly because of impingement on the VSD patch (transvalvular regurgitation), and with revision of the VSD, the AR resolved.

Suggested Reading

1. Shanewise S, Cheung A, Aronson S, et al. ASE/SCA guidelines for performing a comprehensive intraoperative multiplane transesophageal echocardiography examination: Recommendations of the American Society of Echocardiography Council for Intraoperative Echocardiography and the Society of Cardiovascular Anesthesiologists Task Force for Certification in Perioperative Transesophageal Echocardiography. *Anesth Analg.* 1999;89:870-884.
2. Operative Techniques in Thoracic and Cardiovascular Surgery series. Philadelphia: Elsevier; multiple volumes.
3. Seminars in Thoracic and Cardiovascular Surgery series. Pediatric Cardiac Surgery Annual. Philadelphia: Elsevier; multiple volumes.
4. Lai W, Mertens L, Cohen M, Geva T, eds. *Echocardiography for Pediatric and Congenital Heart Disease.* Hoboken, NJ: Wiley-Blackwell; 2009.

APPENDIX: TEE Views

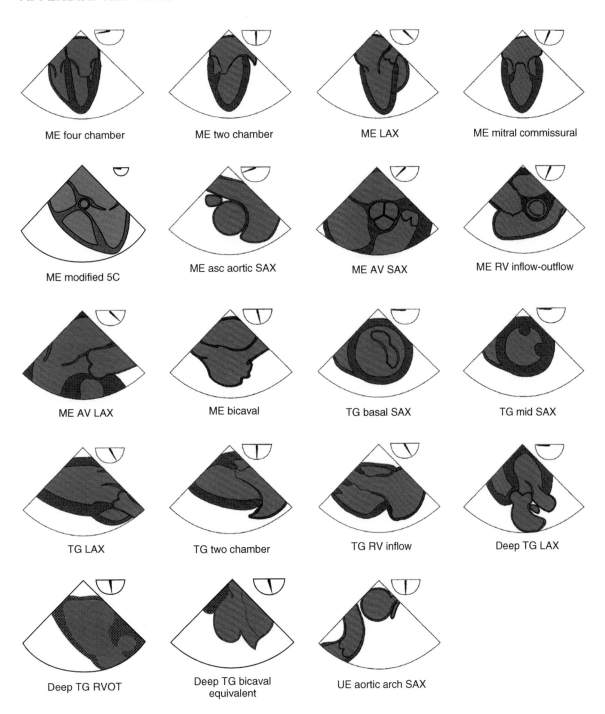

ME four chamber

ME two chamber

ME LAX

ME mitral commissural

ME modified 5C

ME asc aortic SAX

ME AV SAX

ME RV inflow-outflow

ME AV LAX

ME bicaval

TG basal SAX

TG mid SAX

TG LAX

TG two chamber

TG RV inflow

Deep TG LAX

Deep TG RVOT

Deep TG bicaval equivalent

UE aortic arch SAX

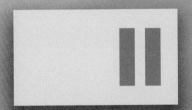

CONGENITAL HEART DISEASE

Shunting Lesions

Brandy Hattendorf

5

Cardiac shunting lesions include atrial septal defects, ventricular septal defects, and patent ductus arteriosus as the most common lesions seen in congenital heart disease. These lesions may be seen in isolation or in association with other congenital heart disease.

Atrial Septal Defects

Atrial deptal defects represent defects in septation of the atria. They are common, representing as much as 10% of cases of congenital heart disease. Anatomic types of defects include (Fig. 5-1):
- Patent foramen ovale (PFO).
- Ostium secundum atrial septal defect (ASD).
- Ostium primum ASD.
- Sinus venosus ASD.
- Coronary sinus (CS) ASD.

Patent Foramen Ovale
- An interatrial communication between the superior limb of the septum secundum on the right side and the septum primum on the left atrial side (Fig. 5-2).
  - The flap of the foramen ovale (FO) can often be seen (Fig. 5-3).
- Functionally closes after birth but may be present in as many as 25% of normal hearts during pathologic evaluation.

> **KEY POINTS**
> - Persists in a normal newborn to 6 months of age.
> - Is not a congenital ASD.

Ostium Secundum Atrial Septal Defect
- Defect in the septum primum.
- Most common type of ASD.
  - 70% of ASDs are secundum defects (Fig. 5-4).

> **KEY POINTS**
> - Many secundum atrial septal defects may be closed percutaneously in the cardiac catheterization laboratory via device.
> - Closure via device depends on the septal rims and size of the defect.
> - A secundum atrial septal defect is best imaged from the subcostal plane.

Ostium Primum Atrial Septal Defect
- Located in the most anterior and inferior aspects of the atrial septum.
- Deficient atrioventricular (AV) septation.

> **KEY POINTS**
> - Associated with trisomy 21.
> - Usually seen in association with AV septal defects with a cleft in the anterior leaflet of the mitral valve, although primum defects can occur in isolation.
> - Both AV valves (AVVs) appear at the same level.
>   - The tricuspid valve (TV) will not be apically displaced.
> - Best imaged in apical view.
>   - Allows for assessment of the atrial septum in relationship to the crux of the heart.

Sinus Venosus Atrial Septal Defects: Two Types
- Superior sinus venosus defects: located in the most superior and posterior region of the atrial septum in close proximity to the right-sided pulmonary veins (PVs) and the entrance of the superior vena cava (SVC) into the right atrium (RA) (Fig. 5-5).
- Inferior sinus venosus defects: located posterior and inferior to the fossa ovalis and adjacent to the inferior vena cava.

> **KEY POINTS**
> - Both types are associated with partial anomalous pulmonary venous return.
>   - Commonly the right upper PVs (Fig. 5-5).

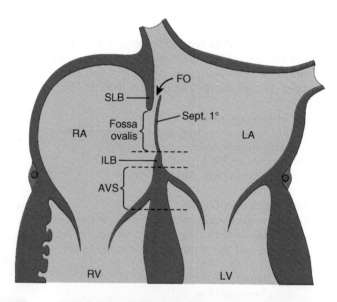

Figure 5-1. Diagram of the atrial septum showing several types of atrial septal defects. *(Adapted from Fyler DC [ed], Nadas' Pediatric Cardiology. Philadadelphia: Hanley & Belfus, 1992.)*

Sinus venosus defect

ASD 1°

ASD 2°

Figure 5-2. Diagram of atrial septal components, showing foramen ovale (FO; *arrow*), septum primum (Sept 1°), left atrium (LA), left ventricle (LV), fossa ovalis, superior limbic bands (SLB) and inferior limbic bands (ILB), atrioventricular septum (AVS), right atrium (RA), and right ventricle (RV). *(From Keane JF, Lock, JE, Fyler DC [eds], Nadas' Pediatric Cardiology, 2nd ed. Philadelphia: Elsevier/ Saunders, 2006.)*

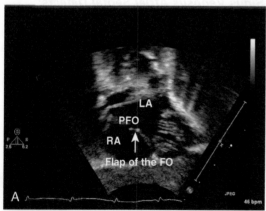
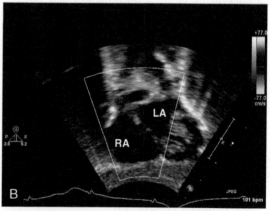

Figure 5-3. Subcostal image of a patent foramen ovale (PFO). **A,** A flap of tissue is seen partially occluding the communication. **B,** Subcostal image a PFO with color Doppler. Left-to-right shunting is seen. The size of the defect is overestimated by the width of the color jet compared with the two-dimensional size of the defect in part A.

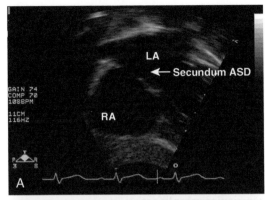

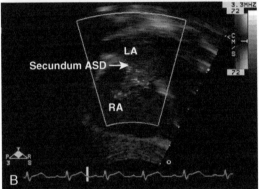

Figure 5-4. Subcostal image of a secundum atrial septal defect (ASD). **A,** In this two-dimensional image, the true size of the atrial septal defect is seen. Septal rims are noted superior and inferior to the defect. Right atrial enlargement is also seen. **B,** With color on the same image, a red color jet is seen representing left-to-right flow across the defect.

Coronary Sinus Atrial Septal Defect
- Least common.
- The left SVC empties into the left atrium.

KEY POINT
• Associated with a persistent left SVC and unroofed CS.

The Echocardiography (Echo) Exam: Step-by-Step Approach

Step 1: Evaluate the Location of the Atrial Septal Defect
- Most ASDs are best imaged from a subcostal view.
- Parasternal short axis view may also be used.
- The apical view is not used for measurements or assessment of most ASDs.
  - The atrial septum is thin, particularly in the region of the fossa ovalis.
  - From an apical view, the septum is parallel to the ultrasound beam, resulting in dropout.
- Evaluate surrounding structures including PVs, the SVC, inferior vena cava, and CS.
- Pulmonary venous anomalies are associated with sinus venosus defects.
  - Agitated saline solution is the preferred contrast used in pediatrics.

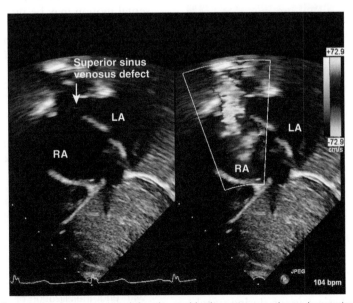

Figure 5-5. Subcostal image of a sinus venosus defect located in the most superior and posterior region of the atrial septum. This defect is associated with partial anomalous pulmonary venous return.

- Contrast echocardiography is performed by rapid injection of agitated saline solution into a peripheral vein.
  - Upper extremity veins are preferred.
  - Filling of the left atrium with contrast echoes confirms the presence of an interatrial communication.

KEY POINTS

- Ostium primum defects are best imaged from an apical four-chamber (4C) view.
- Dropout can occur in the region of the fossa ovalis, giving the impression that an ASD exists in a normal heart or making an existing defect appear larger when imaged from an apical view.
- Evaluate AVV regurgitation, especially in the presence of a primum ASD or a cleft in the anterior leaflet of the mitral valve.
- Injection into the left arm in a patient with a persistent left superior vena caval draining to a CS may cause confusion by resulting in contrast seen in the left atrium.

Step 2: Evaluate the Atrial Septal Defect Dimensions and Position

- A PFO is a defect in the septum primum less than 3 mm in size without associated right atrial or right ventricular dilation and typically with a flap of tissue partially occluding the communication.
- ASD size is quantified as:
  - Small: 3 to 5 mm in size.
  - Moderate: 5 to 8 mm in size.
  - Large: 8 mm or larger.

KEY POINTS

- ASDs may enlarge over time as the right ventricle (RV) becomes more compliant.
- ASDs may also become smaller over time and close spontaneously.
  - Spontaneous closure is more common in the first few years of life.
- Evaluate for additional defects and fenestrated defects.
- In ostium secundum ASDs, septal rims and total septal length should be measured to assess for possible transcatheter device closure.
- Contrast echocardiography (echo) can be used to detect interatrial communications if the atrial septum is not well visualized.

Step 3: Evaluate the Direction of the Shunt

- Can be determined primarily by color Doppler.
- Shunting can be phasic, varying during systole and diastole.

KEY POINTS

- Most shunting is left to right.
- Spectral Doppler may be helpful if the ultrasound beam can be aligned in a parallel fashion. However, velocity of flow is not usually helpful in that a pressure gradient between left and right atria greater than 2 to 3 mm Hg is rare.

Step 4: Determine the Size of the Shunt

- The degree of shunting is determined by ventricular compliance.
- The left-to-right shunt across an ASD is often minimal during infancy as the RV is initially less compliant.

KEY POINTS

- Left-to-right shunt increases with age.
  - Shunting is usually low velocity and biphasic.

Step 5: Evaluate the Effects of Shunting

- In hemodynamically significant shunts, volume overload may result in:
  - Right atrial enlargement.
  - Right ventricular enlargement.
  - Main and branch pulmonary artery (PA) enlargement.
  - Left atrial enlargement.
- The interventricular septum (IVS) may appear flat during diastole.
- Right ventricular dilation with paradoxical septal motion may be present.

Post-Device Atrial Septum Defect Closure Evaluation: Special Considerations

- Evaluate the location of the device monitoring for device migration.
- Evaluate for impingement or distortion of surrounding structures.
  - Aortic erosion is a rare but serious complication after device closure of an ASD.

KEY POINTS

- Determine whether a residual shunt is present.
- "Speckling" may be seen representing blood swirling within the device without the presence of a shunt across the septum.
- Residual shunts may close spontaneously with endothelialization of the device over time after device closure.

Postoperative Evaluation: Special Considerations

- Primary closure: pericardial patch or artificial material such as GORE-TEX may be used to close the defect.
- An intra-atrial baffle may be present for sinus venosus or CS defects.
- Evaluate the atrial septum for any residual shunting as well.
- If a baffle is present, evaluate the baffle for leaks and stenosis.

KEY POINT

- The patch or baffle should appear well placed without dehiscence or impingement of surrounding structures.

Ventricular Septal Defects

A ventricular septal defect is a communication within the interventricular septum that seperates the left ventricle (LV) and RV, allowing for shunting for blood between the ventricles. VSDs represent 20% of congenital heart disease. VSDs can be classified as follows (Fig. 5-6):

- Membranous (Gerbode defect).
- Perimembranous.
  - Also called infracristal.
- Muscular.
- Supracristal.
  - Also called subpulmonic, doubly committed subarterial defect, and/or outlet ventricular septal defects (VSDs).
- Inlet.
  - Also called AV canal (AVC) type defects.

KEY POINTS

- Most common isolated congenital cardiac defect.
- VSDs are frequently associated with more complex cardiac malformations such as:
  - Conotruncal malformations including
    - Double-outlet RV.
    - Truncus arteriosus.
    - Tetralogy of Fallot (TOF).
    - Interrupted aortic arch.
  - Complete AVC defects.
  - Coarctation of the aorta (Ao).
  - Single ventricles.
- VSDs may overlap two or more classifications depending on the size and shape of the defect.

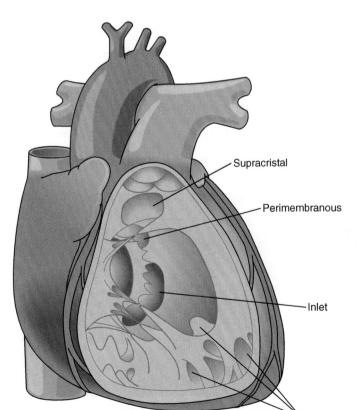

Supracristal

Perimembranous

Inlet

Muscular

Figure 5-6. Diagram of types of VSDs as viewed from the right ventricle. *(Adapted from Fyler DC [ed], Nadas' Pediatric Cardiology. Philadadelphia: Hanley & Belfus, 1992.)*

Membranous

- The membranous septum is a very small area located between the anterior and septal leaflets of the TV.
- The defect is above the TV, which overlaps a small segment of the RA.

KEY POINTS

- Results in a LV-to-RA shunt.
  - Also called a Gerbode defect.

Perimembranous

- A defect in the IVS adjacent to the membranous portion of the IVS and septal leaflet of the TV.
- Most common type of VSD.
  - Malalignment defects are more commonly associated with more complex congenital heart disease such as tetralogy of Fallot.
  - AV conduction tissue is related to the posterior, inferior aspect of the defect.

KEY POINTS

- 80% of all VSDs are perimembranous.
  - There may be malalignment of the ventricles and great arteries.
- May be associated with right ventricular outflow tract obstruction (RVOTO).
- AV conduction tissue is related to the posterior inferior aspect of the defect.
- Best imaged in:
  - Parasternal long axis view (Fig. 5-7).
  - Parasternal short axis (with base-to-apex scanning) view.
  - Apical 4C view (see Fig. 5-11).

Muscular

- Second most common type of VSD.
- Can be located anywhere in the muscular septum, including:
  - Anterior, posterior, mid, and apical.
- Multiple muscular VSDs with a net moderate to large shunt may be referred to as "Swiss cheese" defects.
- Atrioventricular conduction tissue is located superior and anterior to the defect.

KEY POINTS

- Multiple muscular VSDs are commonly seen.
- Best imaged in:
  - Parasternal long axis view (Fig. 5-8).
  - Subcostal and parasternal short axis (anterior/posterior assessment) view.
  - Apical view for base-to-apex assessment.

Supracristal (Subpulmonary)

- Located inferior and anterior to the pulmonary valve (pulmV).
- Defects do not close spontaneously.
- Least common defect, representing 6% of VSDs.
- There is a higher incidence in the Asian population, with supracristal VSDs representing up to 30% of the VSDs in this population.

KEY POINTS

- Associated with aortic valve right cusp prolapse with or without aortic regurgitation (AR).
- Best imaged in:
  - Parasternal long axis view (for imaging aortic valve cusp prolapse) (see Fig. 5-12).
  - Parasternal short axis view: at approximately the 1 o'clock position with the jet aimed toward the PA (Fig. 5-9).
  - Subcostal long axis and short axis views.

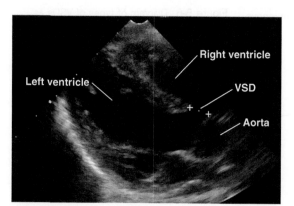

Figure 5-7. Parasternal short axis view of a perimembranous VSD.

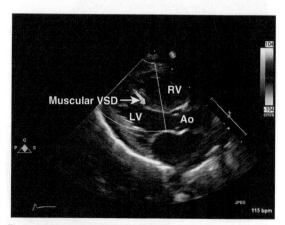

Figure 5-8. Parasternal long axis view of a small midmuscular VSD with left-to-right shunting.

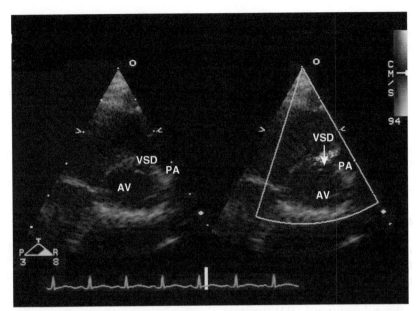

Figure 5-9. Parasternal short axis view of a supracristal VSD. *Left,* The defect is seen at the 1 o'clock position. *Right,* The jet is seen by color Doppler aimed toward the pulmonary artery (PA). Aortic insufficiency, although not seen in this patient, is associated with a supracristal VSD.

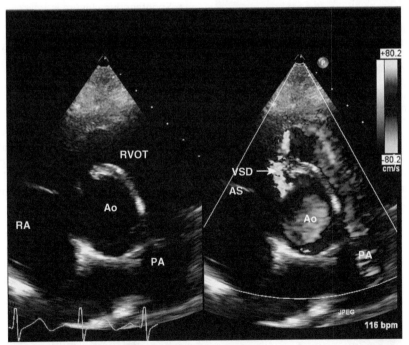

Figure 5-10. Parasternal short axis view of a perimembranous VSD. *Left,* This defect is small, measuring less than one third the aortic diameter. *Right,* The defect is located at the 11 o'clock position on the aorta and does not extend past the 12 o'clock position. There is left-to-right shunting seen with color Doppler.

Inlet

- Located posterior and superior in the inlet septum beneath the septal leaflet of the TV.
- May involve malalignment of the IVS with the atrial septum.

KEY POINTS

- Associated with endocardial cushion defects (also called AVC defects) including AVV defects and primum ASDs.
- Best imaged in:
  - 4C view: apical and subcostal views.
  - Subcostal: long axis and short axis views.

The Echo Exam: Step-by-Step Approach
Step 1: Evaluate the Ventricular Septal Defect Location

- Scan the entire septum from the base of the heart to the apex of the heart.
- The IVS is a three-dimensional (3D) structure contained in many planes. To fully interrogate the septum, the plane of sound must be angulated both anteriorly and posteriorly in all "standard" views.

KEY POINTS

- Evaluation of the septum requires multiple imaging planes with a segmental approach as the septum lies in many planes.
- Use both two-dimensional (2D) and color Doppler mapping to identify ventricular shunting lesions.
  - Defects may be difficult to visualize by color in newborns or infants with increased pulmonary vascular resistance.
- Very small defects such as a tiny apical muscular VSD may only be seen by color Doppler.
  - Such small defects can be obliterated by the cardiac muscle during systole.
- Multiple VSDs are common.

Step 2: Evaluate Ventricular Septal Defect Size

- VSDs are classified as:
  - Small: less than one third the size of the aortic diameter (Fig. 5-10).
  - Moderate: one third to two thirds the size of the aortic diameter.
  - Large: greater than two thirds the size of the aortic diameter.
- Measurements should be obtained on 2D images. Measurements obtained on images with color Doppler overestimate size.
- VSDs do not enlarge in size.
- VSDs may become smaller and/or close spontaneously.

KEY POINTS

- 35% of small perimembranous and up to 80% of small muscular defects close spontaneously.
- Spontenous closure is most likely in the first few years of life.
- Redundant or aneurysmal TV tissue may result in reduction of the effective orifice perimembranous defects and may even result in spontaneous closure (Fig. 5-11).
- Spontaneous closure is unlikely in nonrestrictive defects.
- Supracristal (subpulmonic), inlet, and malalignment VSDs do not close spontaneously.

Step 3: Evaluate the Direction of the Shunt

- Shunting primarily occurs in systole.
- The shunt is left to right in smaller lesions with normal pulmonary resistance.
- Both color Doppler and spectral Doppler evaluation are useful when evaluating shunt direction.

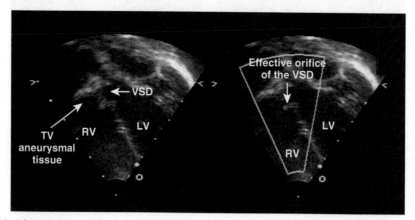

Figure 5-11. Apical four-chamber (4C) view demonstrating a perimembranous VSD partially occluded by tricuspid valve (TV) aneurysmal tissue. When the VSD is interrogated using color Doppler, the left-to-right shunt is quite small with a significant reduction of the effective orifice perimembranous defect by aneurysmal tissue.

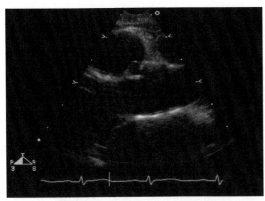

Figure 5-12. Parasternal long axis view of a supracristal VSD. There is distortion of the aortic valve leaflets with prolapse of the right aortic cusp. The aortic cusp is seen filling and nearly obliterating the supracristal defect. Aortic regurgitation may also be present.

Step 4: Determine the Size of the Shunt

- In the absence of increased right ventricular pressure, the severity of left-to-right shunting is proportional to the size of the defect.
  - In an unrestricted defect, equalization of ventricular pressure will occur over time, reflecting the development of pulmonary hypertension.
- The greater the size of the lesion and the lower the pulmonary resistance, the larger the left-to-right shunt.

KEY POINTS

- Align the defect so that the VSD jet is parallel to the cursor to obtain a peak velocity via pulsed or continuous wave (CW) Doppler.
- Right ventricular pressure can be estimated from the modified Bernoulli equation using the peak velocity across a VSD based on blood pressure as an estimate of systemic pressure.
- $4 \times$ (peak velocity across the VSD)^2 = pressure difference between the LV and RV.
- Blood pressure—$4 \times$ (peak velocity across the VSD)^2 = estimated right ventricular pressure.
- With equal ventricular pressure, the size of the shunt is determined by arterial and systemic vascular resistance.
- Use angulation of the plane of sound or alternative imaging rather than using theta (θ) to change your angle of interrogation. Using theta (θ) will provide an inaccurate measurement by altering the Bernoulli equation.

Step 5: Evaluate the Effects of Shunting

- Volume overload is reflected by:
  - Left atrial dilation.
  - Left ventricular enlargement and hypertrophy.

- Pulmonary hypertension may be present reflecting changes from chronic volume overload.
  - Estimate PA pressure (in the absence of pulmV disease) using a tricuspid regurgitation (TR) jet.
    - Use care to avoid contamination of the TR jet from the VSD jet.
  - Indications of possible pulmonary hypertension include:
    - Low-velocity shunting across the VSD.
    - Right-to-left shunting across the VSD.
    - Ventricular septal flattening.
    - Right ventricular hypertrophy.
  - Hypertrophied right ventricular muscle bundles (infundibular stenosis) can occur as an isolated finding or with the development of a double-chamber RV.
    - Occurs in 3% to 7% of patients.
    - Look for distortion of the aortic valve with a supracristal VSD (Fig. 5-12).
  - Malalignment VSDs may be associated with anterior or posterior deviation of the septum with subvalvar outflow obstruction.
    - TOF: anterior deviation of the conal septum results in RVOTO.
    - Interrupted aortic arch: posterior deviation of the Zconal septum results in LVOTO.

KEY POINTS

- Evaluate for volume overload.
- VSD left-to-right shunt may result in an increased spectral Doppler velocity across the pulmonary valve in the absence of pulmonary valve disease (flow-related relative pulmonic stenosis).
- Subaortic membranes and fibrous ridges may form in association with a VSD, resulting in left ventricular tract obstruction (LVOTO).
- Depending on the size and angulation of the jet, shunting across a VSD may cause a hypertrophied right ventricular muscle bundle in the inferior infundibular septal region resulting in RVOTO.
- AR is seen in association with supracristal VSDs due to aortic cusp prolapse from a poorly supported right coronary cusp (RCC).

Postoperative Assessment: Special Considerations

- If the VSD was closed using a patch, this area may appear echo bright.
- The patched portion of the septum will be dyskinetic.
- Postoperatively, residual shunts may occur at the borders of the patch.
- Occasionally closing a large VSD may "unmask" smaller defects not previously detected.

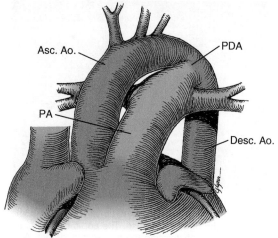

Figure 5-13. Anatomic drawing of a large persistent patent ductus arteriosus. *(Adapted from Fyler DC [ed], Nadas' Pediatric Cardiology. Philaladelphia: Hanley & Belfus, 1992.)*

- Monitor for LVOTO, particularly in malalignment VSDs.
- Evaluate for TR and/or valvular dysfunction.

Patent Ductus Arteriosus

- A patent ductus arteriosus is a persistent patency of a fetal connection between the descending aorta just distal to the origin of the left subclavian artery and PA (Fig. 5-13).
- The ductus is most commonly left sided regardless of the presence of a left or right aortic arch.
- Occasionally in the presence of a right aortic arch, the duct may be right sided.
  - Joins the right aortic arch just distal to the right subclavian artery and the right PA.
- Rarely bilateral ducti are present.

KEY POINT

• Delayed closure may be seen in:
  • Premature infants.
  • Children born at high altitudes.
  • Children with maternal rubella exposure during early pregnancy.

The Echo Exam: Step-by-Step Approach
Step 1: Determine the Presence of a Patent Ductus Arteriosus

- Image using a high left parasternal short axis view (three-finger or three-prong view) (Fig. 5-14).
- The transducer can then be rotated clockwise to see insertion of the ductus into the descending aorta (Fig. 5-15).

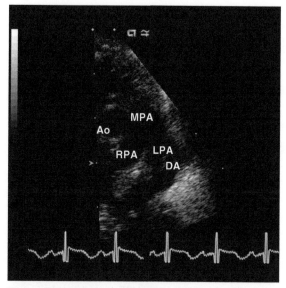

Figure 5-14. High left parasternal short axis view demonstrating the three-finger or three-prong view demonstrating the ductus arteriosus (DA) and left and right branch PAs.

KEY POINTS

• A patent ductus arteriosus (PDA) in the presence of systemic to suprasystemic pulmonary pressures can be very difficult to identify by color Doppler.
  • May only be seen by 2D imaging.
• Assess for the presence of pulmonary hypertension.
  • The tricuspid regurgitant jet can be used to estimate pulmonary arterial systolic pressure.
  • Secondary evidence of increased right ventricular and pulmonary pressures such as a flattened interventricular septal motion suggests the presence of pulmonary hypertension.

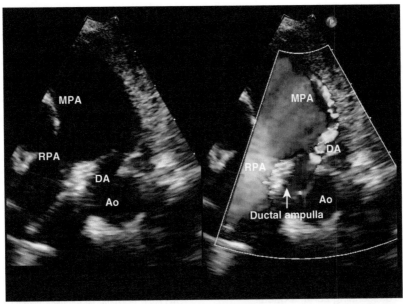

Figure 5-15. Parasternal short axis view with color in the DA. Note the ampulla of the DA is seen originating from the aorta (Ao) with flow from the aorta entering the PA (left-to-right flow).

Step 2: Evaluate the Size of the Patent Ductus Arteriosus

- Quantitative methods may be used, but no single parameter should be used in isolation. These include:
  - The ratio of the smallest duct diameter to the ostium of the left PA calculated using the following equation:

    Ductal diameter (mm)/diameter of the ostium of the left PA (mm)

    - Small: <0.5.
    - Moderate: >0.5 to 1.
    - Large: >1.
  - Percentage of retrograde diastolic flow to antegrade aortic flow in the descending aorta (estimated percentage by CW Doppler).
    - Small: <30%.
    - Moderate: 30% to 50%.
    - Large: >50%.

Step 3: Evaluate the Direction of the Shunt

- Align the PDA flow such that the cursor is parallel to the flow to achieve a complete Doppler signal.

Step 4: Determine Whether the Shunt Is Hemodynamically Significant

- Left ventricular enlargement indicates a hemodynamically significant shunt.

KEY POINTS
• In a patient with a PDA and normal pulmonary resistance, there will be left-to-right shunting (Fig. 5-16).   • In the setting of pulmonary hypertension and/or complex CHD, the ductus may be bidirectional or right to left.

- Measure peak velocity by pulsed wave at the pulmonary end of ductus:
  - >1.5 m/s suggests that the ductus is not hemodynamically significant.
  - <1.5 m/s suggest that the ductus is hemodynamically significant.
- The presence of turbulence in systole and diastole in the main PA suggests a hemodynamically significant shunt.

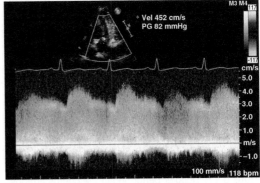

Figure 5-16. Doppler performed in the DA demonstrates continuous left-to-right shunting with a peak velocity of 4.5 m/s.

Step 5: Evaluate for Other Cardiac Disease

- A coarctation of the aorta may be masked in the presence of a ductus arteriosus (DA).
- Coarctation of the aorta is suggested by:
  - Narrowing in the isthmus region of the descending aorta.
  - The presence of a posterior shelf in the juxtaductal region of the aorta.
  - An increased distance from the left carotid and left subclavian arteries.
- Obtain a suprasternal notch "candy cane" view of the aortic arch with alignment of the cursor parallel to the entire descending aorta.

KEY POINTS

- CW Doppler should always be performed in the descending aorta.
  - If the Doppler cursor is not aligned parallel to the entire descending aorta, a ductal dependent coarctation of the aorta may be missed.
- Many cyanotic congenital heart lesions depend on the presence of a DA to maintain circulation before surgical repair (Fig. 5-17).

Surgical Ligation and Device/Coil Closure: Special Considerations

- Ligation of the LPA is a known complication after surgical ligation.

KEY POINTS

- Both branch pulmonary arteries should be assessed by 2D, color Doppler, and spectral Doppler.
- No residual shunting should be present after ductal closure.
- Assess the aortic arch to ensure that a coarctation of the aorta is not present after ligation.

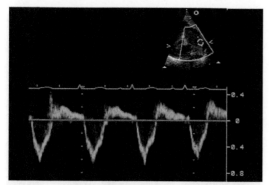

Figure 5-17. Doppler performed in the ductus arteriosus of an infant with a ductal-dependent cardiac lesion. There is bidirectional shunting with primarily right-to-left flow (below the baseline) seen in systole.

Suggested Reading

1. Allen HD, Driscoll DJ, Shaddy RE, Feltes TF, eds. *Moss and Adams' Heart Disease in Infants, Children and Adolescents: Including the Fetus and Young Adult.* 7th ed. Philadelphia: Lippincott Williams & Wilkins; 2007: 632-645, 667-701.
   These chapters review the basic anatomy and physiology of atrial and VSDs and PDA. Clinical presentation and pictures of anatomic specimens are included.
2. Keane JF, Fyler DC, Lock JE. *Nadas' Pediatric Cardiology.* 2nd ed. Philadelphia: Saunders; 2006:527-548, 603-626.
   A concise description and review of ventricular and atrial septal defects and PDA. Images include diagrams and angiograms.
3. Lai W, Mertens L, Cohen M, Geva T, eds. *Echocardiography in Pediatric and Congenital Heart Disease: From Fetus to Adult.* Hoboken, NJ: Wiley-Blackwell; 2009:158-187, 283-296.
   Includes a description of the anatomic lesions and additional imaging techniques.
4. Praagh VS, Carrera ME, Sanders SP, et al. Sinus venosus defects: unroofing the right pulmonary veins—anatomic and echocardiographic findings and surgical treatment. *Am Heart J.* 1994;128:365-379.
   Key paper describing the anatomic findings of a sinus venosus defect seen by echo.
5. Hubail Z, Lemler M, Ramaciotti C, et al. Diagnosing a patent foramen ovale in children: is transesophageal echocardiography necessary. *Stroke.* 2011;42:98-101.
   Describes the key findings for diagnosis of an ASD by transthoracic echo and provides evidence that transthoracic imaging rather than transesophageal echo in children is very effective and less invasive due to better acoustic windows in children.
6. Butera G, Romagnoli E, Carminati M, et al. Treatment of isolated secundum atrial septal defects: impact of age and defect morphology in 1,013 consecutive patients. *Am Heart J.* 2008;156:706-712.
   Demonstrates percutaneous closure via device of ASDs is possible on most patients and associated with a low complication rate.
7. Radzik D, Davignon A, van Doesburg N, et al. Predictive factors for spontaneous closure of atrial septal defects diagnosed in the first 3 months of life. *J Am Coll Cardiol.* 1994;23:851-853.
   101 infants were followed, demonstrating that interatrial defects measuring less than 3 mm in size do not need to be followed and often close spontaneously (hence the definition of a patent foramen ovale). Defects larger than 8 mm do not close spontaneously and are considered large.
8. Berger F, Ewert P, Biornstad P, et al. Transcatheter closure as standard treatment for most interatrial defects: experience in 200 patients treated with Amplatzer Septal Occluder. *Cardiol Young.* 1999;9:468-473.
   Device closure has replaced surgical closure as treatment for most ASDs. This paper validates this practice.
9. Chiu SN, Wang JK, Lin MT, et al. Aortic valve prolapse associated with outlet-type ventricular septal defect. *Ann Thorac Surg.* 2005;79:1366-1371.
   Description of the association of an outlet defect with aortic RCC prolapse as well as the association of perimembranous VSDs with infundibular hypertrophy and a subaortic ridge.
10. Canale JM, Sahn DF, Allen HD, et al. Factors affecting real-time, cross-sectional echocardiographic imaging of perimembranous ventricular septal defects. *Circulation.* 1981;63:689-697.
    This paper effectively describes the multiple imaging planes needed to identify and fully image a VSD. Patients had VSDs proven by angiography. It also correlates the size of the VSD to the diameter of the aorta and correlates this ratio with quantification of interventricular shunting (Qp/Qs) (pulmonary/systemic volume flow rate) data from the cardiac catheterization.

11. Mehta AV, Chidambaram B. Ventricular septal defect in the first year of life. *Am J Cardiol*. 1992;70:364-366. *Description of the isolated VSDs found in 124 infants who were followed over time. Spontaneous closure was seen in both perimembranous and muscular VSDs with a higher incidence of spontaneous closure in muscular VSDs.*

12. Glen S, Burns J, Bloomfield P. Prevalence and development of additional cardiac abnormalities in 1448 patients with congenital ventricular septal defects. *Heart*. 2004; 90:1321-1325.

13. Ramaciotti C, Vetter JM, Bornemeier RA, et al. Prevalence, relation to spontaneous closure and association of muscular ventricular septal defects with other cardiac defects. *Am J Cardiol*. 1995;75:61-65.

14. Turner SW, Hunter S, Wyllie JP. The natural history of ventricular septal defects. *Arch Dis Child*. 1999;81: 413-416. *A group of 1448 patients with VSDs were followed. This article demonstrates the increased association of VSDs with cardiac abnormalities as well as the development of abnormalities over time, including infundibular pulmonary stenosis and AR. This article recommends that patients with VSDs be followed by a cardiologist until at least 30 years of age.*

15. Sutherland GR, Godman M, Smallhorn F, et al. Ventricular septal defects: two dimensional echocardiographic and morphological correlations. *Br Heart J*. 1982;47:316-328. *Validates the use of echo in identifying VSDs.*

16. Minette MS, Sahn DF. Ventricular septal defect. *Circulation*. 2006;114:2190-2197. *This article is a review of VSDs, including the basic anatomy, physiology, treatment, and long-term prognosis, and including findings in adult patients.*

17. Su BH, Watanabe T, Mitsumasa S, et al. Echocardiographic assessment of patent ductus arteriosus shunt flow pattern in premature infants. *Arch Dis Child*. 1997;77: F36-F40. *This article outlines methods of echocardiographic assessment of PDA in premature infants to predict hemodynamically significant shunts.*

18. Sehgal A, McNamara PJ. Does echocardiography facilitate determination of hemodynamic significance attributable to the ductus arteriosus? *Eur J Pediatr*. 2009;168:907-914. *Methods for ductal assessment including echocardiographic markers of hemodynamically shunting.*

Atrioventricular Septal Defect: Echocardiographic Assessment

6

Jeffrey A. Conwell

Background

Atrioventricular septal defects (AVSDs) are a collection of congenital cardiac defects all having a common atrioventricular (AV) junction and a lack of AV septation. Defects can be either complete or partial. A complete AVSD consists of an inlet ventricular septal defect (IVSD), a primum atrial septal defect (ASD), and a single AV valve (AVV). Partial AVSDs have a primum ASD, two separate AVV orifices, and cleft present in the left-sided AVV. AVSDs make up 2.9% to 6.2% of all congenital heart disease. A complete AVSD occurs in 30% to 50% of patients with trisomy 21.

KEY POINTS

- Complete AVSDs are common in patients with trisomy 21. All patients diagnosed with trisomy 21 should undergo echocardiography (echo) to assess their cardiac anatomy shortly after the diagnosis is made.
- Various terms have been used to describe this defect including complete AVSD, complete atrioventricular canal (AVC) defect, common AVC defect, endocardial cushion defect, and atrioventricularis communis. For this chapter, AVSD is used.
- Complete AVSDs are commonly diagnosed in early childhood either as part of the evaluation for trisomy 21 or due to development of signs and symptoms of pulmonary overcirculation associated with shunting from the ventricular component. Partial AVSDs act similarly to ASDs and may be diagnosed later in life.

Anatomy

A complete AVSD has a common AV junction, a primum ASD, an IVSD, and a common AVV (Fig. 6-1). The primum ASD is anterior and inferior to the fossa ovalis, adjacent to the AVVs. The AVV consists of five leaflets: superior and inferior bridging leaflets, a left mural leaflet, a right mural leaflet, and a right anterosuperior leaflet (Fig. 6-2).

A partial AVSD usually has a primum ASD and two separate AVVs, with a cleft in the anterior leaflet of the left-sided AVV (mitral valve [MV]) (Fig. 6-3). The cleft in the left-sided AVV usually results in some degree of regurgitation of the valve. There are rare instances of partial AVSDs with only an IVSD and no primum ASD.

The term transitional AVSD has been used to refer to complete AVSDs in which the IVSD is predominantly occluded by chordal tissue from the AVV, resulting in minimal or no ventricular level shunting (Fig. 6-4). In transitional defects, there are two separate AVV orifices with a cleft in the left-sided AVV.

Associated defects include left ventricular outflow tract obstruction (LVOTO), tetralogy of Fallot (TOF) (5%), dual-orifice left-sided AVV, and hypoplasia of one of the ventricles. Unbalanced AVSDs occur in 10% to 15% of patients, and, when present, two thirds are right ventricular dominant. When an unbalanced AVSD is present, there is the potential for hypoplasia of the nondominant chamber and outflow tract from that chamber. In right ventricular dominance, there can be hypoplasia of the left ventricle (LV) and aorta. In left ventricular dominance, there can be hypoplasia of the right ventricle (RV) and pulmonary artery (PA). Rarely, the AVSD can be severely unbalanced to give a double-inlet ventricle.

KEY POINTS

- LVOTO may occur secondary to chordal attachments from the AVV that cross into the outflow tract.
- Anterior deviation of the infundibular septum may be seen causing right ventricular outflow tract (RVOT) obstruction (RVOTO) and would be consistent with TOF.
- The balance of a complete AVSD is extremely important to determine. If the defect is unbalanced, then attempting to septate the heart for a two-ventricle repair may not be successful and a single-ventricle (Fontan) approach may be needed.

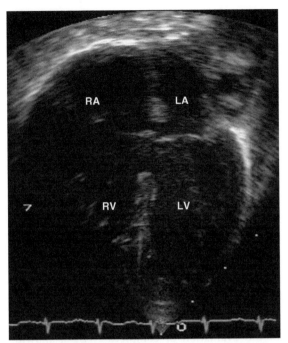

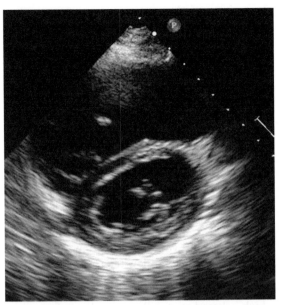

Figure 6-3. Parasternal short axis view showing a cleft in the anterior leaflet of the left-sided AVV.

Figure 6-1. Apical four-chamber (4C) view of complete atrioventricular septal defect (AVSD). The primum atrial septal defect (ASD) can be seen above the common atrioventricular valve (AVV) and the inlet ventricular septal defect is seen below the level of the AVV.

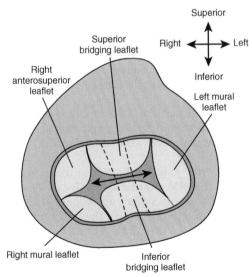

Figure 6-2. The illustration shows the basic arrangement of the leaflets to be found in the valve guarding the common atrioventricular (AV) junction. The *black dotted lines* show the plane of the ventricular septum (VS), and the *double-headed arrow* shows the zone of apposition between the leaflets that bridge the VS. The valve is shown as seen from the cardiac apex, looking up the barrels of the ventricles. *(From Anderson RH, Baker EJ, Redington A, et al., eds.* Paediatric Cardiology, *3rd edition, 2010, Philadelphia: Elsevier, Figure 27-11.)*

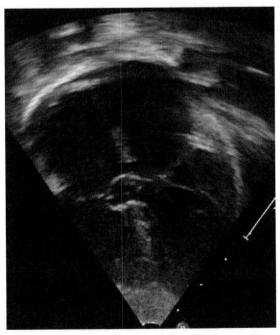

Figure 6-4. Apical 4C view of a transitional AVSD. The chordal attachments of the AVV to the crest of the VS are dense enough to have created only minimal shunting at the ventricular level.

Overview of the Echocardiographic Approach

The echocardiogram (echo) should fully evaluate all the components of the AVSD and assess for any associated abnormalities. Images should define the size of the atrial and ventricular components and demonstrate the direction of shunting. The AVV attachments need to be defined, and function of the AVV should be assessed by pulsed wave (PW) Doppler and color flow Doppler (CFD). The balance of the AVV above the ventricles should be evaluated along with flow across the valve to demonstrate the flow into both ventricles. Additional ASDs or ventricular septal defects (VSDs) can be present, and careful assessment of the atrial septum (AS) and ventricular septum (VS) should be performed. The outflow tracts should be interrogated, looking for any obstruction (Box 6-1).

AVSDs are described by Rastelli classification, which is based on papillary muscle configuration, specifically attachments of the superior bridging leaflet (Box 6-2 and Fig. 6-5):

- Rastelli type A: the superior bridging leaflet has attachments to the crest of the VS.

BOX 6-1 Goals of Echocardiographic Examination

- Atrial component (primum ASD)
  - Size of the defect
  - Direction of shunting
  - Additional ASDs
- Ventricular component (VSD)
  - Size of the defect
  - Direction of shunting
  - Additional VSDs
- Assess anatomy of the common AVV
  - Rastelli classification (type A, B, or C)
  - Presence and degree of valve regurgitation.
    - Note whether on the right or left side of the AVV
  - Additional valve abnormalities
    - Dual-orifice left AVV
- Balance of the defect
  - Distribution of the AVV over the ventricles
  - Assess for ventricular hypoplasia
- Assess for outflow tract obstruction
  - Left ventricular outflow
  - Right ventricular outflow
- Hemodynamics.
  - Flow across the AS and VS
  - Peak velocity across the VSD
  - Severity of AVV regurgitation
  - Assess ventricular function
- Assess for associated lesions
  - Patent ductus arteriosus (PDA)
  - Coarctation of the aorta
  - TOF

BOX 6-2 Rastelli Classification

- Based on papillary muscle configuration
  - Type A: anterior bridging leaflet mostly in the LV with attachments to the crest of the VS
  - Type B: Attachments of the anterior bridging leaflet to the right ventricular side of the septum
  - Type C: No attachments of the anterior bridging leaflet to the VS (free-floating bridging leaflet)

- Rastelli type B: the attachments are to the right side of the VS.
- Rastelli type C: the superior bridging leaflet is free floating with no attachments to the VS.

Anatomic Imaging

An apical four-chamber (4C) view is very useful in the evaluation of complete AVSDs, allowing visualization of the primum ASD, IVSD, and the common AVV. The AVV(s) will be noted to be at the same level as the primum ASD just above the AVV and the IVSD just below. From the apical 4C view, the balance of the AVV above the ventricles can be assessed and CFD can be used to assess for valve regurgitation.

Subcostal views allow evaluation of the primum ASD to determine size and direction of flow (Fig. 6-6). Subcostal short axis view allows an en face view of the AVV and can be used to assess the balance of the valve to the ventricles and look for attachments of the superior bridging leaflet to determine the Rastelli classification (Figs. 6-7 and 6-8).

The parasternal long axis view allows for assessment of the VS and AVV regurgitation (AVVR). In the parasternal short axis view, the VSD can be evaluated.

The aortic valve, which is usually wedged between the MV and tricuspid valve (TV) annuli, is anteriorly displaced or "unwedged" in AVSDs, resulting in elongation of the left ventricular outflow tract (LVOT). LVOTO may occur in all types of AVSDs but is more common in the partial defects. An apical five-chamber (5C) view allows assessment of the LVOT for possible obstruction (Boxes 6-3 and 6-4).

Partial AVSDs will have two separate AVVs noted to be at the same level. A cleft in the anterior leaflet of the left-sided AVV usually results in AVVR. There is also a primum ASD. Rarely a partial AVSD will have no primum ASD, but will have only an IVSD. The best views for evaluation include the subcostal long axis and short axis

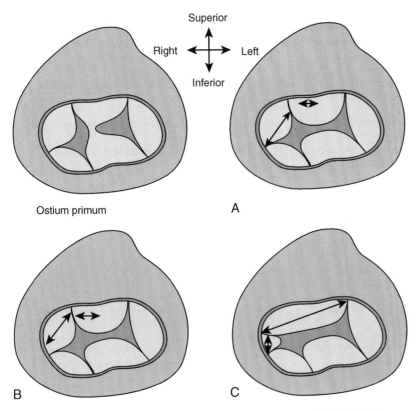

Superior

Right ⟷ Left

Inferior

Ostium primum

A

B

C

Figure 6-5. The illustration shows the essence of the Rastelli classification of variability in the superior bridging leaflet. Although not included by Rastelli et al., it is now evident that the spectrum of malformation can be extended to include the ostium primum defect (*top left*). Then, depending on the commitment of the superior bridging leaflet to the right ventricle (RV) (*wide double-headed arrow*), there is a spectrum with reciprocal diminution in size of the anterosuperior leaflet of the left ventricle (LV) (*narrow double-headed arrow*), as shown in **A** through **C**, which represent the types designated alphabetically in the original description. *(From Anderson RH, Baker EJ, Redington A, et al., eds. Paediatric Cardiology, 3rd edition, 2010, Philadelphia: Elsevier, Figure 27-20.)*

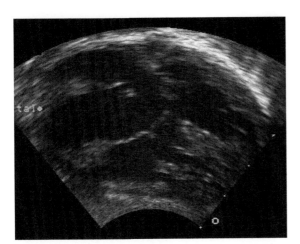

Figure 6-6. Subcostal long axis view shows the primum ASD above the common AVV.

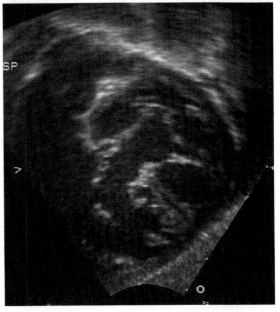

Figure 6-7. Subcostal short axis view of the common AVV. There are attachments of the superior bridging leaflet to the crest of the VS consistent with a Rastelli type A defect.

views to look at the AS and the AVV, the apical 4C view for the AVVs and ventricular shunting, and the parasternal short axis for the VS and the cleft in the MV (see Box 6-3).

A transitional AVSD refers to a complete AVSD in which there are chordal attachments of the AVV to the crest of the VS, resulting in a restrictive VSD or no shunting at the ventricular level. There is a single AVV and a primum ASD. Imaging views are the same as for complete AVSDs (see Box 6-3).

KEY POINTS

- Full definition of the AVSD is needed to assist with surgical planning. The surgeon will use the information from the echo to determine which approach to use in septation of the heart and creating two separate AVVs from the single AVV.
- The atrial component of an AVSD may be quite large, resulting in a "common atrium." In this situation, drainage of the systemic and pulmonary veins should be clearly defined before surgical intervention.
- The VSD may appear to be small in the apical 4C view, at least in a single plane. It is important to sweep the plane of the transducer from posterior to anterior in the heart to determine the extent of the defect.
- The primum ASD is usually moderate to large in size. Occasionally a patient may have a very small primum ASD of a size that is hemodynamically insignificant.
- Transitional AVSDs will often appear to have a significant ventricular component on two-dimensional imaging. There will be prominent chordal attachments to the VS, and when the defect is interrogated with CFD, minimal or no shunting will be detected.

BOX 6-3 Anatomic Imaging

- Diagnostic imaging overview
  - AVVs are at the same level
  - Absence of the AV septum
  - Unwedging and anterior displacement of the aortic valve
  - Elongated LVOT
  - Counterclockwise rotation of left ventricular papillary muscles
  - Cleft of left AVV component directed toward the septum
- Complete AVSD
  - Primum ASD (interatrial communication anteroinferior to fossa ovalis and adjacent to the AVV)
  - VSD (posterior portion of VS at the level of the AVV)
  - Common (single) AVV
- Partial AVSD
  - Primum ASD
  - No VSD
  - Common AVV with two separate orifices (cleft in left-sided AVV)
- Transitional AVSD
  - Chordal attachments of the AVV to the crest of the septum resulting in restrictive VSD
  - Primum ASD

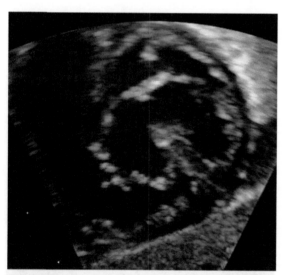

Figure 6-8. Subcostal short axis view of the common AVV. There are no attachments to the crest of the VS consistent with a Rastelli type C defect.

Acquisition

Complete and Transitional Atrioventricular Septal Defect

Step 1: Assess the Atrioventricular Valve

- In the subcostal short axis view, look for attachments of the anterior bridging leaflet to the crest of the septum, to the right of the septum, or if the leaflet is free floating (Rastelli classification type A, B, or C).
- CFD assessment for AVVR. If present, quantify the degree and whether from the right or left side of the AVV (Fig. 6-9).
- Balance of the valve above the ventricles can be determined from the apical 4C view and subcostal short axis view.
  - By drawing an imaginary line from the AS to the VS, does the valve look like it is equally committed to both ventricles?
- With CFD, determine whether there is flow across the valve into both ventricles (part of the assessment of "balance" of the valve).

Step 2: Assess the Inlet Ventricular Septal Defect

- Determine the presence and size of an IVSD.
- Determine direction of flow by CFD and spectral Doppler.
- Assess the remainder of the VS for additional VSDs.
- Apical 4C and parasternal long axis and short axis views allow for good imaging of the VS.

Step 3: Assess the Primum Atrial Septal Defect

- The primum ASD will be at the level of the AVV(s) and can be seen best in the subcostal

BOX 6-4 Overview of Imaging Windows	

Complete AVSD
- Subcostal long axis view
  - AS (primum ASD and additional ASDs)
  - Unwedging of the aortic valve
  - Elongation of the LVOT ("goose-neck" deformity)
- Subcostal short axis view
  - Anatomy of the common AVV
  - Chordal attachments of the superior bridging leaflet
  - En face view of the AVV to assess balance
- Apical 4C view
  - IVSD
  - Balance of common AVV to ventricles
  - Valve regurgitation
- Apical 5C view
  - LVOT
- Parasternal long axis view
  - AVVR
  - VS
  - LVOT

- Parasternal short axis view
  - VSD

Partial and Transitional AVSD
- Subcostal long axis view
  - AS (primum ASD and additional ASDs)
  - "Unwedging" of the aortic valve
  - Elongation of the LVOT ("goose-neck" deformity)
- Subcostal short axis view
  - AVVs
    - Cleft in left-sided AVV
    - Two separate valve orifices
- Apical 4C view
  - AVVs in relation to the septum
  - AVVs at the same level
  - Valve regurgitation
  - Ventricular level shunting
- Parasternal short axis view
  - VSD
  - Cleft in the left AVV

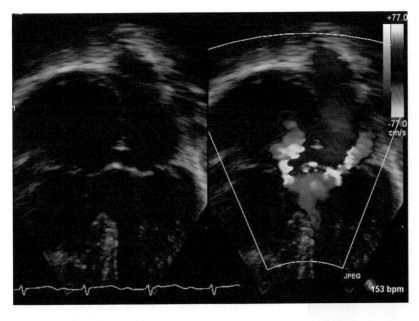

Figure 6-9. Apical 4C color compare image of complete AVSD showing mild right- and left-sided AVVR.

long axis view but may also be seen in the apical 4C view.
- Determine the size of the defect.
- Determine the direction of flow by spectral Doppler and CFD.
- Assess for additional atrial level shunts.

Step 4: Assess for the Presence of Associated Defects
- LVOTO using the parasternal long axis view and apical 5C view.

- If LVOTO is present, need to assess the aortic arch for possible coarctation of the aorta.
- RVOTO, in particular TOF.
- A dilated coronary sinus (CS) suggests the presence of a left superior vena cava to the CS.
- Hypoplasia of one ventricle (Figs. 6-10 and 6-11).
  - Coarctation of the aorta may be present in a right ventricular dominant AVSD.

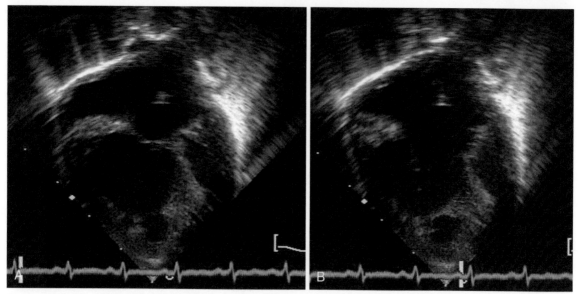

Figure 6-10. Two images from an apical 4C view of a right ventricular dominant complete AVSD. **A**, During systole with the common AVV closed. The valve appears to be predominantly above the RV; also note the small LV. **B**, During diastole showing that the AVV opens predominantly into the RV.

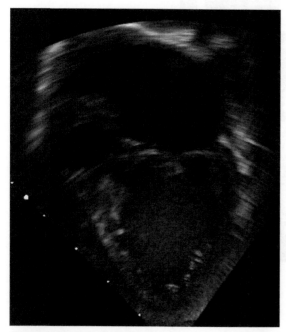

Figure 6-11. Apical 4C view of a left ventricular dominant AVSD with the common AVV predominantly above the LV.

- Pulmonary stenosis or RVOTO may be present in the left ventricular dominant AVSD.
- Patent ductus arteriosus (PDA).

Step 5: Assess the Chamber Size and Function

- Shunting across the primum ASD may cause dilation of the right atrium (RA), RV, and PAs.
- Shunting across the VSD may cause dilation of the LV.
- When there is a large VSD present, the interventricular septal position is flattened.

Partial Atrioventricular Septal Defect
Step 1: Assess the Atrioventricular Valves
- The AVVs will be at the same level in the apical 4C view (Fig. 6-12).
- A cleft will be present in the left-sided (mitral) AVV and is best seen in the parasternal short axis or subcostal short axis view (Fig. 6-13).
- CFD and spectral Doppler evaluation for regurgitation and stenosis. If present, quantify the degree.

Step 2: Assess the Atrial Septum
- The primum ASD will be at the level of the AVV(s) and can be seen best in the subcostal long axis view but may also be seen in the apical 4C view.
- Determine the size of the defect.

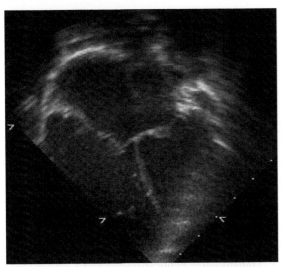

Figure 6-12. Apical 4C view of a partial AVSD. There is a large primum ASD above the AVVs, and the AVVs are at the same level.

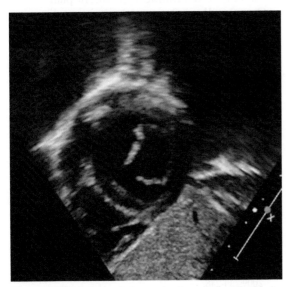

Figure 6-13. Subcostal short axis view of the left-sided AVV showing a cleft in the anterior leaflet.

- Determine the direction of flow by spectral and CFD.
- Assess for additional atrial level shunts.

Step 3: Assess the Ventricular Septum
- Partial AVSDs rarely have ventricle-level shunting.
- Assess for any ventricular shunting.
- Parasternal long axis and short axis views are best.

Step 4: Assess for Associated Defects
- LVOTO from the apical 5C view.

Step 5: Assess the Chamber Size and Function
- Shunting across the primum ASD may cause dilation of right heart structures.
- If there is significant left-sided AVVR, the LV and left atrium may become dilated.

Physiologic Data

Step 1: Atrioventricular Valves
- Assess severity of AVVR by CFD.
  - Severity is a qualitative assessment.
- If there is a restrictive VSD, the right ventricular systolic pressure should be estimated from the TV regurgitation jet velocity by continuous wave (CW) Doppler.

Step 2: Atrial Septal Defect
- Assess the direction of the shunt with CFD.
- Assess the direction of the shunt with spectral Doppler.
  - Spectral Doppler may make it easier to determine whether shunting is bidirectional.

Step 3: Ventricular Septal Defect
- Assess the direction of the shunt with CFD.
- Assess the direction of the shunt with spectral Doppler.
- Record the peak velocity by spectral Doppler.

Step 4: Outflow Tract Obstruction
- Peak velocity across the LVOT by pulsed and CW Doppler.
- Peak velocity across the RVOT by pulsed and CW Doppler.

Step 5: Hemodynamic Load on Ventricles
- Dilation of the RV.
- Dilation of the LV.
- Increased flow across the pulmonary valve.
- Increased left AVV inflow.

Pitfalls

- The IVSDs in complete AVSDs are usually large and nonrestrictive. A low spectral Doppler velocity may be present due to the large defect and should not be interpreted as evidence of pulmonary hypertension (PHTN).

- Right-sided AVVR Doppler velocity is increased if the VSD is nonrestrictive as the pressure from the LV is transmitted to the LV. The increased right heart pressures signifies the expected presence of elevated right ventricular pressure due to the large VSD. However, elevated right ventricular pressure (expected) does not equate to increased pulmonary vascular resistance (PVR), which is typically a late finding associated with pathologic changes in the pulmonary vasculature.
- The balance of an AVSD is often best determined on the initial study done in the newborn period. Later studies may be difficult to interpret due to dilation of chambers that occurs secondary to shunting at the atrial or ventricular level.
- LVOTO may develop after surgical repair and not be evident on preoperative studies.
- AVV regurgitation may be progressive over time before surgery, so follow-up ECGs are needed before surgical intervention.

In older patients with complete AVSDs with no previous surgery, elevation of PVR (also termed Eisenmenger syndrome) will develop. The anatomic findings are the same as those seen before surgery, but with the increased right heart pressures, the shunting at the VSD may be right to left. In unoperated-on patients, significant AVVR may also develop.

Intraoperative imaging by transesophageal echocardiography (TEE) can assist with identifying AVV morphology, AVVR, and other associated defects at the time of the initial surgery. Immediate postoperative assessment of the surgery can be done after cardiopulmonary bypass and should include looking for residual VSDs, ASDs, AVV stenosis or insufficiency, and LVOTO or RVOTO. The finding of a left ventricular-to-right atrial shunt is termed a Gerbode defect. This will be of high velocity due to the pressure difference between these two chambers. This can be confused with residual tricuspid regurgitation jetting into the RA, which will be of low velocity postoperatively if the right ventricular pressure has appropriately decreased.

After surgery, patients will require lifelong follow-up. Echocardiography can be helpful in assessing for residual atrial or ventricular level shunting. The right- and left-sided AVVs should be assessed not only for regurgitation, but also for stenosis. Severe left AVVR may occur in as many as 20% immediately postoperatively, and 10% to 15% of patients will require reoperation. LVOTO may occur in 10% to 15% of patients after repair and is more common in partial AVSDs. Reoperation is required in 5% to 10% of patients to relieve the obstruction. If the repair was performed later

---

BOX 6-5 Postoperative Assessment

- AVVR
- Residual ASD
- Residual VSD
- LVOT
- PHTN
- Ventricular dysfunction
- Stenosis of AVV

in life, patients may be at risk of the development of PHTN and should be assessed for this possibility (Box 6-5).

Alternative Approaches

- Transthoracic echocardiography (TTE) is often the only imaging needed to determine the cardiac anatomy. Older patients may need to undergo TEE to define the anatomy.
- Usually echocardiography will fully define the anatomy to determine a treatment plan. Occasionally patients may require cardiac catheterization to evaluate PA pressures if there is concern about the presence of PHTN.

Suggested Reading

1. Backer CL, Stewart RD, Mavroudis C. Overview: History, anatomy, timing, and results of complete atrioventricular canal. *Semin Thorac Cardiovasc Surg Pediatr Card Surg Annu.* 2007;3-10.
   A review of the history of surgical repair of AVSD, timing of repair, and recent outcomes.
2. Bakhtiary F, Takacs J, Cho MY, et al. Long-term results after repair of complete atrioventricular septal defect with two-patch technique. *Ann Thorac Surg.* 2010; 89:1239-1243.
   A study looking at 121 consecutive patients from 1975 to 1995 with regard to mortality and need for reoperation.
3. Cohen MS. Common atrioventricular canal defects. In: Lai WW, Mertens LL, Cohen MS, Geva T, eds. *Echocardiography in Pediatric and Congenital Heart Disease: From Fetus to Adult.* Hoboken, NJ: Wiley-Blackwell; 2009:230-248.
   A chapter with a discussion of echocardiographic findings in AVSDs.
4. Cohen GA, Stevenson JG. Intraoperative echocardiography for atrioventricular canal: Decision-making for surgeons. *Semin Thorac Cardiovasc Surg Pediatr Card Surg Annu.* 2007;47-50.
   Discussion of the use of pre- and postoperative TEE to assist with surgical planning and evaluation of surgical results.
5. Craig B. Atrioventricular septal defect: from fetus to adult. *Heart.* 2006;92:1879-1885.
   Review of AVSDs including fetal diagnosis.
6. Ebels T, Elzenga N, Anderson RH. Atrioventricular septal defects. In: Anderson RH, Baker EJ, Redington A, et al., eds. *Paediatric Cardiology.* 3rd ed. Philadelphia: Elsevier; 2010:553-589.
   A chapter with a thorough review of anatomy, pathophysiology, evaluation, and treatment discussions.
7. Espinola-Zavaleta N, Munoz-Castellanos L, Kuri-Nivon M, Keirns C. Understanding atrioventricular septal

defect: Anatomoechocardiographic correlation. *Cardiovasc Ultrasound.* 2008;6:33.
Echocardiographic images compared with pathology specimens with similar findings with the conclusion of good correlation between echocardiographic findings and anatomy.

8. Lim DS, Ensing GJ, Ludomirsky A, et al. Echocardiographic predictors for the development of subaortic stenosis after repair of atrioventricular septal defect. *Am J Cardiol.* 2003;91:900-903.
This article looks at 448 patients with AVSDs, finding 10 with subaortic stenosis. Findings suggest that displacement of the AVV into the LV may be a marker of potential subaortic stenosis. In evaluating the LVOT look for displacement of the AVV into the LV as potential indication of development of LVOT after repair.

9. Mahle WT, Shirali GS, Anderson RH. Echo-morphological correlates in patients with atrioventricular septal defect and common atrioventricular junction. *Cardiol Young.* 2006; 16:43-51.
A good review of echocardiographic imaging of AVSDs and the limitations of imaging.

10. Sittiwangkul R, Ma RY, McCrindle BW, et al. Echocardiographic assessment of obstructive lesions in atrioventricular septal defects. *J Am Coll Cardiol.* 2001;38:253-261.
This article looks at 549 patients with AVSDs for left-sided inflow or outflow obstruction with the conclusion that echocardiography provides accurate preoperative information.

Conotruncal Lesions

Amy H. Schultz

7

Tetralogy of Fallot

Background

- The four historically described features of tetralogy of Fallot (TOF) are ventricular septal defect (VSD), overriding aorta (Ao), pulmonary stenosis (PS), and right ventricular hypertrophy (RVH) (Fig. 7-1).
- However, it is better for the echocardiographer to understand the key features:
  - Large VSD of the anterior malalignment type (the conal or infundibular portion of the ventricular septum [VS] is anteriorly displaced).
  - Underdevelopment of the right ventricular outflow (RVO), which can lead to obstruction at the subvalvar, valvar, and supravalvar levels.
  - The aortic override and RVH can be thought of as secondary consequences to these features.
- A continuum of severity exists.
  - "Pink tets" have little in the way of PS, exclusively left-to-right shunting and physiology more akin to a large VSD.
  - The typical patient with TOF has an intermediate degree of obstruction, which usually progresses with time.
  - Toward the severe end of the spectrum, there may be critical degrees of obstruction, requiring ductal patency for adequate oxygenation.
  - In the extreme, there is pulmonary atresia. There may be no identifiable central pulmonary arteries (PAs); the lungs are supplied by multiple collateral vessels, termed major aortopulmonary collaterals (MAPCAs). This anatomy is also termed pulmonary atresia/VSD, distinguishing it from pulmonary atresia with an intact VS.
- A notable variant is TOF with absent pulmonary valve (pulmV) syndrome.
  - The pulmonary valve leaflets are vestigial. In utero, there is free pulmonary insufficiency (PI) and usually a relatively mild degree of stenosis.
  - The ductus arteriosus is usually absent.
  - The branch PAs are often severely dilated and may compress the airways, leading to severe respiratory distress at birth.
- A typical TOF repair involves closing the VSD to provide unobstructed outflow from the left ventricle (LV) to the aorta and relief of all levels of pulmonary valve stenosis, often using a transannular patch.
- Coronary artery anatomy must be clearly defined before placement of a transannular patch to ensure that no important coronary artery crosses the right ventricular outflow tract (RVOT).

Overview of Echocardiographic Approach

- Cardiac segmental connections are normal (two dimensional [2D]).
- Demonstrate the anterior malalignment of the conal septum and the various levels of RVOT obstruction (2D, color Doppler, pulsed wave [PW] Doppler, and continuous wave [CW] Doppler).
- Demonstrate the branch PAs (or lack thereof if not present) (2D, color Doppler).
- Evaluate for DA (2D, color Doppler, PW Doppler, CW Doppler).
- Evaluate for additional VSDs (2D, color Doppler).
- Evaluate coronary artery anatomy (2D, color Doppler).
- Evaluate arch branching pattern; right aortic arch is present in approximately 25% (2D, color Doppler).

Anatomic Imaging
Acquisition

- Transthoracic echocardiography (TTE) is used to establish the diagnosis in neonates.
- Transesophageal echocardiography (TEE) may be used pre- and postoperatively.

- Beginning with the subcostal views, evaluate the segmental anatomy.
  - Perform careful 2D sweeps in the frontal (long axis) and bicaval (sagittal) planes, noting the morphology and relationship of structures. The segmental anatomy is normal (see Chapter 1, The Pediatric Transthoracic Echocardiogram).

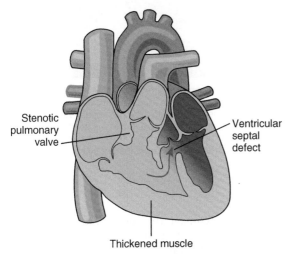

Figure 7-1. Schematic depicting the anatomy of tetralogy of Fallot (TOF).

Labels on schematic:
- Stenotic pulmonary valve
- Ventricular septal defect
- Thickened muscle

- In addition, perform a true subcostal short axis (45 degrees between the frontal and bicaval planes) 2D sweep from base to apex. This can be particularly helpful in visualizing:
  - Atrial septal defect (ASD).
  - Ventricular morphology.
  - Malalignment VSD (the anterior malalignment of the conal septum is well seen).
  - Any additional muscular VSDs.
  - Mitral-aortic fibrous continuity (if no continuity, consider the diagnosis of double-outlet right ventricle [DORV]).
  - RVOT.
- A right oblique view can be obtained by rotating 90 degrees counterclockwise from the short axis view and angling the beam of sound toward the right shoulder. This provides good views of the anterior malalignment VSD and RVOT (Fig. 7-2).
- Apical views
  - Ensure that both ventricles have normal size and function.
  - In the five-chamber view, the main VSD is apparent.
  - Assess for any additional muscular VSDs.

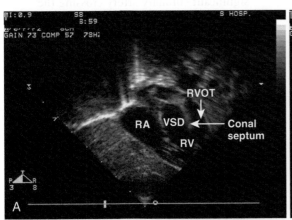

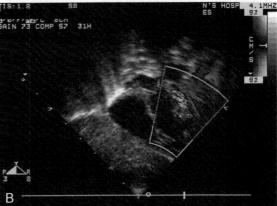

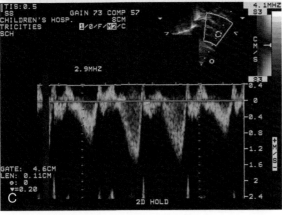

Figure 7-2. Subcostal right oblique views of the right ventricular outflow tract (RVOT) in TOF. **A,** Two-dimensional (2D) image shows the anteriorly malaligned conal septum and the resultant VSD. The RVOT is somewhat narrowed by the deviated conal septum. **B,** The addition of color Doppler shows aliasing of flow in the RVOT. **C,** Pulsed wave Doppler in the RVOT shows only mild acceleration of flow in the RVOT. There is a slightly late-peaking waveform, consistent with dynamic obstruction. In this patient, the obstruction was predominantly higher up, at the valve level.

- Parasternal long axis view (Fig. 7-3)
  - Note mitral-aortic fibrous continuity. If not present, consider the diagnosis of DORV.
  - Note the override of the aortic valve (AV).
  - Optimize image of pulmonary valve for annular measurement.
- Parasternal short axis view (Fig. 7-4)
  - Note the anterior malalignment of the conal septum and the large VSD.
  - Note any evidence of RVOTO, pulmonary valve hypoplasia/stenosis, supravalvar stenosis, and branch PA stenosis.
    - In TOF/absent valve, the main PA and branch PAs will be dilated (Fig. 7-5).
    - In TOF with pulmonary atresia, the main PA (Fig. 7-6) or central PAs may be absent.

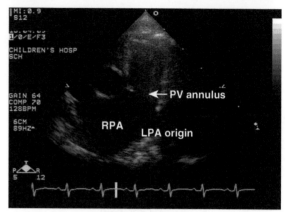

Figure 7-5. Parasternal short axis view of the pulmonary valve and proximal PAs in TOF with absent pulmonary valve syndrome. The hypoplastic pulmonary valve annulus with vestigial pulmonary valve leaflets is seen. The proximal right pulmonary artery (RPA) is massively dilated; the origin of the dilated left pulmonary artery (LPA) is seen.

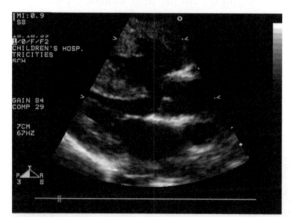

Figure 7-3. Parasternal long axis view of unrepaired TOF: the aorta (Ao) is seen overriding the ventricular septal defect (VSD); fibrous continuity between the aortic valve (AV) and mitral valve (MV) is noted.

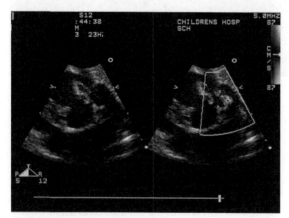

Figure 7-4. Parasternal short axis view of unrepaired TOF: the anteriorly malaligned conal septum is well seen, leaving a large VSD. The RVOT is narrowed, and the pulmonary valve (pulmV) is hypoplastic. A restricted jet of color flow passes through the pulmonary valve, which in this case was unicuspid.

- Carefully image the coronary arteries (Figs. 7-7 and 7-8). In particular, demonstrate the origin and course of the anterior descending coronary and rule out any coronary artery crossing the pulmonary outflow tract. A significant coronary artery crossing the pulmonary outflow tract precludes a transannular patch. Decreasing the dynamic range and appropriate adjustment of focal zone and zoom features facilitates visualization.
- Short axis sweeps of the ventricles are used to evaluate function and any additional VSDs. Additional muscular VSDs may be difficult to detect by color Doppler imaging in the presence of another large VSD; thus, careful attention to the 2D images is mandatory.
- High parasternal short axis images, rotated slightly counterclockwise, may be used to image a patent ductus arteriosus (PDA).
- Suprasternal notch imaging
  - Demonstrate arch sidedness and branching from the suprasternal short axis view. A right aortic arch occurs in about 25%. Some types of right aortic arch constitute a vascular ring. (See Chapter 1, The Pediatric Transthoracic Echocardiogram, for technique.)
  - Branch PAs may be well seen from suprasternal notch short axis view.
  - With variants of TOF with more significant obstruction, the ductus may be tortuous and originate from the underside of the arch. This is best seen with the sagittal view of the arch.

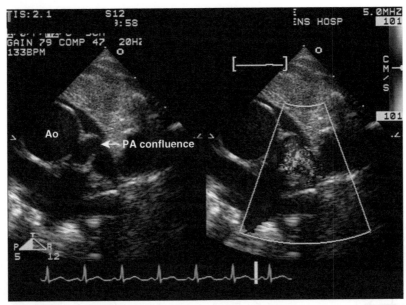

Figure 7-6. Parasternal short axis view of the PAs in TOF with pulmonary atresia. In this case, the central PAs are confluent, but there is no main PA segment. The color panel shows the entry of the ductus (red) into the confluence of the branches.

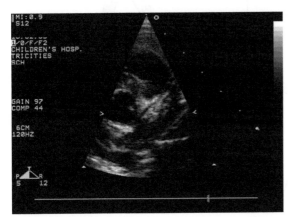

Figure 7-7. Parasternal short axis 2D image showing a normal course of the left anterior descending coronary artery. In this case (not shown), the right coronary artery was also shown to be normal, with no significant branch crossing the RVOT. Color confirmation of the coronary courses is also recommended (not shown).

Analysis

- Measure ASD/patent foramen ovale (PFO) from the subcostal 2D views.
- Measure the malalignment VSD from the parasternal short axis 2D view and another orthogonal view (apical or subcostal).
- Measure any additional VSD in the view in which it is best seen.
- Measure the pulmonary valve annulus, main PA, and branch PAs from the parasternal views. Compare with norms based on body surface area (BSA) (Z scores).
- Measure the PDA at its narrowest point in the view in which it is best seen.

Pitfalls

- In TOF with pulmonary atresia with no central PAs, the left atrial appendage (LAA) can be mistaken for the main PA. Avoid this pitfall by careful attention to the 2D images and use of color Doppler. The LAA will have a to-and-fro flow pattern in it.

Physiologic Data

- Doppler techniques are used to:
  - Assess size, location, and direction of shunting of ASDs and VSDs.
  - Evaluate PDA.
  - Assess RVOTO and PA stenosis.
  - Further visualize coronary arteries.
- Subcostal views
  - Perform color sweeps of the atrial septum (AS) and VS. Be alert for any additional muscular VSDs, which may be difficult to visualize because the ventricular pressures are typically equal due to the large primary VSD. Determine the direction and velocity of shunting across shunts. Generally, VSDs will be unrestrictive.
  - Evaluate RVOT from the subcostal short axis view.
    - This view provides good Doppler alignment for spectral analysis in the subvalvar and valvar region.
    - Perform a careful PW analysis, starting within the right ventricle (RV) below any muscle bundles evident on 2D imaging, marching up through the RVOT and pulmonary valve. Use the 2D image to

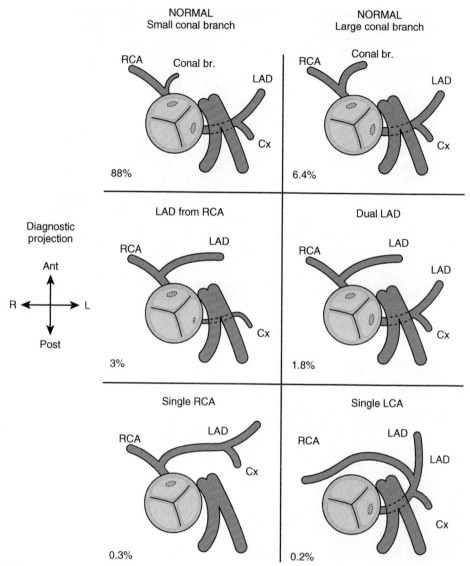

Figure 7-8. Coronary artery patterns observed in TOF. Frequency of occurrence is shown in the lower left-hand corner of each box. Note that approximately 94% of cases of TOF have one of the two "normal" patterns. Although more complex patterns are rare, they are critical to recognize because they preclude indiscriminate transannular patch. Conduit placement or careful, limited transannular incisions are required for repair. *(From Need LR, et al. Coronary echocardiography in tetralogy of Fallot: diagnostic accuracy, resource utilization and surgical implications over 13 years. J Am Coll Cardiol. 2000;36:1371–1377.)*

guide your placement of the Doppler cursor, thus demonstrating the significance of obstruction at the various levels.
- Use CW Doppler to determine the highest velocity.
- Apical views
  - Assess tricuspid valve (TV) and mitral valve (MV) function with color Doppler. Note that obtaining a right ventricular (RV) pressure estimate is irrelevant in the presence of a large VSD. The RV pressure is equal to the left ventricular (LV) pressure.
  - Evaluate the apical muscular septum with color Doppler for additional VSDs.
- Parasternal views
  - Assess valve function with color Doppler.
  - Assess outflow tract obstruction with color Doppler and spectral Doppler. In particular, pulmonary outflow obstruction may be assessed from the parasternal short axis. Use careful PW Doppler to localize various levels of obstruction. Use CW Doppler to assess highest velocity.
  - Evaluate the muscular septum with color Doppler for additional VSDs.

- Use color Doppler with very low Nyquist limit to assess flow in coronary arteries. Confirm that direction of flow is consistent with your understanding of the 2D anatomy. If not, reevaluate 2D anatomy.
- Evaluate for PDA with color Doppler from high parasternal window as described previously. If present, demonstrate velocity and direction of shunting by spectral Doppler.
- Suprasternal sagittal views
  - Evaluate for PDA by color Doppler. If a ductus is present, demonstrate velocity and direction of shunting by spectral Doppler.
  - In TOF with pulmonary atresia, examine the course of the arch and thoracic aorta with color Doppler to identify collaterals.

Alternate Approaches
- Cardiac catheterization with angiography is used:
  - To definitively determine coronary artery anatomy if there is concern about an abnormal pattern or if the coronary arteries were inadequately imaged.

KEY POINTS

- Key anatomic features
  - Large VSD of the anterior malalignment type.
  - Underdevelopment of the pulmonary outflow, which can lead to obstruction at the subvalvar, valvar, and supravalvar levels.
  - The aortic override and RVH can be thought of as secondary consequences to these features.
- Key aspects of the preoperative echocardiogram
  - Define the location and severity of the levels of pulmonary outflow obstruction.
  - Evaluate for any coronary artery crossing the RVOT (present in ~5% of cases) that would preclude a transannular patch repair.
  - Evaluate for additional VSD and PDA.
  - Evaluate arch sidedness and branching pattern.
- Notable anatomic variants include the following:
  - TOF with pulmonary atresia (also known as pulmonary atresia/VSD). In the most severe cases, there may be no identifiable central PAs, and the lung fields are supplied by MAPCAs.
  - TOF with absent pulmonary valve: main PA and branch PAs are typically severely dilated and may cause airway compression; the ductus is usually absent.

- In all cases of TOF with pulmonary atresia with MAPCAs to determine the number, size, and location of collaterals and to define which segment(s) of the lung is perfused by each collateral.

TOF Repaired

Background
- Repair of TOF entails the following:
  - Patch closure of the VSD.
  - Establishment of unobstructed outflow from the RV to the PAs, tailored to the anatomy of the individual patient.
    - In the best case, the pulmonary valve annulus is of adequate size and RV muscle bundles can be resected through the TV and pulmonary valve, avoiding right ventriculotomy (transatrial/ transpulmonary repair).
    - More frequently, the pulmonary valve annulus is hypoplastic, and a transannular patch is required. The surgeon incises from the main PA, across the pulmonary valve and onto the RV and then augments the area with a patch. Free PI results.
    - If a coronary artery crosses the RVOT or if there is pulmonary atresia with no continuity of the main PA to the RV, then an RV-to-PA conduit is placed.
    - If pulmonary blood flow (PBF) is via MAPCAs, the collaterals must first be brought together (unifocalized) before the conduit is placed. In this case, often the VSD is not closed at the first operation.
  - Closure of any large ASD. A PFO is frequently left open to facilitate maintenance of cardiac output in the immediate postoperative period.
- The most important long-term follow-up issue in TOF is the development of RV dilation and dysfunction due to chronic PI and previous ventriculotomy. Serial evaluation of RV size and function is key.
- Branch PA stenosis can be an important issue after TOF repair.
- Aortic root enlargement and aortic insufficiency are observed late after TOF repair.

Overview of Echocardiographic Approach
- Review the history if possible before beginning the study to understand what type of repair was performed.

- Evaluate for residual ASD or VSD (2D, color Doppler, PW Doppler, CW Doppler).
- Evaluate the outflow from the RV to PAs (2D, color Doppler, PW Doppler, CW Doppler).
  - Residual obstruction can occur at any level. Use PW Doppler to localize any area of obstruction.
  - Free PI is often present (color Doppler, PW Doppler).
  - Evaluate for branch PA stenosis (more commonly left).
- Evaluate RV size and function (2D). Estimate RV pressure if possible from the TR velocity (color Doppler, PW Doppler, and CW Doppler).
- Evaluate aortic root size and AV regurgitation (2D, color Doppler).

Anatomic Imaging
Acquisition
- Subcostal views
  - Perform 2D sweeps to evaluate for obvious residual ASD or VSD. Use the short axis subcostal view to visualize the RVOT.
- Apical views
  - Assess the size and function of both ventricles, in particular the RV.
    - TOF repair often leads to long-standing severe PI, which can lead to right heart dilation and RV dysfunction.
    - Previous ventriculotomy also contributes to RV dysfunction.
    - As the right heart dilates, the angle of the TV annulus may tilt, the RV develops a "shoulder" near the free wall TV annulus, and the apex becomes broader (Fig. 7-9).

- Assessment of RV dilation remains a qualitative assessment.
  - Visualize the VSD patch from the five-chamber (5C) view, assess for any obvious residual VSD.
- Parasternal views
  - Optimize long axis 2D image for measurement of aortic annulus, root, sinotubular junction, and ascending aorta.
  - The VSD patch can be visualized from long axis and short axis views; assess for any obvious residual VSD.
  - Visualize the RVOT and branch PAs. Optimize view of branch PAs for measurement. If a conduit is present, pay attention to the motion of the conduit valve leaflets, which can become calcified and immobile over time.
  - Assess the size and function of both ventricles.
    - The RVOT in particular may demonstrate hypokinesis due to a history of ventriculotomy and the presence of a transannular patch.
    - Compare the size of the RV with that of the LV in the short axis view (Fig. 7-10).
    - Note whether RVH is present.
  - Septal wall motion is often paradoxical after TOF repair. This finding is not concerning in and of itself. It may render shortening fraction an inaccurate assessment of LV systolic function.
- Suprasternal notch views: may be used to visualize branch PAs if not well seen from the parasternal short axis view.

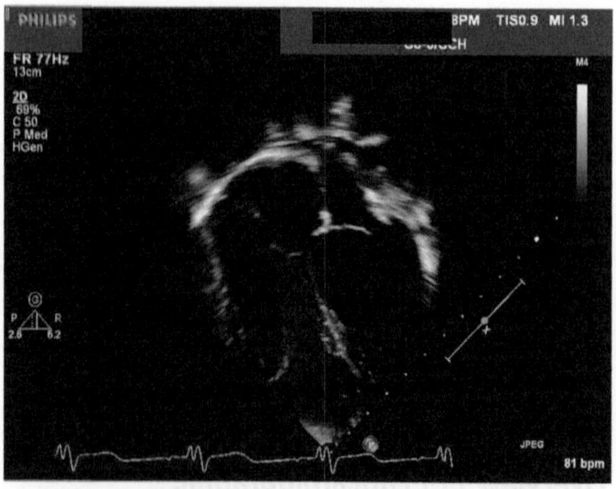

Figure 7-9. Apical view of a dilated right ventricle (RV) after repair of TOF. Note the broad right ventricular apex, the "shoulder" of the RV cavity near the lateral tricuspid annulus, and the tilt of the tricuspid valve (TV) annular plane relative to the plane of the MV.

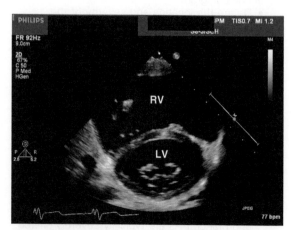

Figure 7-10. Parasternal short axis view of the RV and left ventricle (LV) after repair of TOF in a patient with severe RV dilation.

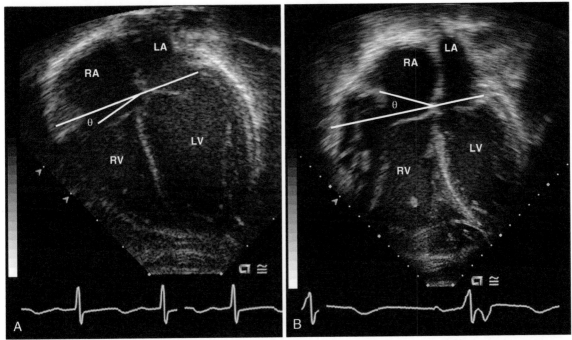

Figure 7-11. Method for calculating TV annular tilt for assessment of RV dilation. *(From Punn R, Behzadian F, Tacy TA. Annular tilt as a screening test for right ventricular enlargement in patients with tetralogy of Fallot. J Am Soc Echocardiogr. 2010;23(12):1297–1302.)*

Analysis

- Measure the size of any residual ASD or VSD from the 2D views where best visualized.
- In the apical view, assess TV annulus angle. An angle greater than 20 degrees has been associated with RV volume greater than 150 mL/m^2 (Fig. 7-11).
- Assess biplane LV ejection fraction in the apical view.
- Measure LV dimensions in the parasternal short axis or long axis view. Calculate shortening fraction if septal wall motion is not paradoxical.
- Measure branch PAs from the parasternal short axis view or the suprasternal notch view. Compare with norms for BSA (Z score) in smaller patients. Usual norms can be used for average adult-sized patients.

Physiologic Data

- Doppler techniques are used to assess the following:
  - Size, location, and direction of shunting of residual ASD and VSD.
  - Atrioventricular valve (AVV) function.
  - RVO and PAs for residual obstruction.
  - Degree of PI.
  - AV function.

Acquisition

- Subcostal views
  - Perform color Doppler sweeps to identify any residual ASD or VSD. If present, assess direction of shunting. Assess velocity of shunting across any residual VSD.
  - Use the subcostal short axis view to assess the RVOT for residual obstruction. Use color Doppler to screen for areas of aliasing and PW Doppler to localize and determine magnitude of obstruction. Obtain overall peak velocity by CW Doppler.
- Apical views
  - Assess MV and TV function. Obtain RV pressure estimate if possible.
  - Some authors have used RV myocardial performance index as an index of RV function.
  - Assess AV function and quantify regurgitation as appropriate.
  - Use color Doppler over the VSD patch to assess for any residual defect.
- Parasternal views
  - Assess AV regurgitation.
  - Assess AVV regurgitation; obtain RV pressure estimate if possible.
  - Assess for residual VSD or additional VSD by color Doppler; obtain peak velocity if present.

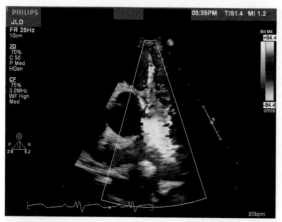

Figure 7-12. Parasternal short axis view with color Doppler of the main and branch PAs in TOF after repair with a transannular patch. This frame is in diastole. Note the reversal of flow (red) all the way to the branch PAs.

KEY POINTS

- Repair entails relief of any obstruction to pulmonary outflow (subvalvar, valvar, or supravalvar levels) and patch closure of the VSD. Frequently, a small PFO is left intentionally.
- Frequently, a transannular patch is performed, resulting in free PI.
- Important postoperative features to evaluate include the following:
  - Residual VSD or ASD.
  - Residual pulmonary outflow obstruction at any level.
  - Branch PA stenosis.
- The most common long-term follow-up issue is RV dilation and dysfunction in the setting of free PI.
- If a conduit is used in the repair, it should be assessed for both insufficiency and stenosis.

- Assess RV outflow from the ventricle through the branch PAs for residual obstruction and assess degree of PI (Fig. 7-12).
  - Screen for aliasing and flow reversal by color Doppler.
  - Note width of PI jet compared with width of RVOT.
  - Use PW Doppler at all levels to localize and quantify obstruction. Also note location of flow reversal (main PA, branch PAs).
  - Note that multiple levels or long segment narrowing in the pathway from the RV to the PAs may be present. In this case, the mean gradient may be more predictive of true peak-to-peak gradient measured invasively.

Alternate Approaches
- Magnetic resonance imaging (MRI) can quantify RV size and systolic function and the pulmonary regurgitant fraction. In addition, anatomic assessment is superior in patients with poor windows.
- Cardiac catheterization is used to accurately measure pressure gradients, particularly in the setting of multiple levels of obstruction. Filling pressures can also be obtained, and angiography can further clarify anatomy. Interventions are possible for branch PA stenosis, and in some select cases for pulmonary valve replacement.
- Nuclear medicine lung perfusion scan can be performed to quantify relative flow to the two lungs to help determine whether cardiac catheterization for branch PA interventions is indicated.

Double-Outlet Right Ventricle

Background
- The diagnosis of DORV is a "grab bag" of lesions that share the common feature that both the aorta and PA arise from the RV.
- It can be difficult to determine when the aorta is "assigned to" the RV.
  - If the aorta is normally located, but the portion of the VS beneath it is missing, the aorta will appear to override the VS.
  - Most forms of DORV include a VSD.
- Features that suggest (controversy exists here) that the aorta should be "assigned to" the RV include the following:
  - Separation of the aortic annulus from the mitral annulus by muscle.
  - The aorta lies more than 50% over the RV.
- Observing the location of the VSD and the relationship of the great vessels (GVs) to each other and the VSD is key.
- It is useful to subcategorize DORV into several recognizable types to aid recognition and management. Traditionally, this has been done based on the relationship of the VSD to the GVs (Fig. 7-13).
  - DORV with subaortic VSD and
    - No pulmonary stenosis (VSD type).
    - Pulmonary stenosis (tetralogy type).
  - DORV with subpulmonary VSD (transposition type).
    - The form of DORV with subpulmonary VSD, side-by-side GVs, and bilateral conus is given the eponym Taussig-Bing anomaly.
  - DORV with doubly committed VSD: in this anatomy, the VSD is very large, often due

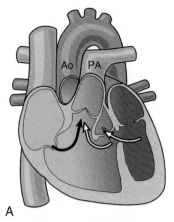
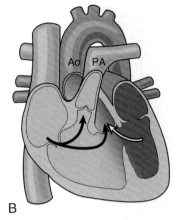
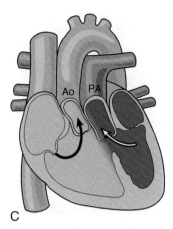

A   B   C

Figure 7-13. Schematic showing the physiology of three major types of double-outlet right ventricle (DORV). **A,** DORV with subaortic VSD and no pulmonary stenosis (PS) (VSD type): oxygenated left ventricular (LV) blood *(open arrow)* is directed through the VSD to the aorta; deoxygenated RV blood (solid arrow) is directed to the PA. **B,** DORV with subaortic VSD and PS (tetralogy type): oxygenated LV blood *(open arrow)* is directed through the VSD to the aorta; due to the presence of PS, deoxygenated RV blood *(solid arrow)* flows partly to the PA and partly across the VSD to the aorta. **C,** DORV with subpulmonary VSD (transposition type): oxygenated LV blood *(open arrow)* is directed preferentially through the VSD to the PA; deoxygenated RV blood *(solid arrow)* is directed preferentially to the aorta. *(Redrawn from Silka MJ. Double outlet right ventricle. In McMillan JA, DeAngelis CD, Feigin RD, Warshaw JB, eds.* Oski's Pediatrics: Principles and Practice, *3rd ed. Philadelphia: Lippincott Williams & Wilkins, 1999, Figure 3-11.)*

to hypoplasia or absence of the conal septum. Both GVs are related to the VSD. Typical repair is similar to that for the VSD type.
- DORV with remote or noncommitted VSD and other more complex forms of DORV need to be managed on an individual basis and are often treated with single-ventricle (SV) palliation.

Overview of Echocardiographic Approach
- A segmental approach to assessing the anatomy is used (2D) to:
  - Establish normal atrial situs.
  - Evaluate ventricular looping: normal for the noncomplex varieties; complex forms of DORV are not further discussed here.
  - Evaluate GVs.
    - Commitment to the LV versus RV.
    - Relationship to each other and the VSD.
    - Note any obstruction to either GV (subvalvar or valvar level).
- Subcostal views are the best for determining the degree of commitment of each GV to the LV versus RV and for visualizing the pathway from the LV to the most proximal GV.
- Parasternal long axis view: useful for identifying a lack of fibrous continuity between the MV and the closest GV.
- Be alert for complicating features such as straddling AVVs.

- Color Doppler and spectral Doppler are used to assess outflow tract obstruction.

Anatomic Imaging
Acquisition
- TTE is used to establish the diagnosis in neonates.
- TEE may be used pre- and postoperatively and may be performed specifically to assess the relationship of the VSD to the GVs.
- Three-dimensional (3D) imaging can be important in helping to understand the size of the VSD and its relationship to the GVs, particularly in cases in which there is concern about the adequacy of the pathway of the LV to the nearest GV.
- As discussed previously, DORV is a "grab bag" of many different lesions. The following discussion applies to the more straightforward forms, characterized by fundamentally normal atrial situs and ventricular looping with various relationships of the GVs to each other and the VSD. There are many more complex hearts that fall under the moniker of DORV but are beyond the scope of this chapter.
- Beginning from the subcostal views, evaluate the segmental anatomy.
  - Perform careful 2D sweeps in the frontal (long axis) and bicaval (sagittal) planes, noting the morphology and relationship of structures.

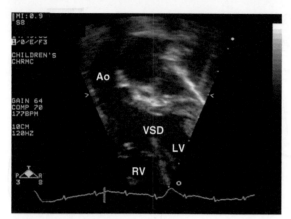

Figure 7-14. Subcostal short axis view of a DORV with a subaortic VSD. The aorta appears to sit completely over the RV. There is no mitral-aortic continuity (the MV is not even apparent in this view). The pathway from the LV through the VSD to the aorta is shown. Chordal attachments to the ventricular septum (VS) are noted on the RV side, consistent with RV morphology.

- In addition, perform a true subcostal short axis (45 degrees between the frontal and bicaval planes) 2D sweep from base to apex. This can be particularly helpful in visualizing ventricular morphology, commitment of the GVs, the VSD, and the potential pathway from the LV to the nearest GV (Fig. 7-14).
- Atrial situs solitus: the inferior vena cava (IVC) enters the right atrium (RA); at least some pulmonary veins (PVs) enter the left atrium (LA). Note any ASD or PFO.
- Ventricular looping: D-looped (normal) in the subset of DORV discussed here:
  - The morphologic RV is on the right, characterized by coarse trabeculations and a morphologic TV with chordal attachments to the septum.
  - The morphologic LV is on the left, characterized by a smooth septal surface and a morphologic MV with no chordal attachments to the septum.
- GV relationships: identify each GV; note the GV relationships to each other and the commitment to each ventricle.
  - The PA is identified as the GV that bifurcates; the aorta does not bifurcate and has coronary arteries arising from it.
  - In the long axis view, note whether there is separation of the MV from the closest GV.
  - In the true short axis view, note the degree of commitment (location over) of each GV, the LV and RV; more than 50% override above the RV suggests commitment to the RV.

- Note the relationship of the GVs to each other: usual spiral relationship with the aorta posterior and to the right is seen in the VSD type and tetralogy types. Parallel relationship with the aorta rightward is seen in the transposition type (see Chapter 8, Transposition of the Great Arteries, for further discussion of imaging).
- Once the segmental anatomy is established, use the subcostal views to further define additional details of the anatomy.
  - Note the relationship of the VSD to the GVs. Optimize images of the potential pathway from the LV to the nearest GV.
  - If the VSD is subaortic, examine for evidence of subvalvar or valvar PS to distinguish between the VSD type and the tetralogy type. The subcostal short axis view is particularly good for evaluation of subpulmonary stenosis.
  - If the VSD is subpulmonary and the GVs are transposed, evaluate for evidence of subvalvar or valvar AS. If present, be alert for evidence of arch obstruction on later views.
  - Be alert for any evidence of straddling AVVs (chordae or leaflets crossing the VSD to attach into the other ventricle).
  - In the transposition type, note the size of the atrial shunt. Although a large VSD is invariably present, an atrial communication may also be needed for effective mixing as streaming from the LV to PA and RV to aorta can occur (see Chapter 8, Transposition of the Great Arteries, for further details).
- Apical views
  - Ensure that both ventricles are apex forming.
  - Examine for any evidence of straddling AVVs.
  - With anterior angulation, evaluation of the outflow tracts is possible.
  - Assess for any additional muscular VSDs.
- Parasternal long axis view (Fig. 7-15)
  - Note muscular separation of the MV from the nearest GV.
  - Visualize potential pathway from the LV to the nearest GV.
- Parasternal short axis view
  - Note the relative positions of the semilunar valves and reconfirm the relationship of the GVs. Evaluate the morphology of the semilunar valves.
  - In the VSD type, the GVs have a usual relationship to one another, with the AV seen in cross section and the pulmonary

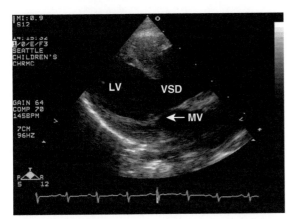

Figure 7-15. Parasternal long axis view of a DORV. In this case (which has a subaortic VSD), the MV is well seen, but the AV is not even visible due to its displacement over the RV. The large VSD is well seen.

valve and main PA in the long axis view wrapping around the AV.

- In the tetralogy type, the relationship of the GVs to each other is usual (as above in VSD type), but the conal septum will be noted to be anteriorly malaligned in the parasternal short axis view.
  - Note any evidence of RVOTO, pulmonary valve hypoplasia/stenosis, and PA stenosis.
  - Carefully image the coronary arteries. In particular, demonstrate the origin and course of the anterior descending coronary and rule out any coronary crossing the pulmonary outflow tract. A significant coronary crossing the pulmonary outflow tract precludes a transannular patch. Decreasing the dynamic range and appropriate adjustment of focal zone and zoom features facilitates visualization.
- In the transposition type, the semilunar valves are usually side by side, AV rightward, but the AV may also be anterior and rightward.
  - Delineation of coronary artery anatomy is key (see Chapter 8, Transposition of the Great Arteries, for details) because management may be by arterial switch operation (ASO).
  - The more side by side the GVs are, the greater the risk of a so-called inverted coronary artery pattern, where the right coronary artery arises from a more leftward sinus and then crosses anteriorly to the native AV. This is of concern if a transannular patch will be needed after ASO to alleviate neopulmonary outflow obstruction.

- Cranial angulation demonstrates the branch PAs arising from the pulmonary valve.
- Short axis sweeps of the ventricles are used to evaluate function and any additional VSDs. Additional muscular VSDs may be difficult to detect by color Doppler imaging in the presence of another large VSD; thus, careful attention to the 2D images is mandatory.
- High parasternal short axis images, rotated slightly counterclockwise, may be helpful in imaging a PDA in the VSD or tetralogy types; the ductus will likely be seen better from the sagittal view of the arch in the transposition type.
- Suprasternal notch imaging
  - Arch sidedness and branching should be established from the suprasternal short axis view due to the significant association between the DORV and right aortic arch. Some types of right aortic arch constitute a vascular ring (see Chapter 1, The Pediatric Transthoracic Echocardiogram, for technique).
  - The transposition type has a significant association with arch obstruction (particularly if subaortic or AV stenosis is noted). Evaluate the arch carefully by 2D imaging. It may be difficult to rule out a coarctation if a large PDA is present.
  - In the transposition type, the PDA is usually best imaged in the sagittal (long axis) view of the arch. In the tetralogy type with more significant obstruction, the PDA may be seen as a tortuous vessel arising from the underside of the arch in this view.

Analysis

- Key measurements include the size of the ASD, VSD, and semilunar valves.
- The ASD is measured from the 2D subcostal images. This is particularly important in the transposition type.
- The VSD is measured from multiple views. Use the subcostal short axis view and the parasternal short axis view in particular. A 3D en face view of the VSD can also be particularly helpful.
- Measure any additional VSD in whichever view it is identified.
- Measure both semilunar valves in systole, typically from the parasternal views. Compare with norms for BSA.

Pitfalls

- The most difficult aspects of imaging a DORV are determining the size of the VSD and determining its relationship to the GVs.

- Use careful subcostal 2D imaging to determine these features. Spend a lot of time on the subcostal views, understanding what you are seeing. Use the subcostal short axis view described above. Do not turn on the color until you understand the 2D anatomy.
- Use 3D imaging of the VSD to further understand its size and shape.

Physiologic Data

- Doppler techniques are used to:
  - Assess size, location, and direction of shunting of ASDs and VSDs.
  - Evaluate PDA.
  - Assess for outflow tract obstruction.
  - Further visualize coronary arteries.
- Subcostal views
  - Perform color sweeps of the AS and VS. Be alert for any additional muscular VSDs, which may be hard to visualize because the ventricular pressures are typically equal due to the large primary VSD. Determine direction and velocity of shunting across shunts. Generally, VSDs will be unrestrictive.
  - Evaluate outflow tracts for evidence of aliasing. Use careful PW Doppler to localize various levels of obstruction. Use CW Doppler to assess highest velocity.
- In the tetralogy type, the pulmonary outflow is well seen from a subcostal short axis, and this provides good Doppler alignment for spectral analysis in the subvalvar and valvar region.
- Apical views
  - Assess TV and MV function.
  - With anterior angulation, additional color Doppler and spectral Doppler evaluation of the outflow tracts can be performed.
  - Evaluate the apical muscular septum with color Doppler for additional VSDs.
- Parasternal views
  - Assess valve function with color Doppler.
  - Assess outflow tract obstruction with color Doppler and spectral Doppler. In particular, pulmonary outflow obstruction may be assessed in the tetralogy type from the parasternal short axis. Use careful PW Doppler to localize various levels of obstruction. Use CW Doppler to assess highest velocity.
  - Evaluate the muscular septum with color Doppler for additional VSDs.
  - Use color Doppler with a very low Nyquist limit to assess flow in coronary arteries. Confirm that direction of flow is consistent with your understanding of the 2D anatomy. If not, reevaluate 2D anatomy.
  - Evaluate for DA with color Doppler from high parasternal window as described earlier

for VSD and tetralogy types. If present, demonstrate velocity and direction of shunting by spectral Doppler.
- Suprasternal sagittal views
  - In transposition type, evaluate arch flow pattern by color Doppler and spectral Doppler.
  - Evaluate for DA by color Doppler. If a DA is present, demonstrate velocity and direction of shunting by spectral Doppler.

Alternate Approaches

- Cardiac catheterization can be used to define coronary artery anatomy if it is not well seen and delineation is important to the repair (tetralogy or transposition types). MRI may also be used to define anatomic relationships.

KEY POINTS

- DORV is a "grab bag" of lesions that share the common feature that both the aorta and PA arise from the RV.
- Features that suggest that the aorta should be "assigned to" the RV include the following:
  - Separation of the aortic annulus from the mitral annulus by muscle.
  - The aorta lies more than 50% over the RV.
- Traditionally, the DORV has been subcategorized into several types based on the relationship of the VSD to the GVs.
  - DORV with subaortic VSD and no PS (VSD type).
  - DORV with subaortic VSD and PS (tetralogy type).
  - DORV with subpulmonary VSD (transposition type).
  - DORV with doubly committed VSD: typical repair is similar to that for the VSD type.
  - DORV with remote or noncommitted VSD and other more complex forms of DORV: managed on an individual basis, often with SV palliation
- Subcostal and parasternal views are most heavily used in assessing the anatomy.
  - The pathway from the LV to the nearest GV must be well demonstrated.
  - Be alert for complicating features such as straddling AVVs.
- Other aspects of the preoperative assessment are analogous to that of other lesions (VSD, tetralogy type, or transposition type), depending on the anticipated type of repair.

Double-Outlet Right Ventricle: Post-Repair

- The repair of DORV, as described here, is determined by the subtype and analogous to the repairs of the lesion with the same name.

The reader is referred to the appropriate sections in this or other chapters.

- In all cases, special attention should be paid in serial follow-up studies to the left ventricular outflow (LVO) pathway because it is at risk of obstruction (early or late).
- For the VSD type of DORV, see Chapter 5, Shunting Lesions.
- For the tetralogy type of DORV, see the section in this chapter on TOF.
- For the transposition type of DORV, ASO with VSD closure is performed; see Chapter 8, Transposition of the Great Arteries. Additional specific issues include the following:
  - For ASO with VSD closure in the setting of side-by-side GVs, a LeCompte maneuver may not be performed. Evaluate the course of the branch PAs carefully to determine whether they straddle the ascending aorta.
  - There is a much more frequent association with subaortic stenosis, AV stenosis, and arch obstruction in the transposition type of DORV than straightforward dextro-transposition of the great arteries (d-TGA).
  - After ASO, aortic outflow obstruction becomes neopulmonary outflow obstruction. Evaluate for this on serial follow-up, or if a transannular patch was performed at any time, evaluate for the secondary consequences of chronic free PI (discussed in the TOF section).
  - If subsequent reoperation for neopulmonary outflow obstruction is needed, the coronary artery pattern must be clarified to rule out a crossing coronary artery. One may not be able to determine this by echo in the postoperative state. Review the preoperative comprehensive echocardiogram or use alternate imaging modalities (angiography, computed tomography angiography, or MRI).
  - Any aortic arch repair needs to be evaluated serially. There is a particular risk of recoarctation in the first few months after initial repair. See Chapter 12, Left Heart Anomalies, section on coarctation of the aorta.
- More complex forms of DORV are likely to be managed by SV palliation; see Chapter 10, Echocardiographic Imaging of Single-Ventricle Lesions, section on surgical repair.

Truncus Arteriosus

Background
Anatomy

- Truncus arteriosus is a cardiac malformation in which a single semilunar valve and GV emerge from the heart, and the GV gives rise to the aorta and the PAs. The truncal valve typically overrides a large VSD (Fig. 7-16).
- Two classification schemes exist (Fig. 7-17):
  - Collett-Edwards types I, II, and III. This classification is more commonly used in clinical practice.
    - Type I: an main PA segment is present.
    - Type II: the branch PAs arise separately but close to each other from the posterior aspect of the truncus.
    - Type III: the branch PAs arise separately from the right and left aspects of the truncus.
  - Van Praagh types A1 to A4.
- The truncal valve is frequently abnormal.
  - The most common number of cusps is three (69%), with four the next most common (22%), followed by two (9%). One or five is rare.
  - 50% of truncal valves have some degree of insufficiency.
  - 5% to 10% of truncal valves are stenotic.
- Secundum ASD is reported in 10% to 20% of cases.
- The PDA is absent in at least 50% of cases.
- Interruption of the aortic arch is present in about 15% of cases, typically type B (between the left common carotid and left subclavian arteries).

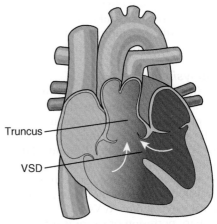

Figure 7-16. Schematic of truncus arteriosus showing a single great vessel (GV) overriding a large VSD. The GV gives rise to the aorta and PAs. Not shown here are the coronary arteries that also arise from the truncal root.

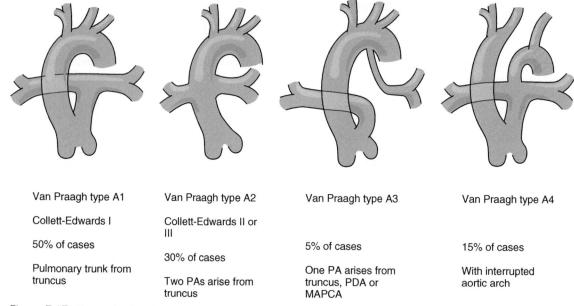

Van Praagh type A1	Van Praagh type A2	Van Praagh type A3	Van Praagh type A4
Collett-Edwards I	Collett-Edwards II or III		
50% of cases	30% of cases	5% of cases	15% of cases
Pulmonary trunk from truncus	Two PAs arise from truncus	One PA arises from truncus, PDA or MAPCA	With interrupted aortic arch

Figure 7-17. Two main classification schemes of truncus arteriosus. *(From Momma K. Tetralogy of the Fallot and truncus arteriosus. In: Crawford MH, DiMarco JP, eds.* Cardiology. *London: Mosby, 2001, Figure 3-12.)*

- The right aortic arch is present in about one third of cases.
- The main anatomic distinctions to be made on the initial echocardiogram are between truncus arteriosus and the following lesions:
  - TOF with pulmonary atresia (pulmonary atresia/VSD). Identification of the origin of at least one branch PA from the base of the truncus makes the diagnosis of truncus arteriosus.
  - Aortic atresia with VSD and normal-size LV. In this case, the obvious large GV is the PA. A tiny aortic root and ascending aorta can be identified giving rise to the coronary arteries, posterior to the pulmonary root.

Pathophysiology

- The Q_p/Q_s (the pulmonary/systemic volume flow rate) is determined by the relative systemic and pulmonary vascular resistance (PVR) and is typically large.
- Low PVR leads to high PBF and a large volume load on the ventricles.
- The ventricular volume load can be aggravated by significant regurgitation of the truncal valve and/or AVVs.
- Coronary perfusion pressure is often low due to low diastolic blood pressure and elevated ventricular end-diastolic pressure.

Overview of Echocardiographic Approach

- A segmental approach to assessing the anatomy is used (2D).
  - Establish normal atrial situs.
  - Establish normal ventricular looping.
  - A single semilunar valve and GV are identified.
- The GV gives rise to the aorta (identify coronaries) and at least one branch PA from the base of the truncus.
  - Evaluate the aortic arch carefully.
    - It can be easy to mistake a large ductus for the aortic arch in the cases of an interrupted aortic arch.
  - Evaluate arch sidedness and branching.
- Evaluate other important aspects of the pathophysiology.
  - Truncal valve function.
  - AVV function.
  - Ventricular function.

Anatomic Imaging
Acquisition

- TTE is used to establish the diagnosis in neonates.
- TEE is used pre- and postoperatively.
- Beginning from the subcostal views, evaluate the segmental anatomy.
  - Perform careful 2D sweeps in the frontal (long axis) and bicaval (sagittal) planes,

noting the morphology and relationship of structures.

- Atrial situs solitus: the IVC enters the RA, at least some PVs enter the LA. Note any ASD or PFO.
- Ventricular looping: D-looped (normal).
  - The morphologic RV is on the right, characterized by coarse trabeculations and a morphologic TV with chordal attachments to the septum.
  - The morphologic LV is on the left, characterized by a smooth septal surface and a morphologic MV with no chordal attachments to the septum.
  - A VSD is noted underneath the GV.
- A single semilunar valve and GV are identified, overriding the VS.
- Look for evidence of the branch PAs as well as coronary arteries arising from this vessel. The vessel should also continue toward the head as the ascending aorta.
- Apical views
  - The four-chamber view appears relatively normal, with perhaps some of the VSD visible.
  - With anterior angulation, the truncal valve and truncus become visible, overriding a VSD.
  - Assess the apical muscular septum for evidence of additional VSDs.
- Parasternal long axis view
  - A single semilunar valve and GV are seen, overriding a large VSD. The degree of override can vary, with some cases predominantly lying over the RV and rarely some predominantly lying over the LV. In most cases, the truncal valve is approximately centered over the VSD.
  - Note any thickening or doming of the truncal valve leaflets.
- Parasternal short axis view
  - Assess the morphology of the truncal valve. Note the number of cusps and any obvious coaptation gap (Fig. 7-18).
  - Identify coronary artery origins from the truncal root. For tips on visualizing coronary arteries, see Chapter 1, The Pediatric Transthoracic Echocardiogram.
  - With cephalad angulation, the origins of the branch PAs from the truncus should become apparent (Fig. 7-19). Note whether a main PA segment is present (type I). Optimize 2D image of branch PAs for measurement.
  - Evaluate the muscular septum for evidence of additional VSDs.
- Suprasternal notch
  - Evaluate arch sidedness and branching from the short axis view. Right aortic arch is seen

in about one third of cases (see Chapter 1, The Pediatric Transthoracic Echocardiogram, for technique).
- In the sagittal view, evaluate the aortic arch carefully for evidence of interruption.
  - Make sure that you see head and neck vessels emanating from what you think is the aortic arch; it is easy to mistake a large PDA for the transverse arch in cases of truncus arteriosus with an interrupted aortic arch.
  - Interruption of the aortic arch in truncus arteriosus typically lies between the left common carotid and left subclavian arteries (type B).
- Also from the sagittal view, evaluate for PDA. The PDA is absent in a large fraction of cases of truncus arteriosus, but not universally so. In truncus arteriosus with an interrupted aortic arch, it is important to evaluate the size and flow pattern of the duct because systemic blood flow to the lower half of the body depends on the duct.

Analysis
- Measure the size of all shunts at the atrial and ventricular levels.
- Measure the branch PAs and compare to norms (Z scores).
- Measure the PDA, if present, at its narrowest point.

Pitfalls
- When only one GV can be identified, the sonographer may jump to the conclusion that the diagnosis is truncus arteriosus.
  - However, to qualify as truncus arteriosus, the GV *must* give rise to the aorta (marked by coronary arteries) and at least one branch PA.

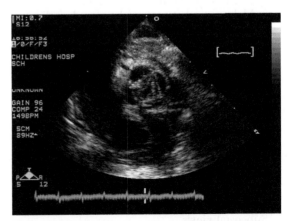

Figure 7-18. Parasternal short axis view demonstrating a quadricuspid truncal valve with markedly thickened leaflets. Note the central coaptation gap.

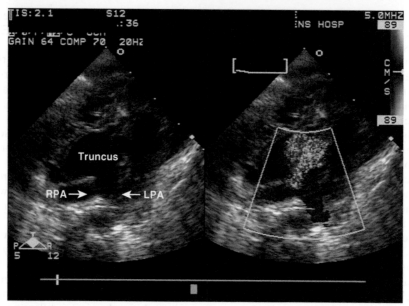

Figure 7-19. Parasternal short axis view of the truncal root showing the branch PA origins. Note the off-axis angulation, which in this case was necessary to visualize the branch PA origins well.

- In TOF with pulmonary atresia (pulmonary atresia/VSD), the single GV is the aorta (coronaries noted), but the branch PAs do not arise from the base of the truncus.
- In aortic atresia with VSD (and a normal-size LV), the single obvious GV is the main PA, but it does not give rise to the ascending aorta or coronary arteries. Rather, on close inspection, a very diminutive ascending aorta (1–2 mm in diameter) giving rise to the coronaries can be identified.
- It is easy to miss interruption of the aortic arch in truncus arteriosus by mistaking the large PDA for the transverse arch.
  - Make sure that you see head and neck vessels emanating from what you think is the aortic arch.
- Do not discontinue prostaglandin until the diagnosis of truncus arteriosus is confirmed, and the aortic arch is determined to not be interrupted.

Physiologic Data
- Doppler techniques are used to:
  - Assess size, location, and direction of shunting of ASDs and VSDs.
  - Assess truncal valve function.
  - Assess arch and, if present, ductal anatomy.
- Subcostal views
  - Perform color sweeps of the AS and VS. Be alert for any additional muscular VSDs,

which may be hard to visualize as the ventricular pressures are equal due to the large primary VSD. Determine the direction and velocity of shunting across shunts.
  - Doppler abdominal aorta. Typically, there is holodiastolic flow reversal due to diastolic flow into the branch PAs. If an interrupted aortic arch is present and there has been constriction of the PDA, poor pulsatility would be seen.
- Apical views
  - Evaluate the truncal valve for evidence of stenosis or regurgitation by color Doppler and spectral Doppler. Some flow acceleration is expected due to the large volume load across the truncal valve (Q_p + Q_s + regurgitant fraction). If the flow acceleration is laminar by PW Doppler and mild in degree, and the valve leaflets appear thin, likely no true stenosis is present.
  - Evaluate the MV and TV for evidence of regurgitation.
  - Evaluate the apical muscular septum by color Doppler for additional VSD.
- Parasternal views
  - Evaluate the truncal valve for regurgitation by color Doppler and examine mechanism.
  - Perform a short axis sweep to evaluate the muscular septum by color Doppler for any evidence of additional VSDs.

- Evaluate branch PAs by color Doppler and spectral Doppler in the short axis view. Some flow acceleration is expected, given the typically high Q_p.
- Suprasternal notch views
  - Evaluate flow in the arch by color Doppler and spectral Doppler.
  - If a PDA is present, evaluate flow pattern by color Doppler and spectral Doppler.

KEY POINTS

- A single semilunar valve and GV emerge from the heart and give rise to the aorta and the PAs. The truncal valve typically overrides a large VSD.
- Distinguish truncus arteriosus from:
  - TOF with pulmonary atresia.
  - Aortic atresia with a VSD and a normal-size LV.
- Evaluate the PA anatomy to subclassify truncus arteriosus.
- The truncal valve is frequently abnormal (50% with some degree of insufficiency, 5%–10% stenotic, 30% with an abnormal number of cusps). Truncal valve stenosis, however, will be overestimated by velocity assessment in the preoperative state when $Q_p + Q_s$ is traversing the valve.
- Evaluate the aortic arch carefully.
  - Interruption of the aortic arch is present in about 15% of cases.
  - It can be easy to miss an interruption by confusing the ductal arch for the true aortic arch.
- Other common features include right aortic arch, a secundum ASD, and absence of the PDA (in cases without interruption of the aortic arch).
- In unrepaired truncus arteriosus, the Q_p/Q_s is typically high, with significant ventricular volume load.

Truncus Arteriosus: Status Post Repair

Background

- Truncus arteriosus is repaired by closing the VSD with a patch such that the LV ejects to the aorta, removal of the PAs from the truncus, and insertion of an RV-to-PA conduit.
- If an interrupted aortic arch is present, the arch is repaired and the ductus is ligated and divided.
- Truncal valvuloplasty may be attempted if the truncal valve is significantly regurgitant. Truncal valve replacement may be required at

some point in the patient's lifetime. Generally, every effort is made to avoid truncal valve replacement in infancy.
- Conduits, especially when inserted in infants, eventually become stenotic and regurgitant.

Overview of Echocardiographic Approach

- Evaluate for residual ASD or VSD (2D, color Doppler, PW Doppler, CW Doppler).
- Right heart issues
  - RV-to-PA conduit regurgitation or stenosis (color Doppler, PW Doppler, CW Doppler).
  - Branch PA stenosis (color Doppler, PW Doppler, CW Doppler).
  - Right ventricular size and function (history of ventriculotomy, volume, and/or pressure load depending on conduit function and branch pulmonary anatomy) (2D).
- Left heart issues
  - Left ventricular outflow tract for obstruction, particularly if the truncal valve was very rightward to begin with. Uncommon in straightforward truncus repair (2D, color Doppler, PW Doppler, CW Doppler).
  - Truncal (functioning as aortic) valve function (2D, color Doppler, PW Doppler, CW Doppler).
  - Left ventricular size and function (especially in the context of truncal valve function) (2D).

Anatomic Imaging

Acquisition

- Subcostal views
  - Evaluate for residual ASD or VSD.
  - Subcostal short axis imaging can often provide good views of the RV-to-PA conduit.
- Apical views
  - Evaluate ventricular function.
  - In 5C view, evaluate LVOT and truncal (aortic) valve.
- Parasternal long axis view
  - Visualize LVOT, truncal valve leaflets, truncal root, and ascending aorta.
  - Evaluate RV and LV function.
  - Visualize RV-to-PA conduit.
- Parasternal short axis view
  - Assess truncal valve morphology; note the number of cusps and any obvious coaptation gap.
  - Assess RV-to-PA conduit and its anastomosis to the branch PAs.

- Pay attention to the motion of the conduit valve leaflets, which can become calcified and immobile over time. Optimize views of branch PAs for measurement of their size.
- Evaluate for residual ASD or VSD.
- Evaluate RV and LV size and function.
- Suprasternal notch
  - If there is a history of an interrupted aortic arch, evaluate arch repair (see Chapter 12, Left Heart Anomalies).
  - Image the branch PAs from the suprasternal notch short axis view if not well seen from the parasternal short axis view.

Analysis
- Measure any residual ASD or VSD on the 2D images from the views in which it is best seen.
- Measure branch PAs in systole from the parasternal short axis view or suprasternal notch short axis view (compare with norms by Z score).
- Evaluate parameters of LV systolic function. There may be paradoxical septal motion after VSD closure, in which case shortening fraction may not be an accurate assessment of systolic function.
- Measure truncal (aortic) root and the ascending aorta in systole on the parasternal long axis views, which are frequently enlarged. Compare with norms and track over time.

Physiologic Data
- Doppler techniques are used to:
  - Assess size, location, and direction of shunting of residual ASD and VSD.
  - Assess truncal valve function.
  - Assess AVV function.
  - Assess arch after repair.

Acquisition
- Subcostal views
  - Perform color Doppler sweeps to identify any residual ASD or VSD. If present, assess direction of shunting. Assess velocity of shunting across any residual VSD.
  - Doppler abdominal aorta to assess pulsatility after arch repair.
- Apical views
  - Assess MV and TV function. Obtain RV pressure estimate if possible.
  - Assess LVOT.

- Assess truncal valve function, quantify regurgitation and/or stenosis as appropriate.
- Parasternal views
  - Assess truncal valve regurgitation.
  - Assess for residual VSD or additional VSD by color Doppler; obtain peak velocity if present.
  - Assess RV-to-PA conduit for stenosis and regurgitation by color Doppler and spectral Doppler. Obtain mean gradient if conduit stenosis is present.
  - Evaluate branch PAs for stenosis by color Doppler and spectral Doppler.
  - Note that multiple levels or long segment narrowing in the pathway from the RV to the PAs may be present. Thus, careful PW Doppler analysis throughout this pathway must be performed to identify sites of obstruction. Mean gradient through the conduit may be more predictive of true peak-to-peak conduit gradient measured invasively.
- Suprasternal notch views
  - If there is a history of interrupted aortic arch repair, assess the aortic arch with color Doppler and spectral Doppler as described in Chapter 12, Left Heart Anomalies.

Analysis
- Measure peak TR velocity to estimate RV pressure.
- Measure peak and mean conduit gradient and branch PA velocities.
- Quantify truncal (aortic) regurgitation as appropriate.
- Calculate arch gradient if present (may need to correct for V_1).

Alternate Approaches
- MRI offers superior visualization of the conduit and branch PAs in postoperative patients with poor echocardiographic windows. In addition, RV size and function, conduit regurgitant fraction, and truncal valve regurgitant fraction can be calculated.
- Cardiac catheterization can provide accurate assessment of pressure gradients across the various levels of potential RVOTO as well as direct measurement of filling pressures. In addition, the option for intervention is available.
- Nuclear medicine lung perfusion scan quantifies relative pulmonary perfusion to the two lungs and can be used to help decide whether cardiac catheterization for branch PA dilation is warranted.

KEY POINTS

- Repair entails patch closure of the VSD, removal of the PAs from the truncus, and insertion of an RV-to-PA conduit. The arch is repaired if interrupted.
- Postoperatively, evaluate for residual ASD or VSD, conduit function, and branch PA stenosis. Reassess truncal valve function; the velocity across the valve will likely have decreased compared with preoperatively due to a reduction in the volume load across the valve.
- On long-term follow-up, serial evaluation of RV size and function, conduit function, branch PA stenosis, truncal (aortic) valve function, and truncal (aortic) root dimensions is performed.
- If the aortic arch was repaired, it should be assessed serially on long-term follow-up.

Suggested Reading

1. Anderson RH, Weinberg PM. The clinical anatomy of tetralogy of Fallot. *Cardiol Young.* 2005;15(Suppl 1):38-47.
2. Hagler DJ. Double-outlet right and left ventricles. In: Eidem BW, Cetta F, O'Leary PW, eds. *Echocardiography in Pediatric and Adult Congenital Heart Disease.* Philadelphia: Lippincott Williams & Wilkins; 2010.
3. Jones FD, Fenstermaker B, Kovalchin JP. Truncus arteriosus. In: Eidem BW, Cetta F, O'Leary PW, eds. *Echocardiography in Pediatric and Adult Congenital Heart Disease.* Philadelphia: Lippincott Williams & Wilkins; 2010.
4. Lewin MB, Salerno JC. Truncus arteriosus. In: Lai WW, Mertens LL, Cohen MS, Geva T, eds. *Echocardiography in Pediatric and Congenital Heart Disease.* Hoboken, NJ: Wiley-Blackwell; 2009.
5. Lopez L. Double-outlet ventricle. In: Lai WW, Mertens LL, Cohen MS, Geva T, eds. *Echocardiography in Pediatric and Congenital Heart Disease.* Hoboken, NJ: Wiley-Blackwell; 2009.
6. Miller-Hance WC, Silverman NH. Transesophageal echocardiography in congenital heart disease with focus on the adult. *Cardiol Clin.* 2000;18(4):861-892.
7. Srivastava S, Parness IA. Tetralogy of Fallot. In: Lai WW, Mertens LL, Cohen MS, Geva T, eds. *Echocardiography in Pediatric and Congenital Heart Disease.* Hoboken, NJ: Wiley-Blackwell; 2009.
8. Mahle WT, Martinez R, Silverman N, Cohen MS, Anderson RH. Anatomy, echocardiography, and surgical approach to double outlet right ventricle. *Cardiol Young.* 2008;18(Suppl 3):39-51.
9. Vyas H, Eidem BW. Tetralogy of Fallot. In: Eidem BW, Cetta F, O'Leary PW, eds. *Echocardiography in Pediatric and Adult Congenital Heart Disease.* Philadelphia: Lippincott Williams & Wilkins; 2010.

Transposition of the Great Arteries

8

Amy H. Schultz

d-TGA: Preoperative Imaging

Background
- In this lesion, the atria and ventricles are aligned normally, but the great arteries are transposed, with the aorta (Ao) arising from the right ventricle (RV) and the pulmonary artery (PA) arising from the left ventricle (LV) (Fig. 8-1).
- The aortic valve (AV) is typically anterior and rightward of the pulmonary valve (pulmV).
- Deoxygenated systemic venous blood circulates to the right atrium (RA) to the RV to the aorta and thus back to the body.
- Oxygenated pulmonary venous blood circulates to the left atrium (LA) to the LV to the PA and thus back to the lungs.
- Mixing between the two circuits is required to sustain life. This can occur via an atrial septal defect (ASD), ventricular septal defect (VSD), or patent ductus arteriosus (PDA).
- Mixing is generally most effective and reliable at the atrial level. Thus, assessment of the size of the ASD is key for acute management.
- Major associated lesions are
  - Dextro transposition of the great arteries (d-TGA) with VSD.
  - d-TGA with VSD and pulmonary stenosis (PS) (typically at both the valvar and subvalvar levels).

Overview of Echocardiographic Approach
- Identify the segmental anatomy (two dimensional [2D]).
  - Normal atrial situs.
  - Normal ventricular looping.
  - d-TGA
    - The aorta arises from the RV.
    - The PA arises from the LV.
  - The segmental anatomy can be abbreviated {S,D,D}.
- Presence or absence and size of shunts at the atrial, ventricular, and ductal levels (2D, color Doppler).

- Relative size, morphology, and function of the AV and pulmV (2D, color Doppler, pulsed wave [PW] Doppler, continuous wave [CW] Doppler).
- Coronary artery anatomy (2D, color Doppler).
- Transthoracic echocardiography (TTE) is essentially always the first study in neonates.

Anatomic Imaging
Acquisition
- Subcostal frontal (long axis [LAX]) sweep, posterior to anterior.
  - Establish normal visceroatrial situs: visualize the inferior vena cava within the liver on the right, connecting to the right-sided atrium. The left-sided atrium should have some pulmonary veins (PVs) visible by 2D imaging.
  - Establish normal atrioventricular alignments: two separate atrioventricular valves (AVVs) are visualized. Two ventricles of good size are visualized.
  - Demonstrate transposed ventriculoarterial connections.
    - The more posterior great vessel (GV) arising from the LV bifurcates, identifying it as the PA (Fig. 8-2A).
    - The more anterior GV arising from the RV does not bifurcate and is thus the aorta; coronary artery origins may be seen from it.
    - Note also that the GVs do not cross each other (as is the case in normally related GVs).
  - Take note as to whether a coronary artery is seen running posterior to the pulmonary root as you sweep anterior from the mitral valve (MV) to the pulmV. This will be useful information to integrate with later parasternal short axis imaging of the coronary arteries.
- Subcostal short axis sweep, base to apex.
  - Atrial morphology is again noted to be normal with the systemic veins entering

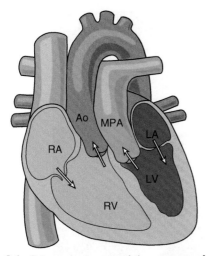

Figure 8-1. Schematic diagram of the anatomy of dextro transposition of the great arteries (d-TGA). Note that the systemic venous return (blue) and pulmonary venous return (red) circulate separately unless a shunt at the atrial, ventricular, and/or ductal level permits mixing between the two circuits.

the RA and at least some PVs visualized entering the LA. Assess the size of interatrial communication (patent foramen ovale [PFO] or ASD).

- Ventricular morphology is examined and is consistent with normal ventricular looping. The left-sided ventricle has a smooth septal surface and AVV morphology consistent with an MV (no chordal attachments to the septum). The right-sided ventricle is trabeculated, with chordal attachments of the AVV to the septum. Assess for VSD (size, location).
- GVs are noted to be transposed with the bifurcating PA arising posteriorly from the LV and the aorta arising anteriorly from the RV. Their parallel relationship is well seen (see Fig. 8-2B).
- Apical views
  - Four chambers, of proportionate size, are seen. Confirm that the ventricular morphology appears usual (right-sided ventricle with moderator band, left-sided ventricle with smooth septal surface).
  - Note any evidence of VSD or outflow tract obstruction.
  - With anterior angulation, the bifurcating PA is seen arising from the LV. If present, a retropulmonary coronary artery may be seen by angling anteriorly from the MV to the pulmV.
  - With further anterior angulation, the aorta may be seen arising from the LV.

- Parasternal long axis view
  - Parallel outflow tracts and proximal GVs are seen (Fig. 8-3).
  - Optimize image of each semilunar valve for measurement of annulus diameter.
  - There is mitral-pulmonary fibrous continuity. If not present, consider the diagnosis of double-outlet RV.
  - Note any evidence of VSD and/or outflow tract obstruction.
- Parasternal short axis view
  - Note the relative orientation of the semilunar valves (Fig. 8-4). Typically, the AV is anterior and rightward of the pulmV, but can range from directly anterior to rightward and side by side.
  - Note morphology of the semilunar valves. The intercoronary commissure of the AV should align with a commissure of the pulmV. If the commissures are not aligned, coronary transfer may be more difficult.
  - Note any evidence of VSD. If one VSD is present, be sure to examine the remainder of the muscular septum for additional defects.
  - Evaluate coronary artery anatomy: origins from the sinuses and proximal courses must be clearly visualized.
    - Many variants are known, although the two most common patterns are present in about 80% of cases.
    - Complex coronary artery patterns may substantially increase the risk of the arterial switch operation (ASO). Rarely, a complex coronary artery pattern precludes ASO.
    - There are two major conventions for nomenclature, the Leiden convention (Fig. 8-5 and Table 8-1) and the descriptive approach advocated by cardiologists at Children's Hospital Boston (Fig. 8-6).
    - Typically, the coronary arteries arise from the two sinuses of the AV that are adjacent to or "face" the sinuses of the pulmV (see Fig. 8-4).
    - In the most common pattern (1L, Cx; 2R) or "usual," the left coronary artery (LCA) arises from the leftward facing sinus and gives rise to the anterior descending artery and circumflex artery (Cx) (Fig. 8-7). The right coronary artery (RCA) arises from the rightward facing sinus.
    - In the second most common pattern (1L; 2R, Cx) or "circumflex from RCA," the leftward facing sinus gives rise solely to

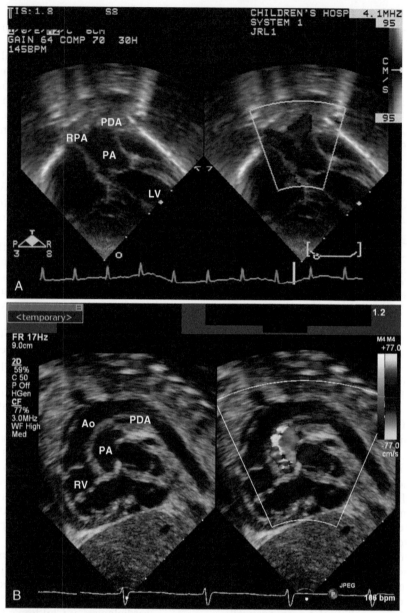

Figure 8-2. **A,** This subcostal frontal image shows the branching pulmonary artery (PA) arising from the left ventricle (LV). The color Doppler panel shows flow into the PA (red), consistent with a patent ductus arteriosus (PDA). The left PA is not seen in this view. **B,** This subcostal sagittal view shows the entire course of the aorta (Ao), arising anteriorly from the right ventricle (RV). The PA parallels the aorta posteriorly. The ductus is patent with color Doppler seen from the aorta to the PA.

the anterior descending, whereas the RCA, arising from rightward facing sinus, also gives rise to the Cx. The circumflex passes posterior to the pulmonary root to reach the left atrioventricular groove; this segment can often be visualized from the subcostal or apical four-chamber (4C) views (Fig. 8-8).

- Visualization of the coronary arteries is facilitated by decreasing the dynamic

range and careful adjustment of focal zone and zoom features.
- Be alert for any evidence of intramural coronary artery (passing between the two GVs), which is rare, but can significantly complicate an ASO (Fig. 8-9). A "double border" appearance of the posterior aortic root is noted when a coronary artery passes between the aortic and pulmonary roots.

Transposition of the Great Arteries

TABLE 8-1	ABBREVIATION CONVENTION USED IN THE LEIDEN CONVENTION FOR DESCRIBING CORONARY ARTERY ANATOMY

Symbols used are as follows:

1 = sinus 1

2 = sinus 2

R = right coronary artery

L = left anterior descending coronary artery; also designated by some authors AD, as it may not arise from the left.

Cx = circumflex coronary artery

Comma = major branches originate from a common vessel

Semicolon = major branches originate separately

Supplemental terms may be used to describe epicardial course and unusual origins.

The series of assigned symbols for any given anatomy are enclosed in parentheses. For example: "normal" or "usual" coronary arteries for d-TGA are designated (1L, Cx; 2R), meaning the left anterior descending and circumflex originate from a common vessel from sinus 1, whereas the right coronary artery arises separately from sinus 2.

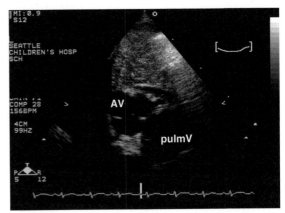

Figure 8-4. Parasternal short axis (SAX) view showing the orientation of semilunar valves. In this case, the aortic valve (AV) is anterior and rightward, which is typical. The origins of the right and left coronary arteries are seen from the two sinuses "facing" the pulmV, although the origin of the circumflex coronary artery (Cx) is not demonstrated here.

- Short axis suprasternal notch views can sometimes be used to supplement coronary artery imaging, if the patient is positioned with a shoulder roll and significant neck extension.
- Transesophageal echocardiography (TEE)
  - Given typically excellent transthoracic windows in neonates, TEE is essentially never used for initial diagnosis of d-TGA. TTE is superior for visualization of the GVs and PDA, which are key in this diagnosis.
  - Depending on institutional practice, a preoperative TEE may be performed in the operating room. See Chapter 4, Intra-operative Transesophageal Echo-cardiography, for discussion.
  - Three-dimensional (3D) imaging generally adds little information to the study, unless a complex muscular VSD is present, in which case 3D imaging can be used to evaluate its size and location.

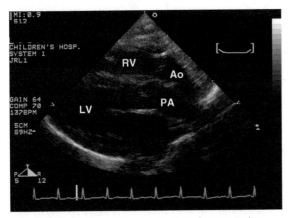

Figure 8-3. Parasternal long axis view demonstrating the parallel great vessels characteristic of d-TGA. There is fibrous continuity between the mitral valve and pulmonary valve.

- Suprasternal notch views
  - The usual assessment of arch sidedness and branching is performed. A right aortic arch is uncommon in d-TGA.
  - Coarctation is rare unless evidence of right ventricular outflow tract (RVOT) (subaortic) obstruction (RVOTO) is present.
  - A PDA is best seen in d-TGA in the sagittal view of the arch due to the parallel orientation of the GVs (Fig. 8-10). The PDA should be assessed for size, direction of shunting, and gradient.

Analysis

- Quantitative analysis consists of measuring sizes of shunts and semilunar valves.
- Atrial shunts (ASD or PFO) should be measured from the subcostal long axis or short axis views.
- VSDs should be measured in whichever view they are seen best, ideally in two orthogonal planes.
- The PDA should be measured at its narrowest point, in the suprasternal notch sagittal view of the arch.
- The pulmV and AV are measured from the parasternal long axis view in systole; compare with norms for body surface area (Z scores).

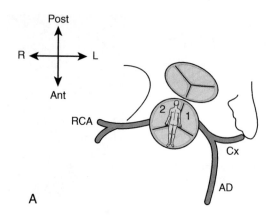

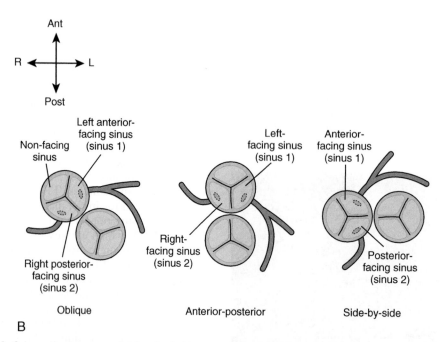

Figure 8-5. **A,** Schematic diagram explaining the Leiden convention for numbering the sinuses of the AV to describe coronary artery anatomy. From the perspective of standing in the noncoronary sinus, looking from the AV toward the PA, the sinus on the right-hand side is 1 and that on the left-hand side is 2. Note that this convention is easily applied by the surgeon standing on the right-hand side of the patient. **B,** Schematic with numbering in echo view. The convention of diagnostic image display is such that cranial is behind the screen, and thus it can become confusing trying to envision oneself standing in the noncoronary sinus. It is easier to remember that sinus 1 is the more leftward and/or anterior facing sinus (depending on the relative orientation of the great vessels) and sinus 2 is the more rightward and posterior sinus. This figure shows the numbering of the sinuses from the parasternal short axis view of the two semilunar valves. RCA, right coronary artery; Cx, circumflex coronary artery; AD, anterior descending artery.

Pitfalls
- The coronary arteries are the most difficult aspect of d-TGA to image.
- The most common pitfall is identifying an RCA and LCA from the two facing sinuses and assuming that the coronary pattern is (1L, Cx; 2R) or "usual," when in fact the Cx has not been imaged. The second most common pattern, (1L; 2R, Cx) or "circumflex from RCA," has a retropulmonary Cx, which can generally be well imaged from the subcostal long axis or the apical view. A slow, careful sweep in one of these views from the plane of the MV to the plane of the pulmV should identify this structure. However, the clinical consequence of this mistake is generally not important because both of the two most common patterns are readily amenable to ASO.
- Failure to identify a more complex coronary artery pattern, in particular, one involving an

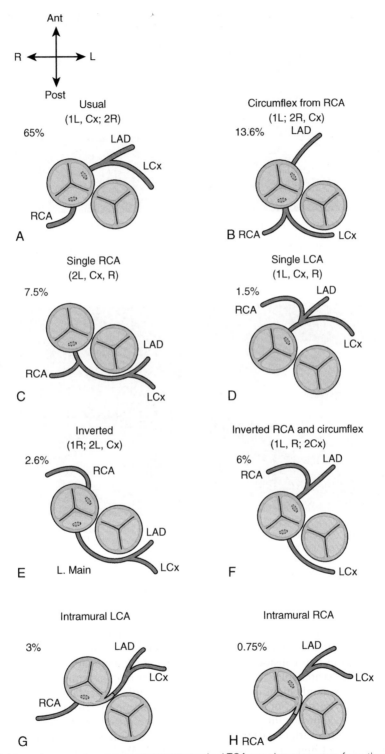

Figure 8-6. The eight most common coronary artery patterns in d-TGA are shown as seen from the parasternal short axis echocardiographic view. The frequency of occurrence is shown in the corner of each panel. The Leiden convention symbols and the eponym assigned by the Boston convention are shown in each panel. *(Adapted from Figure 24.5 in Mertens LL, Vogt MO, Marek J, Cohen MS. Transposition of the great arteries. In: Lai WW, Mertens LL, Cohen MS, Geva T, eds.* Echocardiography in Pediatric and Congenital Heart Disease, *Hoboken, NJ: Wiley-Blackwell; 2009.)*

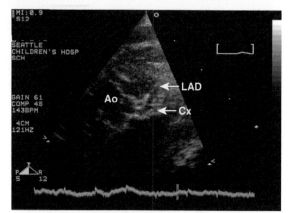

Figure 8-7. The left main coronary artery and its bifurcation into the anterior descending artery and Cx are shown in this modified parasternal short axis view. Often some off-axis angulation is needed to demonstrate the course and bifurcation of the coronary arteries.

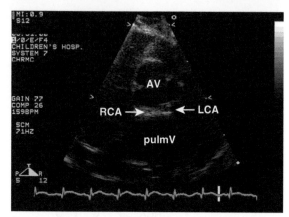

Figure 8-9. Intramural coronary artery in d-TGA: this parasternal short axis view shows the RCA and left coronary artery (LCA) running between the AV and pulmV, consistent with an intramural course. Both coronary arteries originated high and close together, adjacent to the commissure that faced the pulmV.

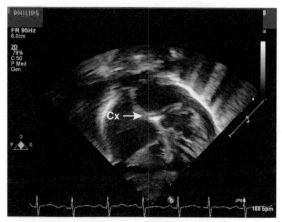

Figure 8-8. As demonstrated in Figure 8-6, when the Cx arises from the RCA (1L; 2R, Cx, or Cx from right coronary artery [RCA]), it reaches the left atrioventricular groove by a retropulmonary course. This may be difficult to see from the parasternal short axis view, but is usually readily evident from the subcostal frontal (shown here) or apical view.

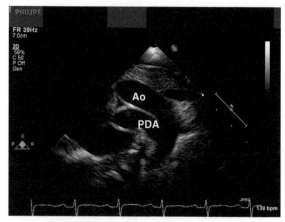

Figure 8-10. Suprasternal sagittal two-dimensional (2D) image showing the PDA arising from the aorta in d-TGA.

intramural coronary artery, will result in inaccurate counseling as to the risk of the operation. Many surgeons now consider all coronary patterns to be "switchable," but the risk of the operation is certainly higher with a complex coronary artery pattern. Some surgeons will alter their operative approach due to an extremely complex coronary artery pattern.

- Also note any evidence of high or juxtacommissural origin.
- Avoid these pitfalls by careful 2D imaging with optimization of focal zone, zoom, and dynamic range settings with confirmation of structures believed to be coronary arteries with color flow imaging. Follow-up imaging may be needed if the pattern is not

determined on the first study. Inspect the area between the two semilunar valves carefully for evidence of a "double border" of the posterior aortic root, which actually represents the coronary passing between the aortic and pulmonary roots. Keep an open mind as to what the coronary artery pattern might be rather than assuming it to be "usual."

- Multiple muscular VSDs, which occur uncommonly with d-TGA, can be easy to miss in the presence of equal ventricular pressures due to either a large primary VSD or a large PDA. Without a pressure gradient across the ventricular septum (VS), color Doppler across such a defect will not produce an aliased jet. Careful inspection of 2D sweeps of the muscular septum from the subcostal short axis, apical, and parasternal short axis views can identify muscular defects, which can then be confirmed by color Doppler imaging.

Physiologic Data
Acquisition
- Subcostal views
  - Perform frontal or short axis color Doppler sweeps of the atrial septum to identify shunts. The mean gradient across the atrial septum is determined by spectral Doppler.
  - Short axis color Doppler sweeps of the VS are used to identify any VSD present and determine direction of shunting. Carefully assess any area that the 2D imaging suggests may have a defect (see Pitfalls). Shunting will not be aliased if ventricular pressures are equal due to a large VSD or PDA.
  - Acquire peak velocity/peak instantaneous pressure gradient across any VSD in the view that most aligns the Doppler angle with the jet.
  - RVOT and left ventricular outflow tract (LVOT) and the semilunar valves may be evaluated for evidence of stenosis or regurgitation by color and spectral Doppler from the subcostal views.
- Apical views
  - Assess the apical muscular septum by color Doppler for evidence of VSD.
  - Assess the RVOT, LVOT, and semilunar valve function by color Doppler and spectral Doppler.
- Parasternal short axis view
  - Color sweep of the VS is used to identify any VSD present and determine the direction of shunting. Carefully assess any area that the 2D imaging suggests may have a defect (see Pitfalls). Shunting will not be aliased if ventricular pressures are equal due to a large VSD or PDA.
  - Acquire peak velocity/peak instantaneous pressure gradient across any VSD in the view that most aligns the Doppler angle with the jet.
  - Use color Doppler to confirm the presence and direction of blood flow in the coronary arteries (Fig. 8-11).
- Suprasternal notch view
  - Use color Doppler and PW Doppler to determine direction of shunting in the PDA. Use CW Doppler to determine peak velocity and peak instantaneous pressure gradient (PIPG) across the PDA.

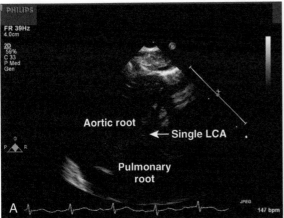

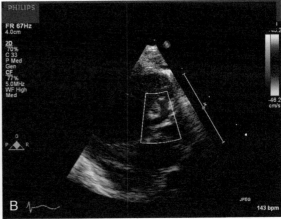

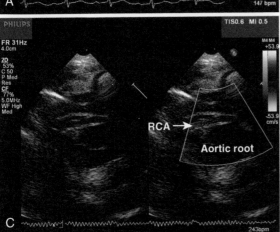

Figure 8-11. Single LCA (1L, R, Cx). **A,** A single LCA seen from the parasternal short axis view with 2D imaging. **B,** Color imaging of the single LCA. **C,** 2D and color Doppler imaging showing the RCA branch coursing anterior to the aortic root.

- Assess the flow in the aortic arch carefully by color Doppler and spectral Doppler if there is evidence of RVOTO.

Pitfalls
- Color Doppler in a PDA is frequently interpreted as being left to right when it is in fact bidirectional because the eye tends to focus on the red jet in diastole. Use of PW Doppler in the PDA easily identifies the directionality of shunting.

Alternate Approaches
- If TTE is unable to define the coronary artery pattern, cardiac catheterization is recommended.

KEY POINTS

- Establish the diagnosis of d-TGA by demonstrating the segmental anatomy: normal atrial situs, normal ventricular looping, and d-TGA.
- Mixing between the systemic and pulmonary circuits is required to sustain life. This can occur via an ASD, VSD, or PDA, but is most effective at the atrial level.
- Thus, assessment of the size of the ASD is key for acute management.
- Major associated lesions are VSDs and PS.
- Coronary artery anatomy can be highly variable and can influence surgical management, although the two most common patterns account for 83% of cases of d-TGA.
- Intramural coronary arteries are most problematic and should not be missed.

Transposition of the Great Arteries: Status Post Arterial Switch Operation

Background
- The ASO became the standard operative approach for management of d-TGA in the late 1980s.
- In this operation:
  - The great arteries are transected above the sinotubular junctions.
  - The coronary arteries are transferred from the native aortic root to the "neo-aortic" (native pulmonary) root.
  - The ascending aorta is anastomosed to the neo-aortic (native pulmonary) root.
  - The branch PAs are brought anterior to the ascending aorta (LeCompte maneuver).
  - The main PA (MPA) is anastomosed to the neo-pulmonary (native aortic) root.

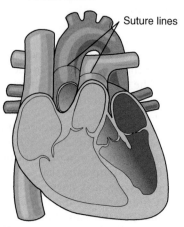

Arterial switch

Suture lines

Figure 8-12. Schematic depicting the anatomy of d-TGA after arterial switch operation (ASO). Note the suture lines in each GV.

- Any associated ASD or VSD is closed.
- The resulting anatomy is depicted in Figure 8-12.

Overview of Echocardiographic Approach
- Evaluate for complications related to the repair.
  - Residual ASD or VSD (2D, color Doppler, PW Doppler, CW Doppler).
  - Supravalvar PS at the anastomosis (color Doppler, PW Doppler, CW Doppler).
  - Branch PA stenosis due to the branch PAs being stretched across the ascending aorta (color Doppler, PW Doppler, CW Doppler).
  - Supravalvar aortic stenosis at the anastomosis (color Doppler, PW Doppler, CW Doppler).
  - Coronary artery patency and secondary effects of coronary artery occlusion (regional wall motion abnormalities [RWMAs]) (2D).
- In addition, the abnormal natural history of the native pulmV and root functioning as the systemic outflow can result in:
  - Neo-AV regurgitation (color Doppler).
  - Neo-aortic root dilation (2D).
- TTE is the standard modality for assessment. TEE may be used in the case of poor transthoracic windows or pre- and postoperatively.

Anatomic Imaging
Acquisition
- Subcostal views
  - Assess for residual ASD or VSD.
  - In addition, in patients with good windows, subcostal short axis imaging provides

excellent views of the RVOT and supravalvar pulmonary region.
- Apical views
  - Assess the regional wall motion and evidence of supravalvar aortic stenosis in the five-chamber (5C) view.
- Parasternal views
  - Long axis view: visualize neo-AV and root; neo-pulmV and root; supravalvar aortic and pulmonary anastomoses; assess regional wall motion.
  - Short axis view: assess for residual ASD or VSDs; assess regional wall motion; evaluate proximal branch PAs, which now straddle the ascending aorta (may be better seen in the suprasternal notch view). If the windows are good, the reimplanted coronary arteries may be imaged, typically arising from the two sinuses of the neo-AV that "face" the neo-pulmV (native aortic).
- Suprasternal notch views
  - Short axis view: visualize the branch PAs straddling the ascending aorta (Fig. 8-13).
  - Sagittal view of the arch: evaluate supravalvar aortic anastomosis.
- TEE: intraoperative TEE is often used to assess the repair. In patients with poor transthoracic windows, TEE can be used for later follow-up as well.
  - Assess for evidence of residual ASD or VSD (use two views).
  - Assess the regional wall motion from standard views given coronary transfer. Keep in mind original coronary artery pattern.
  - The reimplanted coronary artery buttons can be visualized in the short axis view of the neo-AV.

- Assess the supravalvar aortic and pulmonary anastomoses in long axis mid-esophageal views (generally between 90 and 120 degrees).
- Visualize the branch PAs straddling the ascending aorta. This can generally be done from the midesophageal (ME) long axis view of the RVOT, withdrawing slightly and then rotating right and left to see the respective branch PAs and also by withdrawing from the short axis view of the neo-AV.
- 3D imaging: generally not a standard part of a routine evaluation, but could be used to further assess the neo-AV and root or left ventricular (LV) systolic function.

Analysis
- Measure any residual ASD or VSD noted on 2D imaging in whichever view it is best visualized, ideally two orthogonal planes.
- Measure neo-aortic root in the parasternal long axis view. Measure supravalvar aortic and pulmonary anastomoses in the parasternal long axis view if any concern for narrowing. Pediatric norms for these measurements are taken in systole (valve maximally open).
- Measure LV chamber dimensions (LV end-diastolic dimension, LV end-systolic dimension) and parameters of LV systolic function (ejection fraction [EF], shortening fraction).

Pitfalls
- Branch PAs can be difficult to visualize. Try the suprasternal notch view in addition to the parasternal short axis view.

Physiologic Data
Acquisition
- Subcostal views
  - Use color Doppler to assess for residual ASDs or VSDs. Obtain peak velocity/PIPG across any residual VSD.
  - Subcostal short axis views of the RVOT, neo-pulmV, and supravalvar pulmonary region can be very useful in identifying and localizing obstruction. Use color Doppler to screen for aliasing of flow or significant regurgitation. Use PW Doppler to "march" through these levels of pulmonary outflow to identify the site of flow acceleration, most commonly in the supravalvar pulmonary region at the anastomosis. Use CW Doppler to identify the highest velocity, once the site of flow acceleration has been identified.

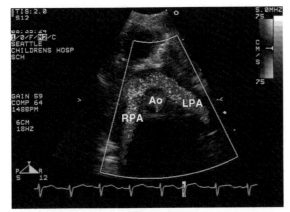

Figure 8-13. LeCompte maneuver: the branch PAs are seen straddling the ascending aorta from this suprasternal notch image.

- The LVOT, neo-AV, and supravalvar aortic region can be similarly evaluated from the subcostal views, but supravalvar aortic stenosis is less common than supravalvar PS.
- Apical views
  - Assess for tricuspid regurgitation (TR) or mitral regurgitation (MR) with color Doppler; further quantify as appropriate.
  - Assess the LVOT, neo-AV, and supravalvar aortic region in the 5C view, using color Doppler to screen for aliasing of flow or significant regurgitation. Use PW Doppler to "march" through these levels of outflow to identify the site of acceleration. Use CW Doppler to identify the highest velocity.
- Parasternal views
  - Assess the RVOT, neo-pulmV, supravalvar pulmonary region, and branch PAs with a combination of color Doppler, PW Doppler, and CW Doppler as above to identify any obstruction or significant valve regurgitation.
  - Perform a short axis color Doppler sweep to assess for residual ASD or VSD. Obtain peak velocity/PIPG across any residual VSD.
- Suprasternal notch view
  - Assess branch PAs with color Doppler (see Fig. 8-13), PW Doppler, and CW Doppler for degree of stenosis.

Alternate Approaches
- Magnetic resonance imaging (MRI) may be used to evaluate aspects of the anatomy, particularly branch PAs, if windows are poor.
- Cardiac catheterization and angiography can be used to evaluate coronary artery patency as well as severity of obstruction to RV or LV outflow.
- Nuclear medicine pulmonary perfusion scans can be used to quantify the percentage of blood flow to each lung, in the setting of suspected asymmetric branch PA stenosis.

KEY POINTS

- Understand how the operation is performed (see text) to guide the postoperative study.
- The most notable difference from normal anatomy is that the branch PAs are translocated anterior to the ascending aorta (LeCompte maneuver).
- Assess for major complications related to the repair, including residual shunts, supravalvar pulmonary or aortic stenosis, branch PA stenosis, and coronary stenosis or occlusion.
- Evaluate the abnormal natural history of the native pulmV and root in the systemic circulation: neo-AV regurgitation and neo-aortic root dilation.

Transposition of the Great Arteries: Status Post Atrial Switch Operation (Senning/Mustard)

Background

- The Senning and Mustard operations baffle systemic and pulmonary venous return within the atria such that the systemic venous return is directed to the left-sided tricuspid valve (TV) and RV. Pulmonary venous return is directed to the right-sided MV and LV (Fig. 8-14).
- The correction is physiologic, not anatomic.
- The RV remains the systemic ventricle.
- In the Mustard operation, the atrial septum is excised and the baffle is constructed with other tissue, typically pericardium.
- In the Senning operation, atrial septal and free wall flaps are used to construct the baffle.

Overview of Echocardiographic Approach

- Evaluate for complications related to the repair.
  - Residual shunts: baffle leaks or residual VSD (2D, color Doppler, PW Doppler, CW Doppler).
  - SVC or IVC stenosis or occlusion (contrast, color Doppler, PW Doppler, CW Doppler).
  - Baffle stenosis (color Doppler, PW Doppler, CW Doppler).
- In addition, the abnormal natural history of the right ventricle (RV) functioning in the systemic circulation can result in:
  - TR (color Doppler).
  - RV dysfunction (2D).

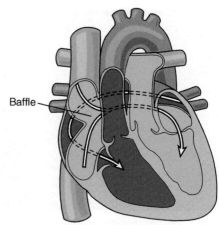

Intra-atrial baffle (Mustard or Senning procedure)

Baffle

Figure 8-14. Schematic depicting the anatomy of d-TGA after atrial switch operation (Mustard or Senning).

- Left ventricular outflow tract obstruction (LVOTO) due to compression (2D, color Doppler, PW Doppler, CW Doppler).
- TTE is the standard modality for assessment. TEE may be used in the case of poor transthoracic windows or pre- and postoperatively.

Anatomic Imaging
Acquisition
- Subcostal view
  - Given the predominantly adult age of this patient population, windows may be limited. However, in cases with good windows, the SVC and IVC and their entry into the baffle should be imaged to the full extent possible.
- Apical 4C view
  - Assess RV and LV size and function.
  - Focus on the atria and use careful posterior and anterior angulation to demonstrate the systemic venous baffle (the portion in the LA is best seen) and the course of the PVs to the TV, respectively (Figs. 8-15 and 8-16).
- Parasternal views
  - Long axis
    - Compression of the LV outflow by the enlarged RV may be seen.
    - The SVC is seen along its course to the MV by angling somewhat toward the RV inflow.

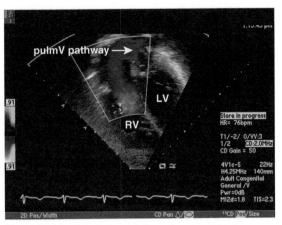

Figure 8-16. Apical view of the pulmonary venous pathway coursing toward the pulmV after a Mustard operation.

- Short axis
  - Assess RV and LV size and function.
  - Evaluate IVC limb of the baffle (Fig. 8-17).
  - Evaluate pulmonary venous pathway.
- Suprasternal notch view
  - Visualize SVC.
  - If occlusion of the SVC is suspected, use saline solution contrast injection in an upper extremity while imaging the IVC and SVC in turn to evaluate.
  - IVC complications are less common, but an analogous technique can be used.
  - Saline solution contrast injections can also be used to identify baffle leaks.

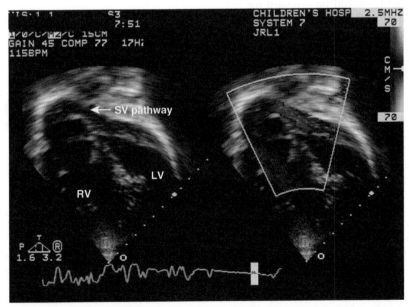

Figure 8-15. Apical view of the systemic venous pathway coursing toward the MV after a Mustard operation.

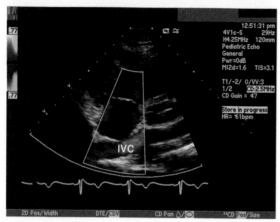

Figure 8-17. Parasternal short axis view demonstrating the course of the inferior vena cava to the MV after a Mustard operation.

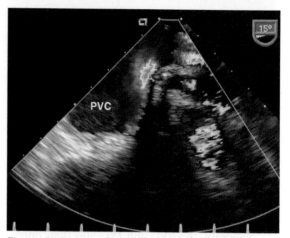

Figure 8-18. Transesophageal echocardiography with color flow Doppler demonstrates unobstructed flow through the pulmonary venous pathway toward the tricuspid valve.

- TEE is particularly useful in better assessing atrial anatomy. It may also be used to guide procedures such as stenting of stenosis or baffle leak closure.
  - Assess for baffle leak along the entirety of the interatrial baffle, with both 2D and color Doppler.
  - Stenosis of the SVC or IVC limb may be seen, particularly if pacemaker or implantable cardioverter-defibrillator leads traverse the SVC limb.
  - The pulmonary venous pathway may be assessed for obstruction (Fig. 8-18).
  - For patients with atrial arrhythmias requiring TEE cardioversion, both atria and the baffle should be assessed for thrombus or baffle leak that would serve as a source of potential paradoxical emboli.
  - The mechanism of TR and pulmonary or subpulmonary stenosis and location of residual VSD may all be identified.
- 3D imaging
  - With appropriate applications, 3D imaging may develop a role in quantification of systemic RV function.
  - 3D imaging could be used by a skilled operator to assess baffle anatomy.

Analysis
- Measure any residual VSD or baffle leak in whichever view it is best seen (ideally two orthogonal views).
- Although RV EF and other standard measures of systolic function are not as accurate in the assessment of the LV, area of fractional shortening, RV end-diastolic

diameter and end-systolic dimension, and RV EF may be useful measures, particularly when comparing with previous studies in the same patient.

Pitfalls
- The main challenge is usually visualization of complex baffle anatomy in patients with poor windows due to older age and history of cardiac surgery.
- Learn to visualize the baffles from as many windows as possible so that the sonographer can take advantage of whatever window is best in an individual patient.

Physiologic Data
Acquisition
- Subcostal view
  - Assess the SVC and IVC with color Doppler and spectral Doppler.
  - Follow the cavae through the baffle to the MV as permitted by the windows.
  - Identify any aliasing or flow acceleration suggestive of stenosis.
  - PW Doppler is best for localizing obstruction.
- Apical views
  - Assess TR and MR; quantify as appropriate.
  - Angle posteriorly to assess the systemic venous baffle for evidence of leak or obstruction by color Doppler (see Fig. 8-15). PW Doppler throughout course of cavae to MV to identify obstruction.
  - Angle anteriorly to visualize course of PVs to TV. Use color Doppler and PW Doppler to identify any obstruction (see Fig. 8-16).

- Apical 5C: assess for LVOTO with color Doppler and spectral Doppler.
- Parasternal views
  - Long axis
    - Assess for MR and TR.
    - Assess the SVC along its course to the MV with CF Doppler and PW Doppler by angling somewhat toward the RV inflow.
  - Short axis
    - Evaluate the IVC limb of the baffle with color Doppler (see Fig. 8-17) and PW Doppler.
    - Assess the course of PVs to the TV with color Doppler and PW Doppler.
    - Assess for any residual VSD with color Doppler; if present, obtain peak velocity/ PIPG.
- Suprasternal notch view
  - Assess the SVC flow pattern with spectral Doppler, which should appear normal.
  - Little flow at all may suggest occlusion.
  - Accelerated, nonphasic pattern may suggest significant SVC stenosis.

Alternate Approaches
- MRI may be used for anatomic and functional assessment in patients with poor windows. RV function and TR can be quantified.
- Cardiac catheterization can be used to assess hemodynamics and anatomy. Interventions can be performed to close baffle leaks and to dilate and/or stent a stenotic SVC or IVC.

Transposition of the Great Arteries, Ventricular Septal Defect, and Pulmonary Stenosis: Status Post Rastelli or Nikaidoh Procedure

Background
- If the LVOT or pulmV is sufficiently obstructed to preclude ASO, in the presence of a VSD, two operative techniques are available for repair.
- Rastelli procedure: the long-standing surgical approach to this lesion (Fig. 8-19).
  - The VSD is closed such that LV outflow is baffled to the AV.
  - The PA is transected and the pulmV is oversewn.
  - Continuity between the RV and the PAs is established with a conduit.
- Nikaidoh procedure (aortic translocation): newer, more complex surgical technique; argued to produce a more anatomically normal result, no conduit.
  - The MPA is divided, and the pulmV leaflets are excised.
  - The conal septum separating the aortic and pulmV is divided.
  - The AV and root are mobilized from the RV and translocated posteriorly into the pulmV annulus. The coronary arteries may or may not be harvested and reimplanted.
  - The VSD is closed with a patch.

KEY POINTS

- The Senning and Mustard operations restore normal physiology by redirecting blood flow at the atrial level: systemic venous return to the LV and pulmonary venous return to the RV.
- Anatomically, connections remain abnormal.
- The RV functions as the systemic ventricle and the TV as the systemic AVV.
- Assess for complications related to the repair, including residual shunts (baffle leaks or residual VSD), SVC or IVC stenosis/occlusion, and baffle obstruction.
- Use multiple views to visualize the systemic and pulmonary venous pathways, as well as careful color Doppler and PW Doppler analysis.
- Saline solution contrast injection can be very helpful in identifying SVC or IVC stenosis or occlusion and baffle leaks.
- The abnormal natural history of the RV functioning in the systemic circulation can result in RV dysfunction, TR, and LVOTO due to compression by the RV.

Rastelli repair

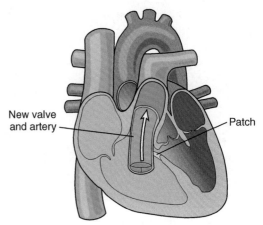

New valve and artery

Patch

Figure 8-19. Schematic depicting Rastelli repair of d-TGA with VSD and pulmonary stenosis (PS). Note that continuity between the RV and PAs is achieved with the insertion of a conduit.

- The aorta is transected, and the branch PAs are brought anterior to the aorta (LeCompte maneuver).
- A segment of ascending aorta is excised to reduce its length, and then the ascending aorta is reanastomosed.
- The MPA is sutured posteriorly to the opening in the RV and then augmented anteriorly with a patch.

Overview of Echocardiographic Approach

- Evaluate for complications related to the repair.
  - Residual ASD or VSD (2D, color Doppler, PW Doppler, CW Doppler).
  - Rastelli procedure
    - LVOTO (2D, color Doppler, PW Doppler, CW Doppler).
    - Conduit stenosis or insufficiency (color Doppler, PW Doppler, CW Doppler).
    - Right ventricular dilation and dysfunction secondary to ventriculotomy and chronic conduit dysfunction (2D).
  - Nikaidoh procedure
    - LVOTO: theoretically less likely than in Rastelli procedure (2D, color Doppler, PW Doppler, CW Doppler).
    - RVOTO or branch PA stenosis (2D, color Doppler, PW Doppler, CW Doppler).
    - Coronary complications as manifested by RWMAs (2D).
    - Supravalvar aortic stenosis (2D, color Doppler, PW Doppler, CW Doppler).
    - RV dilation and dysfunction secondary to free pulmonary insufficiency (2D).

- TTE is the standard modality for assessment. TEE may be used in the case of poor transthoracic windows or pre- and postoperatively.

Anatomic Imaging
Acquisition

- Subcostal views
  - Assess for residual ASD or VSD.
  - In addition, in patients with good windows, subcostal short axis imaging provides excellent views of the RVOT and proximal MPA or conduit.
- Apical views
  - Assess the regional wall motion.
  - Assess for any LVOTO.
  - Nikaidoh procedure: assess for evidence of supravalvar aortic stenosis in the 5C view.
- Parasternal views
  - Long axis
    - Assess the LVOT (Fig. 8-20); evaluate for residual VSD; visualize the AV and root; assess for supravalvar aortic anastomosis (Nikaidoh procedure); assess the RV-to-PA conduit (Rastelli procedure); assess regional wall motion.
  - Short axis
    - Assess for residual ASD or VSD; assess regional wall motion; assess RV size and function; evaluate conduit (Rastelli procedure); evaluate the proximal branch PAs (Nikaidoh procedure: branches now straddle the ascending aorta, may be better seen from the suprasternal notch view).

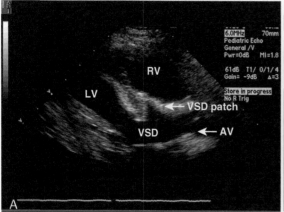
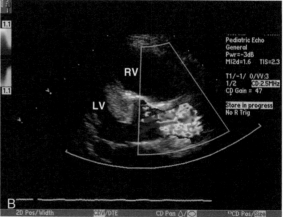

Figure 8-20. Left ventricular outflow tract obstruction after baffling of left ventricular (LV) outflow through a VSD to the AV (Rastelli). **A,** 2D parasternal long axis view shows the long pathway from the LV to the AV through the VSD. Not well seen on this image is a subaortic membrane within the tunnel. **B,** Parasternal long axis color Doppler imaging shows aliasing within the tunnel, at the level of the membrane, proximal to the AV. Spectral Doppler interrogation from other planes demonstrated a peak velocity of 4.9 m/s, mean gradient 49 mm Hg.

- Suprasternal notch views
  - Visualize the branch PAs in a short axis view (for Nikaidoh procedure: straddling the ascending aorta).
  - Nikaidoh procedure: evaluate supravalvar aortic anastomosis.

Analysis
- Measure any residual ASD or VSD noted on 2D imaging in whichever view it is best visualized, ideally two orthogonal planes.
- Measure LV chamber dimensions (LV end-diastolic dimension, LV end-systolic dimension) and parameters of LV systolic function (EF, shortening fraction).

Physiologic Data
Acquisition
- Subcostal views
  - Use color Doppler to assess for residual ASD or VSD. Obtain peak velocity/PIPG across any residual VSD.
  - Subcostal short axis views of the RVOT and proximal conduit/PA: use color Doppler and spectral Doppler to evaluate for obstruction or significant regurgitation.
  - The LVOT, AV, and supravalvar aortic region can be evaluated in the subcostal views; use color Doppler and spectral Doppler to document obstruction.
- Apical views
  - Assess for TR or MR with color Doppler; further quantify as appropriate.
  - Assess the RV pressure estimate by TR velocity given the potential for conduit or PA stenosis.
  - Assess the LVOT, AV, and supravalvar aortic region from the 5C view, using color Doppler to screen for aliasing of flow or significant regurgitation. Use PW Doppler to "march" through these levels of outflow to identify the site of acceleration. Use CW Doppler to identify the highest velocity.
- Parasternal views
  - Assess the LVOT with color Doppler (see Fig. 8-20).
  - Assess the RVOT, conduit or PA anastomosis, and branch PAs with a combination of color Doppler, PW Doppler, and CW Doppler as above to identify any obstruction or significant conduit regurgitation. Mean gradients are likely to be a more accurate assessment of true gradients in a conduit.
  - Use color Doppler to assess for residual ASD or VSD. Obtain peak velocity/PIPG across any residual VSD.

- Assess the RV pressure estimate by TR velocity as above.
- Suprasternal notch views
  - Assess the branch PAs with color Doppler, PW Doppler, and CW Doppler for the degree of stenosis.
  - Nikaidoh procedure: assess the ascending aortic velocity to rule out anastomotic narrowing.

Alternate Approaches
- MRI is used to quantify RV size and function and pulmonary regurgitation and is instrumental in determining appropriate timing of pulmV replacement. MRI may also be used for anatomic assessment if TTE windows are poor.
- Cardiac catheterization and angiography can be used to evaluate coronary artery patency (Nikaidoh procedure) as well as severity of obstruction to RV or LV outflow.
- Nuclear medicine pulmonary perfusion scans can be used to quantify percentage of blood flow to each lung, in the setting of suspected asymmetrical branch PA stenosis.

KEY POINTS

- Two different surgical techniques can be used for repair of this defect; the complications are somewhat different.
- The Rastelli operation baffles the LV outflow through the VSD to the AV and uses an RV-to-PA conduit. Assess for evidence of LVOTO, residual VSD, conduit stenosis, or regurgitation and their effect on RV size and function, and branch PA anatomy.
- The Nikaidoh operation translocates the aorta into the pulmonary annulus before closing the VSD, and thus LVOTO is thought to be less likely. Continuity is established between the RV and PAs without a conduit but with obligate free pulmonary insufficiency. A LeCompte maneuver is performed, bringing the branch PAs anterior to the aorta. Assess for evidence of LVOTO, residual VSD, RVOTO, branch PA stenosis, RV size and function, and coronary complications.

L-TGA (Congenitally Corrected TGA)

Background
- This lesion is also known as congenitally corrected TGA.
- Demonstration of the segmental anatomy is key (Fig. 8-21).
  - Visceroatrial situs is normal.

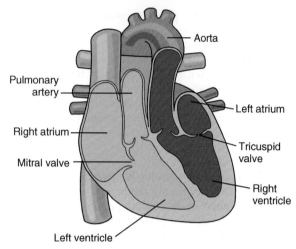

Figure 8-21. Schematic depicting the anatomy of L-TGA, also known as congenitally corrected TGA. Note that although the anatomy is abnormal, the physiology is normal.

- Ventricular looping is abnormal, with the morphologic LV being right sided and aligned with the morphologic RA. The morphologic RV is left sided and aligned with the morphologic LA.
- The PA arises from the right-sided morphologic LV, and the aorta arises from the left-sided morphologic RV. However, the GVs have an abnormal orientation to each other, with the aorta being leftward and anterior of the PA.
- The blood flow is normal, with systemic venous return passing through the right side of the heart to the lungs and pulmonary venous return passing through the left side of the heart to the body.
- The morphologic RV functions as the systemic ventricle, and thus patients are at risk of systemic ventricular dysfunction.
- The AVVs are derived, embryologically, from the ventricles. Thus, the left-sided AVV in this case is a TV and the right-sided AVV is a MV.
- Frequently associated lesions include
  - Ebstein's anomaly of the left-sided morphologic TV.
  - VSD.
  - PS.
  - Various degrees of heart block.
- Whether any surgery is required depends on the associated lesions.

Overview of Echocardiographic Approach
- Identify the segmental anatomy (2D).
  - Normal atrial situs.
  - Levo (L)-looped ventricles (ventricular inversion).

- The morphologic LV and MV are on the right, receiving inflow from the RA.
- The morphologic RV and TV are on the left, receiving inflow from the LA.
- A morphologic RV has a moderator band, coarse trabeculations, chordal attachments to the septum, and a morphologic TV. A morphologic LV has a smooth septal surface, lack of chordal attachments to the septum, and a morphologic MV (2D).
- L-transposed GVs
  - The aorta arises anterior and leftward from the left-sided morphologic RV.
  - The PA arises posterior and rightward from the right-sided morphologic LV.
- Segmental anatomy can be abbreviated {S,L,L}.
- Presence or absence and size of shunts at the atrial and ventricular levels (2D, color Doppler).
- Morphology and function of the AVVs; in particular, assess the left-sided TV for evidence of Ebstein's anomaly and regurgitation (2D, color Doppler, PW Doppler, CW Doppler).
- Evaluate for outflow obstruction; in particular, assess for PS or subpulmonary stenosis (2D, color Doppler, PW Doppler, CW Doppler).

Anatomic Imaging
Acquisition
- Subcostal frontal (long axis) sweep, posterior to anterior.
- Establish normal visceroatrial situs: visualize the IVC within the liver on the right, connecting to the right-sided atrium. The left-sided atrium should have some PVs visible by 2D imaging.
- Demonstrate abnormal ventricular looping: in this view, the main clue is that the VS has a smooth septal surface on the right side.
- Demonstrate L-transposed ventriculoarterial connections.
  - The more posterior GV, arising from the right-sided (morphologic left) ventricle, bifurcates, identifying it as the PA.
  - The more anterior GV arising from the left-sided (morphologic right) ventricle does not bifurcate; coronary artery origins may be seen from it.
- Note any evidence of outflow tract obstruction.
- Note also that the GVs do not cross each other (as is the case in normally related GVs).

- Subcostal short axis sweep, base to apex.
  - Atrial morphology is again noted to be normal with the GVs entering the RA and at least some PVs are visualized entering the LA. Assess for evidence of ASD.
  - Ventricular morphology is examined and is consistent with L-looping (ventricular inversion). The right-sided ventricle has a smooth septal surface and AVV morphology consistent with an MV (no chordal attachments to the septum). The left-sided ventricle has coarse trabeculations, with chordal attachments of the AVV to the septum (Fig. 8-22). Assess for VSD (size, location).
  - GVs are noted to be L-transposed with the bifurcating PA arising posteriorly from the right-sided (morphologic left) ventricle and the aorta arising anteriorly from the left-sided (morphologic right) ventricle. Note any evidence of outflow tract obstruction. Their parallel relationship is well seen.
- Apical views
  - Ventricular morphology is inverted; the moderator band is seen within the left-sided (morphologic right) ventricle. The morphologic RV is dilated and hypertrophied compared with a normal RV (Fig. 8-23). Assess systolic function.
  - Inspect the left-sided TV for evidence of Ebstein's anomaly.
  - Note any evidence of VSD or outflow tract obstruction.
  - With anterior angulation, the PA is seen arising from the right-sided (morphologic left) ventricle.

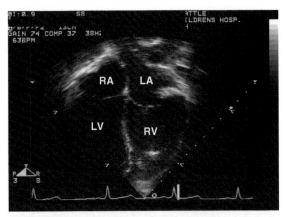

Figure 8-23. Apical 2D view of L-TGA. Note the presence of the moderator band in the left-sided morphologic RV. This patient does not have Ebstein's anomaly of the left-sided TV, although that is a common association.

  - With further anterior angulation, the aorta may be seen arising from the left-sided (morphologic right) ventricle.
- Parasternal long axis view
  - The parasternal long axis view can be confusing in L-TGA.
  - The ventricles are located more side by side than usual.
  - The long axis view is more parallel to the long axis of the body.
  - If the transducer is aligned more conventionally, it is possible to align the pulmV with the left-sided TV.
  - The AV is not seen in the long axis view of the TV and RV.
  - Other windows are recommended for understanding the spatial relationships.
- Parasternal short axis view
  - Relative orientation of the semilunar valves is seen.
  - Typically, the AV is anterior and leftward of the pulmV (Fig. 8-24).
  - Coronary arteries arise from the aortic root most commonly, as depicted in Figure 8-25.
  - Note morphology and relative sizes of the semilunar valves.
  - Sweeping toward the head, the posterior PA can be noted to branch.
  - Note any evidence of VSD.
  - Assess ventricular function.
  - The coronaries can be visualized; most commonly, the RV coronary arises by itself from the leftward posterior sinus, and the anterior descending and Cx arteries arise from a common trunk from the rightward sinus. As in d-TGA, the coronary pattern can be variable.

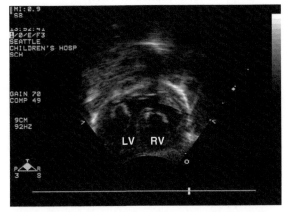

Figure 8-22. Subcostal short axis view at the level of the ventricles in a patient with L-TGA. Note the right-sided morphologic LV with its smooth septal surface. There are no attachments of the MV to the septum. In contrast, note the chordal attachments of the left-sided tricuspid valve within the RV. This patient also has a VSD, seen here, and PS.

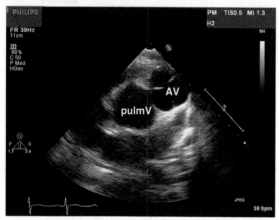

Figure 8-24. Parasternal short axis view showing the typical orientation of GVs in L-TGA. The AV is anterior and leftward of the pulmV.

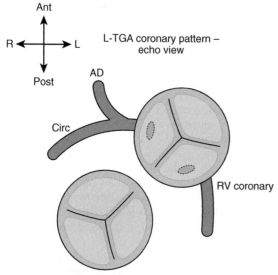

Figure 8-25. Schematic showing typical anatomy of the coronary arteries in L-TGA, parasternal short axis echo view.

- The aortic arch, which runs more anteroposterior than usual, is often better imaged in a high left parasternal window than from the suprasternal notch.

Analysis
- Quantitative analysis consists of measuring sizes of shunts and semilunar valves.
- Atrial shunts (ASD or PFO) should be measured from the subcostal long axis or short axis view.
- VSDs should be measured in whichever view they are seen best, ideally in two orthogonal planes.
- The pulmV and AV are measured from the parasternal long axis view.

Pitfalls
- As noted above, the parasternal long axis views can be particularly confusing. Align the plane of sound more parallel to the long axis of the body. Use other views to understand anatomic relationships.

Physiologic Data
Acquisition
- Subcostal views
  - From the subcostal frontal or short axis view, color Doppler sweeps of the atrial septum identify shunts.
  - Short axis color Doppler sweeps of the VS are used to identify any VSD present and determine the direction of shunting. Carefully assess any area that the 2D imaging suggests may have a defect.
  - Acquire peak velocity/PIPG across any VSD in the view that most aligns the Doppler angle with the jet.
  - The RVOT, LVOT, and the semilunar valves may be evaluated for evidence of stenosis or regurgitation by color Doppler and spectral Doppler (PW Doppler and CW Doppler) from the subcostal views. In particular, there is an association between L-TGA and PS, either at the valvar or subvalvar level.
- Apical views
  - Assess AVV function, in particular, the left-sided TV, which has a high likelihood of regurgitation due to its association with Ebstein's anomaly and function in the systemic ventricle.
  - Assess the apical muscular septum by color Doppler for evidence of VSD.
  - Assess the RVOT, LVOT, and semilunar valve function by color Doppler and spectral Doppler.
- Parasternal views
  - Color sweep of the VS is used to identify any VSD present and determine the direction of shunting. Carefully assess any area that the 2D imaging suggests may have a defect.
  - Acquire the peak velocity/PIPG across any VSD in the view that most aligns the Doppler angle with the jet.
  - Further assess valve function with color Doppler.

Alternate Approaches
- MRI is used for quantification of RV function and TR and can also be used for anatomic definition in patients with poor TTE windows.

KEY POINTS

- Establish the diagnosis of L-TGA by demonstrating the segmental anatomy: normal atrial situs, abnormal (L) ventricular looping, and L-transposed GVs.
- The morphologic RV and TV are on the left; the morphologic LV and MV are on the right.
- A morphologic RV has a moderator band, chordal attachments to the septum, and a morphologic TV. A morphologic LV has a smooth septal surface, lack of chordal attachments to the septum, and a morphologic MV.
- Although the anatomy is abnormal, physiology is normal.
- Frequently associated lesions are Ebstein's anomaly of the left-sided morphologic TV, VSD, PS, and various degrees of heart block.
- The segmental anatomy is best understood from subcostal and apical views. Parasternal long axis views, in particular, can be confusing. The ventricles are more side by side than usual, and the AV is separated by conus from the TV.
- On long-term follow-up, systemic RV and TV function are of greatest importance.

Suggested Reading

1. Earing MG, Ayers NA, Cetta F. Congenitally corrected transposition of the great arteries. In: Eidem BW, Cetta F, O'Leary PW, eds. *Echocardiography in Pediatric and Adult Congenital Heart Disease*. Philadelphia: Lippincott Williams & Wilkins; 2010.
2. Mahle WT, Marx GR, Anderson RH. Anatomy and echocardiography of discordant atrioventricular connections. *Cardiol Young*. 2006;16(suppl 3):65-71.
3. Mertens LL, Vogt MO, Marek J, Cohen MS. Transposition of the great arteries. In: Lai WW, Mertens LL, Cohen MS, Geva T, eds. *Echocardiography in Pediatric and Congenital Heart Disease*. Hoboken, NJ: Wiley-Blackwell; 2009.
4. Miller-Hance WC, Silverman NH. Transesophageal echocardiography in congenital heart disease with focus on the adult. *Cardiol Clin*. 2000;18(4):861-892.
5. Oechslin E. Physiologically "corrected" transposition of the great arteries. In: Lai WW, Mertens LL, Cohen MS, Geva T, eds. *Echocardiography in Pediatric and Congenital Heart Disease*. Hoboken, NJ: Wiley-Blackwell; 2009.
6. Pasquini L, Parness IA, Colan SD, et al. Diagnosis of intramural coronary artery in transposition of the great arteries using two-dimensional echocardiography. *Circulation*. 1993;88:1136-1141.
7. Schultz AH, Lewin MB. D-Transposition of the great arteries. In: Eidem BW, Cetta F, O'Leary PW, eds. *Echocardiography in Pediatric and Adult Congenital Heart Disease*. Philadelphia: Lippincott Williams & Wilkins; 2010.

Venous Anomalies

9

Brian D. Soriano

Background

- Isolated congenital anomalies of large systemic veins such as persistent left-sided superior vena cava (SVC) or interrupted inferior vena cava (IVC) have no hemodynamic impact and are usually found incidentally.
- Totally anomalous and partially anomalous pulmonary venous connections are two conditions in which one or more pulmonary vein (PV) segments do not connect directly to the left atrium (LA). Instead, the PV connects with a systemic vein, mixing with deoxygenated blood before returning to the right atrium (RA).
  - The anomalous connections, whether total or partial, can occur at any level of systemic venous return: supracardiac such as the innominate veins, cardiac level such as the coronary sinus (CS), or infracardiac such as the IVC (Fig. 9-1).
  - Right-sided cardiac or systemic venous dilation will occur in the regions where the anomalous connections occur. With supracardiac connections, for example, the SVC and innominate veins may be dilated.
- In normal anatomy, four separate PVs are the most common arrangement, although normal variations in this number also exist. An entire lung can join a single confluent vein before connecting to the LA. Likewise, each lobe of the right lung can have its own vein connect, leading to five total connections.
- In total anomalous pulmonary venous connection (TAPVC), a right-to-left shunt, typically interatrial, is necessary to supply left ventricular preload.
- In repaired TAPVCs, the incidence of PV stenosis is approximately 11%.

Overview of Echocardiographic Approach

- Direct visualization of PV connections to the LA is typically easier for younger and smaller patients.
- All available transthoracic echocardiography (TTE) windows should be used to evaluate and demonstrate pulmonary or systemic venous connections, whether normal or abnormal. Optimal windows depend on which specific PV is being imaged (Table 9-1).
- Color Doppler maps are useful in confirming an individual systemic or PV connection. Low Nyquist settings, 50 cm/s or less, should be used to ensure adequate color signals. The use of higher settings may lead to a low-signal or even absent color map. PV flow is low velocity, and with some TTE windows, the angle of interrogation can be occasionally perpendicular to the vein.
- For any patient with a history of anomalous PV surgical repairs, individual veins should be evaluated for stenosis (Box 9-1, Fig. 9-2).

Anatomic Imaging
Pulmonary Veins

- A high parasternal short axis (SAX) view, angled inferiorly toward the LA, creates the "crab" view (Fig. 9-3). In this plane, four PVs can be visualized at once. Care must be taken to ensure the left atrial appendage is not confused for the left upper PV (LUPV).
- Right parasternal and subcostal views can help confirm the presence of a normal right upper PV (RUPV) connection; the SVC serves as the anatomic landmark because the RUPV courses directly posterior to it (Fig. 9-4). Other, less commonly used windows can be applied to identify normal connections. For example, from the parasternal long axis (LAX) view, a left-sided PV connection can be detected by

Total anamolous pulmonary venous return: cardiac

Total anamolous pulmonary venous return: infracardiac

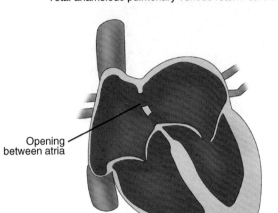

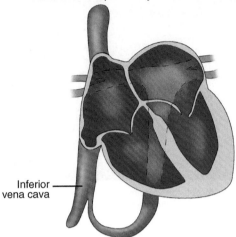

Opening between atria

Inferior vena cava

Total anamolous pulmonary venous return: supracardiac

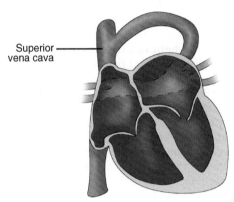

Superior vena cava

Figure 9-1. Schematic diagram of total anomalous pulmonary venous connections and their most common arrangements: cardiac (typically to the coronary sinus), infracardiac (vertical vein passes the diaphragm and inserts to the inferior vena cava), and supracardiac (with connection to the innominate vein).

TABLE 9-1	RECOMMENDED VIEWS TO EVALUATE PULMONARY VEIN ANATOMY
View	**Best-Viewed Pulmonary Veins**
High parasternal short axis (crab view)	RLPV, LUPV, LLPV More challenging: RUPV
Apical 4 chamber	RLPV More challenging: Left lower pulmonary vein origin is adjacent to the left atrial appendage ostium
Apical 5 chamber / LVOT	RUPV, LLPV
Parasternal long axis	Left pulmonary veins (upper and lower can be difficult to distinguish)
Subcostal long axis	RUPV, RLPV, LUPV, LLPV
Subcostal short axis	RUPV

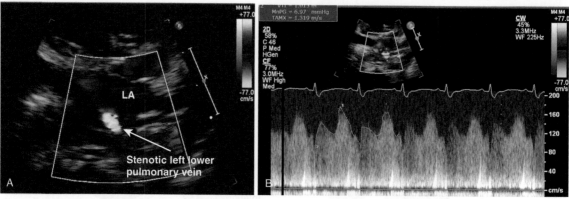

Figure 9-2. **A,** Left lower pulmonary vein (PV) stenosis. Aliased flow and a narrow vena contracta are present. **B,** Spectral Doppler of the stenosis showing continuous flow and a mean gradient of 7 mm Hg.

BOX 9-1 Postoperative Evaluation of Patients with Repaired TAPVC/PAPVC

- Evaluate individual PV connections.
- Evaluate systemic venous connections and the presence or absence of stenosis.
- Assess for the presence or absence of PHTN.
- In repaired scimitar syndrome patients, evaluate the right PVs as they course from the IVC into the LA.

---

two-dimensional (2D) and color imaging (Fig. 9-5).
- Size discrepancy between the IVC and SVC can be a subtle sign of anomalous connections; the systemic vein receiving the PV connection will be dilated out of proportion to the remaining systemic veins.
- In scimitar syndrome, part or all of the right-sided PVs connect anomalously to the IVC. The PVs are oriented more vertically and become more dilated as they approach the heart, creating a curved swordlike ("scimitar") appearance on a chest radiograph (Fig. 9-6).
- In unrepaired TAPVC
  - Obstruction can occur in the PV pathways and is more likely associated with infracardiac and supracardiac types. Cardiac-level TAPVC is less likely to be obstructed.
  - An obligate and unrestricted right-to-left interatrial shunt is almost always present in any form.

Systemic Veins
- Table 9-2 provides an overview of how systemic venous anomalies may be identified.

- A dilated CS should raise the suspicion for the presence of a left-sided SVC (LSVC). Left parasternal views and suprasternal notch views can be used to help visualize the LSVC. The LSVC can be visualized by starting along the left clavicle and angling inferiorly. Low Nyquist (20 cm/s) color Doppler will aid in visualization.
  - The presence or absence of a CS septal defect should be evaluated. Intravenous microbubble contrast can be injected in the left arm to evaluate for a right-to-left shunt via the LSVC and directly into the LA by way of this rare systemic venous anomaly.
  - If an LSVC is present, usually a normal right-sided SVC (RSVC) is also present.
  - A bridging innominate vein may be present between the two vessels.
  - Rarely, an isolated LSVC to dilated CS can exist simultaneously with an absent RSVC.
- Interrupted IVC
  - Congenital anomaly where the hepatic IVC segment is absent. Lower body systemic veins drain via a hemiazygos vein that eventually drains to the SVC.
  - From a transverse abdominal view, a dilated azygos vein can be viewed in cross section and will typically be located adjacent to the vertebral bodies of the spine (Fig. 9-7).
  - The azygos arch and SVC may appear dilated due to the extra blood flow (Fig. 9-8).
- The retroaortic innominate vein (Fig. 9-9)
  - Courses underneath the aortic arch, instead of superiorly.
  - Is best viewed from a suprasternal notch view.

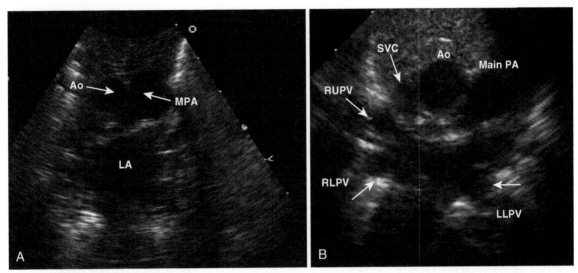

Figure 9-3. Crab view of the left atrium (LA) (**A**) and views of the individual venous connections (**B**).

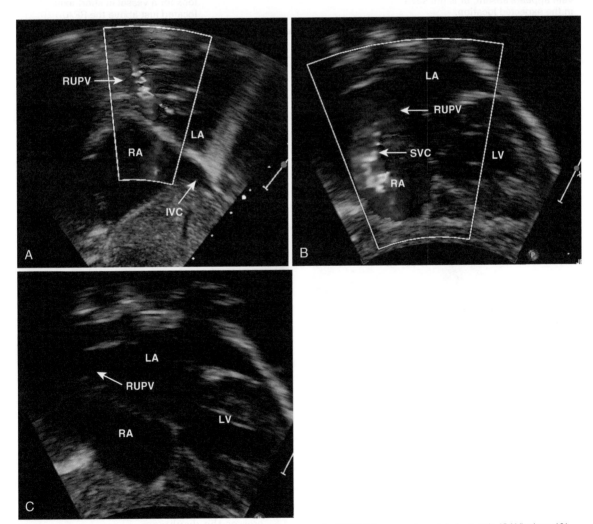

Figure 9-4. Two different views of the right upper pulmonary vein (RUPV) from a subcostal short axis (SAX) plane (**A**) and subcostal long axis (LAX) plane (**B**). The SVC is located just outside the scan plane. **C**, RUPV from a two-dimensional view.

TABLE 9-2   ECHOCARDIOGRAPHIC CUES FOR CONGENITAL SYSTEMIC VEIN ANOMALIES

Anatomic Imaging Problem*	Possible Congenital Diagnosis	To Confirm, Look for
No inferior vena cava present in subcostal views. Only hepatic veins are seen. Azygos arch, as it connects to the SVC, appears dilated or flow appears prominent.	Interrupted inferior vena cava with azygos vein continuation.	• Dilated azygos vein—large venous channel just lateral to the vertebral body. • Prominent flow in the SVC. • Dilated azygos arch, located and connecting posterior to the SVC.
Coronary sinus appears dilated.	Persistent LSVC draining to coronary sinus.	• Suprasternal notch view, aligned along left clavicle—search for a vertical vein than drains from head-to-foot. • Left parasternal window with marker at 12 o'clock should show a LSVC in its long axis.
No centrally located innominate vein present in suprasternal notch, and coronary sinus appears dilated.	Bilateral superior vena cavae without a bridging innominate vein.	The presence of a normal right-sided SVC connection and persistent LSVC (see above).
Innominate vein or left subclavian vein appears absent, or is not seen in the expected location.	Retroaortic innominate vein.	In the long axis aortic arch view, look for a vessel in short axis, located just above the RPA.

*Acquired venous anomalies such as deep vein thrombosis should always be considered if these anomalies are present.

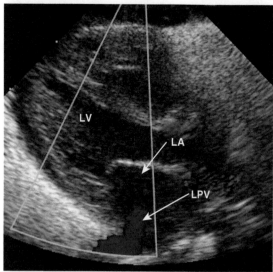

Figure 9-5. View of a left-sided sided PV from a parasternal long axis view.

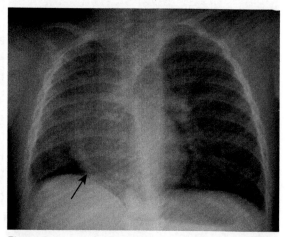

Figure 9-6. Chest radiograph of a patient with scimitar syndrome. The *arrow* indicates the scimitar vein, which anomalously drains right PV flow to the IVC.

Physiologic Data

• Isolated systemic venous anomalies are almost always asymptomatic and require no intervention.
  • The CS septum should be evaluated for any defects.
  • Interrupted IVC or persistent LSVC is sometimes found incidentally, for example, when a central venous catheter is placed and takes an unexpected course.
• Estimation of pulmonary artery (PA) pressures and right ventricular performance is an important element for both pre- and postoperative assessment of either partial anomalous pulmonary venous connection (PAPVC) or TAPVC.
• In unrepaired TAPVC, pulmonary hypertension (PHTN) should prompt the search for a PV obstruction or a restrictive patent foramen ovale.
  • For infracardiac, obstruction usually occurs within the liver or where the vertical vein crosses the diaphragm.
  • For supracardiac, obstruction occurs usually when the vein crosses between the left

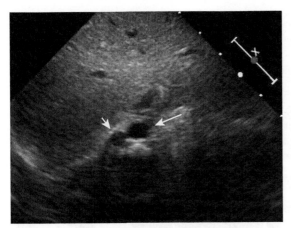

Figure 9-7. Transverse abdominal view of a patient with interrupted IVC with azygos continuation to the superior vena cava (SVC). The *long arrow* shows a midline abdominal aorta, and the *short arrow* shows a dilated azygos vein as it courses just laterally to the vertebral body.

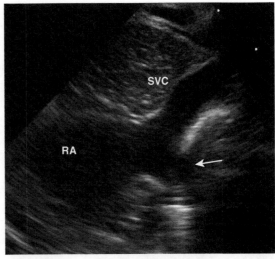

Figure 9-8. High right parasternal view of the SVC and dilated azygos arch (*arrow*). Such an appearance should raise the index of suspicion for an interrupted IVC or PAPVC.

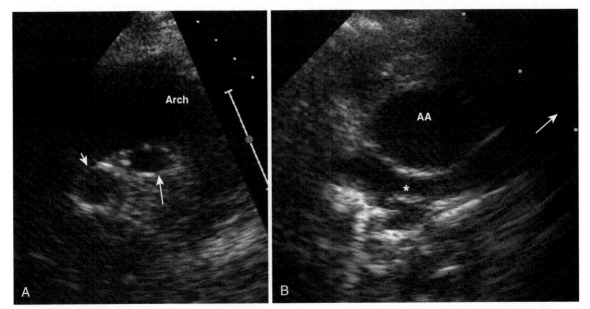

Figure 9-9. **A,** Suprasternal notch view showing two vessels located underneath the aortic arch: a retroaortic innominate vein (*long arrow*) and the right pulmonary artery (*short arrow*). **B,** Suprasternal notch view with the dot of the transducer positioned at the 3 o'clock position. The *arrow* indicates the off-screen location of the left subclavian vein. It continues to run below and posterior to the aorta as a retroaortic innominate vein (*asterisk*).

mainstem bronchus and the left pulmonary artery.

- Doppler imaging, including pulsed wave and color maps, demonstrates a continuous flow pattern. The usual phasic pattern or venous respiratory variations are not present.
- In repaired anomalous connections, PV stenosis is the most common late complication

that requires reintervention or reoperation. To evaluate for vein stenosis, the mean gradient should be estimated by using spectral Doppler averaged over at least two cardiac cycles. Mean gradients of 3 mm Hg or more are a sign of significant stenosis. Peak velocities and maximum instantaneous gradients are less useful and have no applicable clinical correlates.

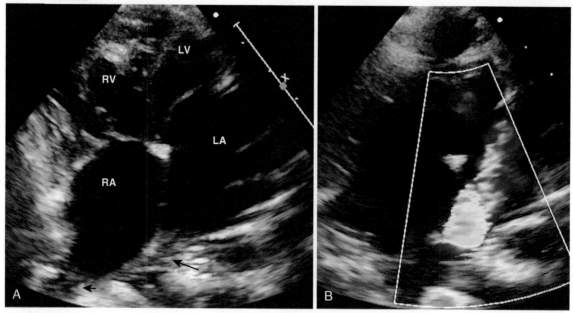

Figure 9-10. A, Oblique parasternal short axis view of all four cardiac chambers. The IVC (*short arrow*) is shown partially in its long axis to show the parallel course of a patient's scimitar repair. The course of the pulmonary venous baffle (*long arrow*) is seen as it empties to the LA. **B,** Aliased color map of the left atrial end of the baffle. Mean gradient in this patient was estimated to be 3 mm Hg.

- In repaired scimitar syndrome, the repaired area is best viewed by imaging the IVC in its long axis (Fig. 9-10). The atrial end of the repaired scimitar vein baffle can typically be located as a "vessel" parallel to the IVC.

Alternate Approaches

- Alternate imaging should be strongly considered when there is unexplained right atrial or right ventricular dilation, or upper-to-lower systemic vein size discrepancy. In addition, an alternate imaging modality should be used when PV anatomy is not completely demonstrated by TTE.
  - In patients with poor acoustic windows, TTE may not identify all PV connections.
  - Magnetic resonance (MR) angiography or computed tomography (CT) angiography can reliably resolve pulmonary venous anatomy.
  - Transesophageal echocardiography (TEE) is also a useful alternate, but is limited to visualizing the proximal venous connections to the RA and LA. It is unlikely that TEE would be able to directly visualize anomalous connections unless they occur at the cardiac level.
- CT angiography or MR angiography can be used when TTE windows are limited or if additional visualization of systemic venous pathways is required.

- Cardiac catheterization can be considered in unrepaired and repaired patients, especially when there is concern for restenosis.

KEY POINTS

- Abnormal systemic venous connections such as persistent LSVC are usually benign and have no hemodynamic impact.
  - An exception is the presence of a CS septal defect, which creates an intracardiac right-to-left shunt.
- Anomalous pulmonary venous connections should be included in the differential diagnosis whenever there is unexpected right atrial and right ventricular dilation and/or if there is unexplained dilation of the systemic veins.
- Large-volume right-to-left shunts across the atrial septum should increase the suspicion for TAPVCs.
- Traditional echocardiography can typically result in complete identification of normal pulmonary venous connections in younger, smaller patients, but may be more challenging in larger patients.
- If TTE is unable to resolve anatomic questions, alternate imaging modalities such as cardiac MR imaging or CT can more definitively identify anomalous connections.
- Approximately 11% of patients who undergo TAPVC repair require reintervention for PV stenosis.

Suggested Reading

1. Fulton DR. Partial anomalous pulmonary venous connection. In: Basow DS, eds. *UpToDate*. Waltham, MA, 2010.
   More detailed review of this condition.
2. Vida VL, Padalino MA, Boccuzzo G, et al. Scimitar syndrome: a European Congenital Heart Surgeons Association (ECHSA) multicentric study. *Circulation*. 2010;122:1159.
   Large series of patients in Europe. Given the low prevalence of this disease, multicenter studies produce the most useful information.
3. Alsoufi B, Cai S, Van Arsdell GS, et al. Outcomes after surgical treatment of children with partial anomalous pulmonary venous connection. *Ann Thorac Surg*. 2007;84:2020.
4. Seale AN, Uemura H, Webber SA, et al. Total anomalous pulmonary venous connection: morphology and outcome from an international population-based study. *Circulation*. 2010;122:2718-2726.
   Perhaps the largest cohort of patients, which was gathered across 19 centers in Europe.
5. Saxena A, Fong L, Lamb R, et al. Cardiac arrhythmias after surgical correction of total anomalous pulmonary venous connection: late follow-up. *Pediatr Cardiol*. 1991;12:89.
6. Soriano BD. Total anomalous pulmonary venous connection. In: Basow, DS, eds. *UpToDate*. Waltham, MA, 2010.
7. Tanel R, Kirshbom P, Paridon S, et al. Long-term noninvasive arrhythmia assessment after total anomalous pulmonary venous connection repair. *Am Heart J*. 2007;153:267.
   Important series that documents that a high proportion of these patients have arrhythmias.

Echocardiographic Imaging of Single-Ventricle Lesions

10

Nadine F. Choueiter and Raylene M. Choy

KEY POINTS

- Echocardiography (echo) is essential in delineating the anatomy, physiology, and postoperative management of single-ventricle (SV) lesions.
- Most common are the lesions that comprise the hypoplastic left heart syndrome (HLHS):
  - HLHS is a spectrum of cardiac defects that result in underdevelopment of the left ventricle (LV) and left ventricular-to-aortic outflow axis.
  - The aortic valve (AV) and mitral valve (MV) are either hypoplastic or atretic with no flow across the valve by color Doppler.
  - The small non-apex-forming LV is best seen from the subcostal apical or parasternal short axis view.
  - The atrial septum (AS) is inspected for restrictive flow from subcostal sagittal views.
  - The aortic arch is most commonly hypoplastic, and systemic flow is ductal dependent.

SV lesions are complex heart defects that result in one of the ventricles being hypoplastic or absent. The most common of these lesions are those that comprise HLHS. SV lesions are divided into three categories based on the adequacy of pulmonary blood flow (PBF) and systemic blood flow (SBF).

- Lesions with unobstructed PBF and SBF:
  - Double-inlet left ventricle (DILV) with Levo (L)-malposition of the great arteries.
  - Double-outlet right ventricle (DORV) with normally related great vessels (GVs).
  - Unbalanced atrioventricular canal (AVC) with a dominant right ventricle (RV).
- Lesions with obstructed PBF:
  - Tricuspid atresia (TA).
  - Pulmonary atresia with intact interventricular septum.
- Unbalanced AVC with a dominant LV.
- DILV with D-malposition of the GVs and subpulmonary stenosis or pulmonary stenosis (PS) (Holmes heart).
- Dextro transposition of the great arteries (d-TGA) and PS or subpulmonary stenosis.
- Lesions with obstructed SBF:
  - HLHS syndrome.
  - Interrupted aortic arch with hypoplastic LV.
  - DILV with L-malposition of the GVs and aortic or subaortic stenosis.
  - DORV with D-malposed GVs and PS or subpulmonary stenosis.
  - d-TGA with aortic or subaortic stenosis.

This chapter discusses in detail the imaging of these three lesions:
- HLHS.
- DILV.
- TA.

Hypoplastic Left Heart Syndrome

Definition and Prevalence

- Underdevelopment of the LV with associated hypoplasia or atresia of both/either of the AV and MV resulting in the inability of the left heart to support systemic circulation.
  - 1% to 2% of all congenital heart disease (CHD) and occurs twice as often in boys as in girls.
  - Fourth most common congenital cardiac anomaly.
  - Most common cause of death from CHD within the first week of life.

The goals of the initial echocardiogram in HLHS are to provide a complete anatomic survey and assess the underlying physiology, which play a critical role in determining the initial management of the patient. In addition to identifying the degree of hypoplasia of the left ventricular (LV) chamber and that of the MV and AV, it is important to assess the function of the RV and tricuspid valve (TV), the size and the direction of flow across the AS, ductal physiology, and associated findings such as ventriculocoronary communications or fistulae and anomalous pulmonary venous return.

Pertinent information is obtained from each of the standard views by two-dimensional (2D) and Doppler.

Parasternal Long Axis View (Fig. 10-1)

- Size discrepancy between the two ventricular chambers: the hypoplastic LV posteriorly and the dilated RV anteriorly.
- Endocardial fibroelastosis echobright areas on the endocardial surface of the LV and the MV papillary muscles.
- Hypoplasia of left atrium (LA). A dilated LA raises the suspicion of an intact AS or a restrictive atrial-level communication.
- Presence of a ventricular septal defect (VSD).
- Patency and mobility of the MV and AV leaflets.
  - The MV is usually hypoplastic with thick doming leaflets and abnormal submitral apparatus or a completely atretic MV replaced by a platelike structure. A supravalvar mitral ring might also be present.
  - Similarly, AV hypoplasia or atresia may be present and might be associated with subaortic obstruction.
  - If patency of the AV or MV is not well defined by 2D imaging, color Doppler with low color scale might help identify antegrade or retrograde valve flow (regurgitation). However, this is best

performed from the apical four-chamber (4C) view.

- Measure hypoplastic ascending aorta (Ao) and AV (typically <4 mm).
- Right ventricular (RV) and TV function by angling transducer toward the right hip. Color Doppler interrogation will reveal the presence of tricuspid regurgitation (TR). Significant TR is a poor prognostic indicator in HLHS.
- Assess right ventricular outflow tract (RVOT) and dilated main pulmonary artery (MPA) by angling the transducer toward the left shoulder.

Parasternal Short Axis View

- Size discrepancy between the large anterior RV and hypoplastic posterior LV (Fig. 10-2).
- Ventricular function.
- Assess size of the aortic root and ascending aorta in cross section (Fig. 10-3).
- Ascertain the presence and position or absence of two papillary muscles. The MV is often a "parachute" (a single papillary muscle).
- Normal relationship of the GVs with the hypoplastic aorta posteriorly and to the right of the MPA.
- Evaluate the size and direction of flow across the patent ductus arteriosus (PDA). This is usually obtained from a high left parasternal view moving the transducer superiorly toward the left shoulder and rotating it counterclockwise to about the 1 o'clock position. The branch pulmonary arteries (PAs) are seen from this view (also known as the "three pant leg view" or the trifurcation view).

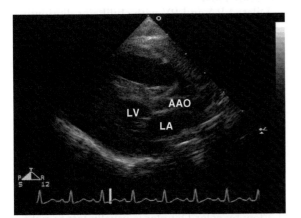

Figure 10-1. Hypoplastic left heart syndrome (HLHS). Parasternal long axis view. Markedly hypoplastic left ventricle (LV), aortic arch obstruction (AAO), left atrium (LA).

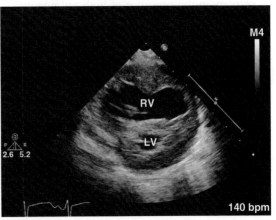

Figure 10-2. HLHS. Parasternal short axis view. Note the size discrepancy between the small LV posteriorly and the right ventricle (RV) anteriorly.

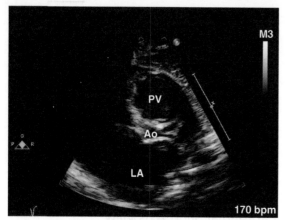

Figure 10-3. HLHS. Parasternal short axis view. The image was taken at the base of the heart. A tiny aortic valve is seen with the left main coronary arising from the left coronary cusp. A dilated pulmonary valve is seen anteriorly.

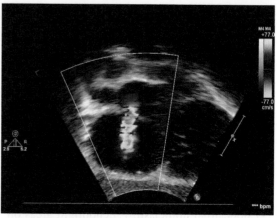

Figure 10-4. HLHS. Subxyphoid long axis color compare image profiling a restricted interatrial communication with aliasing of the jet by color Doppler.

- Doppler interrogation of the PDA is best done from this view. It shows right-to-left flow across the ductus in systole. The direction of flow in diastole is usually dependent on the resistance in the pulmonary vascular bed. The systolic gradient should be assessed for signs of early ductal restriction.
- Presence of ventriculocoronary fistulous connections in the LV myocardium (commonly seen in HLHS with mitral and aortic atresia). This is best performed with color Doppler interrogation of the LV myocardium scanning from base to apex while lowering the color scale because fistulous flow is of low velocity.
- Presence of a VSD using 2D imaging as well as color Doppler interrogation with low color scale to identify small VSDs with low flow velocity in the presence of high pulmonary pressures.
- Evaluate pulmonary valve anatomy and function for stenosis or regurgitation.

Apical Four-Chamber View
- Size discrepancy between the two ventricles: a non-apex forming LV and a hypoplastic LV. The RV is dilated and hypertrophied. Move the transducer into the axilla (i.e., into a far posteroinferior and lateral position) to optimize the visualization of the hypoplastic LV.
- Degree of MV hypoplasia (thick doming stenotic leaflets) or atresia (platelike structure). In the presence of concomitant aortic stenosis or atresia, MV leaflet excursion may be limited secondary to markedly elevated LV end-diastolic pressure.

- MV inflow and regurgitation. If flow by color Doppler is present, pulsed wave (PW) Doppler and continuous wave (CW) Doppler interrogation of the gradient across the MV will assess the degree of stenosis. The transmitral gradient will be underestimated in the presence of a large atrial communication. Degree of AV hypoplasia or atresia in addition to subaortic stenosis.
- Aortic antegrade flow (if flow present) or regurgitation by color Doppler and spectral Doppler interrogation.
- TR by color Doppler interrogation.
- Pulmonary regurgitation by color Doppler interrogation.

Subcostal Four-Chamber or Coronal View
- Dilated RA and RV with slitlike or diminutive LV prompting the evaluation of left-sided structures (MV, AV, and aortic arch).
- Size discrepancy between the GVs with a dilated MPA and hypoplastic ascending aorta. If ascending aorta is severely hypoplastic, this region may be difficult to visualize.
- Optimal view to evaluate the AS and the number, size, location, and degree of restriction across the atrial communication. Bulging of the AS into the RA or a dilated LA suggests restriction of flow at the atrial level (Figs. 10-4 and 10-5).
- Flow by color Doppler is usually left to right but can be bidirectional in the presence of severe TR or anomalous pulmonary venous connections.

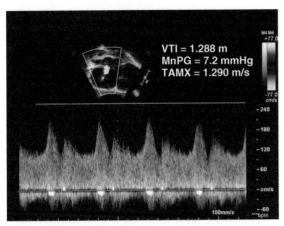

Figure 10-5. HLHS: atrial septal pulsed wave (PW) Doppler interrogation demonstrates continuous waveform without returning to baseline throughout the cardiac cycle, suggestive of a restricted interatrial communication.

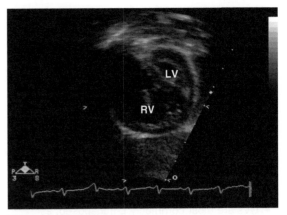

Figure 10-6. HLHS. Subxyphoid short axis view at the mid-ventricular level demonstrating the size discrepancy between the ventricles.

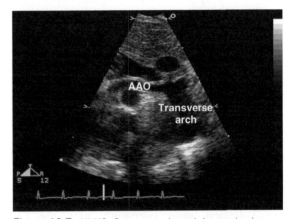

Figure 10-7. HLHS. Suprasternal notch long axis view. Markedly hypoplastic ascending aorta.

- The spectral Doppler cursor is often parallel to the direction of flow across the AS, allowing accurate measurement of the mean pressure gradient across the AS. Tracing of the gradient over three cardiac cycles is usually done to account for respiratory variation.
- Posterior deviation of the superior aspect of the septum primum.
- Septum primum attaching directly to the posterosuperior left atrial wall far to the left of the septum secundum.
- Assess for anomalous pulmonary venous return.
- TR.

Subcostal Short Axis or Sagittal View
- Ventricular size and GV discrepancy (Fig. 10-6).
- Assessment of the AS (same as subcostal 4C view).
- Visualizing the PDA as a continuation of the dilated MPA by angling the transducer toward the patient's left for 2D and Doppler imaging.
- The entire arch can be visualized from this view if the transducer is angled further to the left of the patient's abdomen. This proves to be useful if suprasternal notch (SSN) imaging is not possible.
- Pulsatility of the abdominal aorta by color Doppler and spectral Doppler. A decrease in pulsatility indicates a coarctation. Flow reversal is seen in the presence of a PDA.

Suprasternal Long Axis View
- Define aortic arch anatomy (Fig. 10-7).
  - Size of the ascending aorta, transverse arch, and the upper descending aorta.
- Presence of a coarctation, and, in the case of severe coarctation, a juxtaductal posterior shelf is seen with an increased distance between the left carotid artery and the left subclavian artery. Doppler interrogation might not be very helpful in detecting the degree of coarctation in the presence of a large PDA.
- Presence of retrograde flow in the transverse arch and ascending aorta by Doppler interrogation in the presence of critical AV stenosis or atresia.
- Presence of a PDA and confirmation of ductal flow can also be performed from this view.

Suprasternal Short Axis View
- Arch sidedness and branching.
- Anomalous pulmonary venous return, especially to a vertical vein. In the presence of an intact AS and mitral atresia, the only egress of blood from the LA might be a levoatrial cardinal vein that crosses posterior to the left PA and most commonly drains into the left innominate vein. Other forms of anomalous pulmonary venous drainage are also seen in HLHS (6%).

- Any color flow from the venous system toward the transducer from the SSN view should prompt comprehensive investigation of anomalous pulmonary venous drainage.

Double-Inlet Left Ventricle

KEY POINTS

- Both atria connect through separate right and left atrioventricular valves (AVVs) to a ventricle of LV morphology.
- GVs are most commonly L-transposed, as seen from subcostal sagittal or apical sweep with the PA arising from the LV and the aorta arising from a bulboventricular foramen (BVF) located posteroinferiorly to the dominant ventricle seen.
- The BVF tends to restrict with time, leading to either systemic or pulmonary outflow tract obstruction.

Definition and Prevalence

The most common form of univentricular AV connection. It is defined as the presence of two AVVs committed to one ventricular chamber of LV morphology. DILV is associated with a rudimentary outlet chamber, the BVF. The inlet septum is absent, and both AVVs lie in fibrous continuity with a semilunar valve. The ventricles are L-looped, most commonly with the LV being the more posteroinferior and rightward chamber. The bulboventricle is thus located anterosuperiorly.

- Comprises less than 1% of CHD.
- Associated with situs ambiguous, asplenia/polysplenia.
- Associated with:
  - TGA (85%) typically L-looped (aorta anterior and leftward in relation to the PA).
  - Outflow tract obstruction.
- Aortic arch anomalies (25%) in TGA and a restrictive BVF.
- PS (25%) not associated with a restrictive BVF.
- Holmes heart refers to DILV with:
  - BVF located posteroinferior to the dominant ventricle.
  - Normally related GVs.

The purpose of the initial echocardiogram is to provide a complete anatomic survey and assess the underlying physiology. The basic anatomy of atrial and visceral situs and location of the cardiac apex must be defined. This information is best obtained from subcostal views. It is important to determine the presence of a straddling, atretic, or

stenotic AVV; the relationship of the GVs; the position and degree of restriction of the BVF leading to either systemic or pulmonary outflow tract obstruction; and the physiology of the PDA and other associated anomalies such as abnormal pulmonary or systemic venous connections.

Pertinent information is obtained from the standard views by 2D and Doppler.

Parasternal Long Axis View

- In the majority of cases, the LV will be the posterior chamber. In a Holmes heart, the LV is the more anterior chamber.
- With rightward or leftward angulation of the transducer, both AVVs are seen entering the LV. Note the presence of AV atresia or straddling of chordal attachments. It is important not to mistake this lesion for a large VSD and a dilated LV. In this case, the atrioventricular connection can be further elucidated by rotating to a parasternal short axis view.
- One great artery is seen arising from the LV and the other from the BVF. The latter might be difficult to visualize if it is severely hypoplastic. If the GVs are transposed, many of the echocardiographic findings of TGA can be seen. The GVs are in parallel with the PA posterior.
- The size of and degree of restriction across the BVF should be evaluated by 2D imaging and Doppler interrogation.

Parasternal Short Axis View

Assess relationship between the dominant LV and the BVF. As mentioned, in the majority of cases of DILV, the BVF is the more anterosuperior and leftward chamber. This is best seen as the transducer is angled toward the base of the heart.

- Commitment of both AVVs to the dominant ventricular chamber, architecture of the papillary muscles and the chordae tendineae.
- Relationship of the GVs. Usually seen as two circles as the transducer is angled toward the base if they are transposed. If the GVs are normally related as in a Holmes heart, then the aorta is seen in cross section, and the PA is seen to the right of the aorta in a longitudinal plane.
- Presence of size discrepancy between the AV and pulmonary valve.
- Presence of aortic/pulmonary atresia.
- Confluence of the PAs.
- Presence and physiology of the PDA from a high left parasternal view.
- Size and degree of restriction of the BVF. It is important to measure the BVF in two

orthogonal views to calculate cross-sectional area (major diameter × minor diameter × Π/4) because it is usually elliptical in shape. Patients with a BVF cross-sectional area of less than 2 cm^2/m^2 are at a higher risk of late obstruction.
- Ventricular systolic function.

Apical Four-Chamber Views (Fig. 10-8)
- This is the best view with which to evaluate the crux of the heart and to visualize the salient features of DILV: the two AVVs are connected to the LV without any intervening septum. Presence of a straddling, atretic, or stenotic AVV. The characteristic features of the LV are seen with fine apical trabeculations, smooth basal septal surface, and no septal chordal attachments.
- Right/left and anterior/posterior relationships between the LV and BVF.
- Relationship of the great arteries.
- Evaluate for systemic and pulmonary outflow tract obstruction.
- Degree of restriction across the BVF if the angle of interrogation can be aligned parallel to the flow.
- Stenosis of the AVVs. It is important to note that the degree of stenosis by spectral Doppler across the AVV is underestimated in the presence of an atrial-level communication. In this situation, stenosis can best be assessed by 2D imaging and the degree of mobility of the AVV leaflets.

Subcostal Four-Chamber Coronal View
- Situs, position of apex, atrioventricular connections.
- Ventricular morphology and the characteristic features of the dominant ventricle.
- Position and size of the BVF.
- Relationship of the GVs.
- Commitment of the AVVs.
- Presence and size of atrial-level communication, which is only important in the presence of an atretic or stenotic AVV.
- Evaluate systemic venous return (presence of interrupted inferior vena cava [IVC]).
- Evaluate pulmonary venous return and document the normal connections of four pulmonary veins (PVs) to the LA.

Subcostal Short Axis Sagittal View
- Information obtained from this view is similar to that obtained from the orthogonal coronal views. In addition, the short axis allows the evaluation of the AVVs in a short axis view.

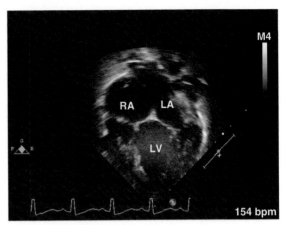

Figure 10-8. Double-inlet LV apical four chamber (4C) view. Both the RA and LA connect to the dominant LV through two separate AVVs. No inlet septum is seen between the two AVVs.

Suprasternal Notch View
- The aortic arch is assessed for obstruction or hypoplasia, especially when the aorta arises from the BVF and there is significant BVF obstruction.
- Aortic arch branching.
- Pulmonary venous return from the "crab" view.

Tricuspid Atresia

KEY POINTS

- Apical views show fibrous tissue replacing TV.
- Atrial septal defect (ASD)/patent foramen ovale (PFO) with right-to-left flow is necessary for survival.
- Varying degrees of RV hypoplasia seen from apical or short axis view.
- Most commonly the GVs are normally related and a perimembranous VSD is present.
- The physiology depends on the relationship of the GVs, the size of the VSD, and the degree of RVOT obstruction (RVOTO).
- Associated cardiac findings are coarctation of the aorta and left juxtaposition of the right atrial appendage (RAA).

In postoperative SV management, the echocardiogram is an important diagnostic tool in evaluating the adequacy of PBF and SBF (PA band gradient, aortic arch flow), ventricular function, atrioventricular regurgitation, restriction across the atrial-level communication, Glenn, Fontan pressures, and branch PA stenosis.

Definition and Prevalence
Absence of a direct connection between the RA and the RV. The atretic valve is usually muscular and rarely fibrous. An atrial-level communication,

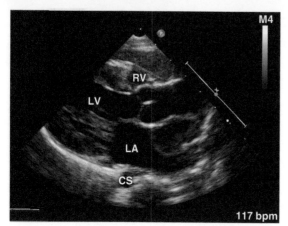

Figure 10-9. Tricuspid atresia (TA). Standard parasternal long axis view. Severely hypoplastic RV. Dilated coronary sinus (CS) suggestive of a persistent left superior vena cava.

either a secundum ASD or a PFO, is necessary for survival.

- TA is classified based on the relationship of the GVs and the degree of obstruction across the VSD.
  - I: normally related GVs (69%).
  - Ia: pulmonary atresia/intact ventricular septum.
  - Ib: PS/small VSD.
  - Ic: no PS/large VSD.
  - II: d-TGA.
  - IIa: pulmonary atresia/VSD.
  - IIb: PS/VSD.
  - IIc: no PS/VSD
  - III: L-TGA.
- Third most common form of cyanotic CHD (0.3%–0.7%).

The goal of the initial echocardiogram in TA is to provide a comprehensive evaluation of the anatomy and physiology, paying special attention to the absence of a direct communication between the RA and RV, the size of the VSD, relationship of the GVs, the size of the atrial-level communication, and the physiology of the PDA. In addition, associated anomalies should be ruled out such as left superior vena cava (LSVC), left juxtaposition of the RAA, and coarctation of the aorta. Associated findings are more common with transposed great arteries.

Pertinent information is obtained from the standard views.

Parasternal Long Axis View
- Size discrepancy between the two ventricles with a hypoplastic anterior RV and large posterior LV (Fig. 10-9).
- The TV is seen as a bright shelf or a plate in the floor of the right-sided atrium in

D-ventricular loop or the left-sided atrium in L-ventricular loop.
- Absence of antegrade flow across the TV can be documented using color Doppler with a low color scale.
- Size and position of the VSD.
- If the VSD is conoventricular, then deviation of the conal septum can best be seen from this view. Anterior deviation is usually seen with normally related GVs, whereas posterior deviation is seen with transposed GVs. In both cases, this may produce subpulmonary obstruction.
- Features of transposition are seen if TGA is present with the GVs in parallel. In d-TGA, the PA sweeps or dives posteriorly.
- In the case of left juxtaposition of the RAA, the AS is perpendicular to the posterior great artery.
- A dilated coronary sinus should raise the suspicion of a persistent LSVC.

Parasternal Short Axis View
- Further characterization of the hypoplastic RV. The RV is located superior to the LV and best seen at the papillary level.
- Size and degree of restriction across the VSD.
- Scan the ventricular septum (VS) from base to apex to assess for the presence of additional VSDs by 2D imaging and color Doppler. If additional VSDs are present, flow will be of low velocity because of the equal pressures in both ventricles. In this case, use a low Nyquist setting.
- Determine the presence of subpulmonary obstruction (in normally related GVs or L-TGA) or subaortic obstruction (in d-TGA).
- In the case of transposed GVs, the aorta and MPA can be seen in cross section with the aorta anterior and to the right of the MPA (d-TGA) or anterior and to the left of the MPA (L-TGA).
- Assess for hypoplasia of the PA and confluence of the branch PAs.
- Presence and physiology of the PDA from a high left parasternal view.
- Ventricular function.

Apical Four-Chamber View (Fig. 10-10)
- Appreciate the lack of direct connection between the RA and the RV and, by angling the transducer posteriorly, demonstrate the type of TA, i.e., muscular, echodense plate of tissue in the floor of the RA, or a fibrous fat-filled sulcus across the TV position.
- Evaluate the degree of RV hypoplasia and the size of the VSD.

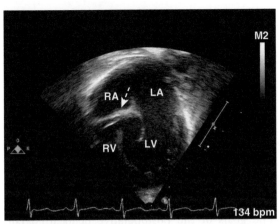

Figure 10-10. TA. Apical 4C view. Size discrepancy between the RV and LV. Severely hypoplastic RV. The tricuspid valve is replaced by fibrofatty tissue in the right atrioventricular sulcus seen as a thick plate of echoes (*arrow*).

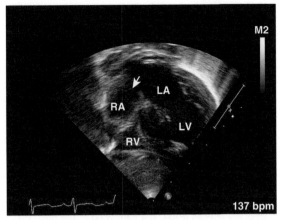

Figure 10-11. TA. Subxyphoid 4C view. Moderate-sized interatrial communication (*arrow*), platelike right atrioventricular junction, and a diminutive RV.

- Assess the relationship of the GVs by sweeping posterior to anterior at the level of the AVVs into the RVOT. A posterior GV that branches should raise the suspicion for TGA.
- Determine the presence of subpulmonary obstruction (in normally related GVs or L-TGA) or subaortic obstruction (in d-TGA) by sweeping anteriorly into the outflow tracts.
- Presence of abnormal septal configuration in the case of left juxtaposition of the RAA.

Subcostal Four-Chamber Coronal View
- Excellent view to determine abdominal viscera, atrial situs, ventricular looping, and relationship of the GVs. A posterior GV that branches should raise the suspicion for TGA.
- The AS is usually perpendicular to the transducer, allowing adequate visualization of the ASD; color Doppler will show right-to-left flow across the ASD. It is unusual for the ASD to be restrictive.
- Visualize the TV as a platelike structure with a hypoplastic RV (Fig. 10-11).
- Determine the size and presence of the VSD.
- Findings consistent with left juxtaposition of the RAA (if present).
  - Convexity of the RA to the left.
  - Superiorly, the AS wraps around the RA.
  - Small RA.
  - RAA courses from right to left posterior to the great arteries and anterior to the LA.

Subcostal Short Axis Sagittal View
- Careful sweeping from right to left allows assessment of the ASD, size of the RV, the VSD, and the degree of RVOTO (if present, secondary to anterior deviation of the outlet septum, muscular hypertrophy, or anomalous muscle bundles).
- Assess the degree of RVOTO by color Doppler and spectral Doppler; the Doppler beam will be parallel to RVOT flow.
- Evaluate ventricular function.

Suprasternal Long Axis View
- Evaluate the aortic arch by 2D imaging: ascending aorta and transverse arch dimensions, especially when there is associated TGA.
- Color Doppler interrogation of the arch may show retrograde filling of the arch with severe arch hypoplasia. Spectral Doppler interrogation will underestimate the gradient across a coarctation due to ductal filling distal to the coarctation.
- A large ductus is seen in the presence of a coarctation with mainly right-to-left flow from the MPA into the arch in systole and left-to-right flow in diastole.
  - In cases of pulmonary obstruction or atresia, the ductus is long and narrow, directed superior and posterior from the MPA to the aorta rather than its usual inferior and posterior direction.
- Pulmonary atresia with severe RV hypoplasia; there is loss of the typical isthmic narrowing.

Suprasternal Short Axis View
- Arch sidedness.
- Confluence and size of the branch PAs.
- Assess pulmonary venous drainage.
- Evaluate for persistent LSVC.

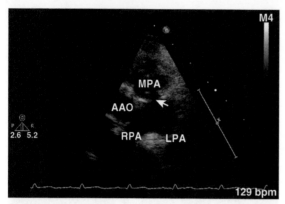

Figure 10-12. Parasternal short axis view of the branch pulmonary arteries (PAs). The narrowing at the main PA indicates the presence of a PA band (arrow).

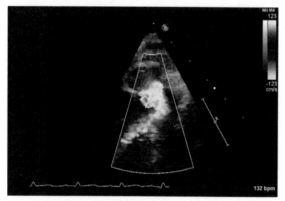

Figure 10-13. PA band. Parasternal short axis view of the branch PAs. Color Doppler shows aliasing of the jet at the site of the PA band.

Postoperative Evaluation

Echocardiographic evaluation following first-stage palliation includes the following:

Post-PA Band Placement

Evaluation of patients after PA banding involves the following.

* Visualizing and documenting appropriate placement of the band: echobright density across the MPA (Fig. 10-12).
* Assessing for migration of the band.
  * Most commonly toward the right PA, causing distortion of this branch.
  * Toward the pulmV encroaching on the valve leaflets.
* Assessing the tightness of the band:
  * Marked poststenotic dilation of the MPA.
  * PulmV leaflets may be echobright and thickened.
  * Assess the gradient across the PA band by color Doppler and spectral Doppler (Fig. 10-13).

* Systolic PA pressure (PAP) can be estimated in the case of a large VSD and no systemic outflow tract obstruction. Systolic blood pressure equals RV systolic pressure. Systolic PAP is obtained by subtracting the systolic blood pressure from the PA band gradient.

Post-PA Band Removal Assessment
* Residual narrowing may be seen by 2D imaging.
* Swirling is seen by color Doppler.

Norwood and Damus-Kaye-Stansel Procedures

The goals of the postoperative echocardiogram after a Norwood or Damus-Kaye-Stansel (DKS) procedure and before a bidirectional Glenn/Hemi-Fontan procedure are to evaluate for the following.

* Restriction of the interatrial communication.
  * Subcostal views.
  * Mean velocity across the atrial communication greater than 1 mm Hg.
* Obstruction across the DKS or the newly created aortic arch (Figure 10-14 shows the DKS procedure).
  * 2D images and Doppler of arch from the SSN view.
  * Assess pulsatility of the abdominal aorta from subcostal views.
* Obstruction or stenosis of the RV-PA conduit or the modified Blalock-Taussig (m-BT) shunt.
  * Proximal aspect of the RV-PA conduit is best seen from the parasternal long axis view angling toward the RVOT or from an apical 4C view.

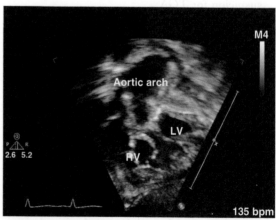

Figure 10-14. Damus-Kaye-Stansel (DKS) procedure. Subxyphoid short axis view demonstrating the patency of the DKS procedure into the aortic arch reconstruction.

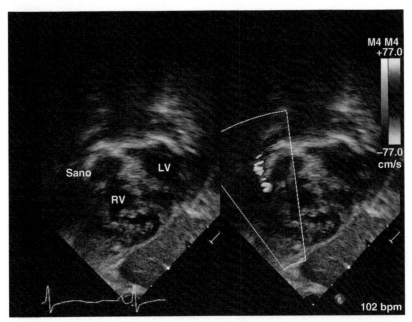

Figure 10-15. Sano shunt. Subxyphoid short axis view at the mid-ventricular level profiling the origin of the Sano shunt from the RV with color Doppler demonstrating aliasing through the proximal shunt.

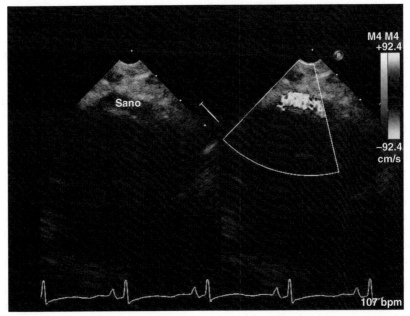

Figure 10-16. Sano shunt. High parasternal long axis view of the right ventricular outflow tract (RVOT) allows visualization of the proximal-to-mid Sano shunt.

- Optimal angle of interrogation for Doppler apical 4C view.
  - Distal aspect of the RV-PA conduit is best seen from a subcostal short axis view (Fig. 10-15), subxyphoid short axis view (Fig. 10-16), or high parasternal long axis view.
- Optimal angle of interrogation for Doppler SSN view.
  - The m-BT shunt is well visualized and traced from the SSN short axis view as it usually originates from the right innominate or right subclavian artery and connects distally to the right PA (Fig. 10-17).
- Optimal angle of interrogation: SSN.
- Distortion or stenosis of the branch PAs.
  - Optimal visualization and angle of interrogation: parasternal short axis, SSN short axis views.
- AVV regurgitation (AVVR).
  - Parasternal short axis, apical 4C views.

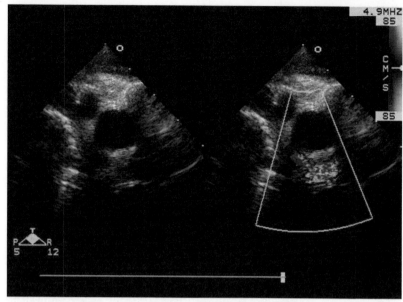

Figure 10-17. Modified Blalock-Taussig (m-BT) shunt. Suprasternal notch (SSN) cross-sectional view of the aorta. The insertion of the distal end of the m-BT shunt into the right PA is seen.

- Neo-AV insufficiency.
  - Parasternal long axis, apical 4C views.
- Ventricular systolic function.
  - Parasternal short axis, subcostal short axis views.

Hybrid Procedure

Hybrid palliation consists of surgical bilateral PA banding, combined with transcatheter balloon atrial septostomy and ductal stenting. It was recently introduced as a less invasive alternative to the Norwood procedure. It avoids the use of cardiopulmonary bypass, which may be associated with adverse neurologic events in the neonatal period. Experience with the hybrid procedure is limited but encouraging.

Post-Hybrid Procedure Assessment
- PA bands
  - As previously mentioned in the Post-PA Band Placement section.
- Ductal stent.
  - SSN and high left parasternal views (Fig. 10-18).

Echocardiographic Evaluation After Bidirectional Glenn/Hemi-Fontan Procedure

The goals of the echocardiogram after a bidirectional Glenn/Hemi-Fontan procedure and before a Fontan procedure completion are to evaluate for the following.

- Superior vena cava (SVC)/cavopulmonary anastomosis obstructions and PA branch distortion or obstruction.
  - High parasternal view, SSN.
  - Flow in the SVC and branch PAs by color Doppler and spectral Doppler is low velocity and phasic (decrease the Nyquist limit) (Figs. 10-19 and 10-20).
- Residual antegrade flow from the ventricle to the PA if the central PA was oversewn or tightly banded.
  - Parasternal views.
- Thrombi in the PA stump, especially if the pulmV leaflets have not been oversewn.
  - Parasternal views.
- Venovenous collaterals and aortic-to-pulmonary collaterals.
  - Detected by color Doppler mapping in the SSN views (decrease Nyquist limit).
  - By spectral Doppler flow is continuous throughout the cardiac cycle.
- Similar to the post-Norwood or DKS palliation echocardiogram, it is important to assess for restriction at the level of the atrial communication, AVVR, aortic arch obstruction (AAO), and ventricular function.

Echocardiographic Evaluation After Fontan Procedure Completion

The goals of the echocardiogram after completion of the Fontan procedure are to evaluate for the following.

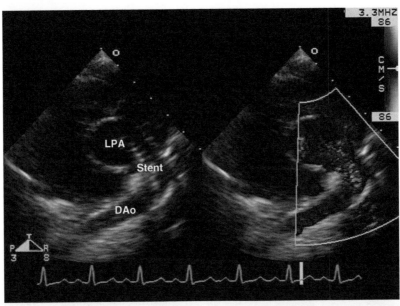

Figure 10-18. Bidirectional Glenn. Modified suprasternal notch imaging with the indicator at approximately the 12 o'clock position off slightly to the right side of the neck demonstrates color flow in the Glenn-PA anastomosis.

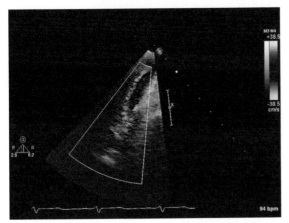

Figure 10-19. Bidirectional Glenn. Doppler profile of the bidirectional Glenn demonstrating low-velocity phasic flow.

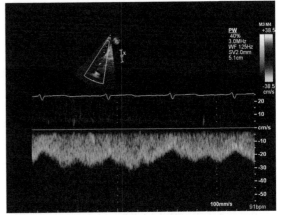

Figure 10-20. Fontan. Subxyphoid long axis image profiling the inferior vena cava connection to the Fontan pathway. The color Doppler interrogation demonstrates low-velocity laminar flow.

- Patency of the Fontan conduit (lateral or extracardiac).
  - Subcostal view can demonstrate the dilated IVC and the IVC-to-PA pathway (Fig. 10-21).
    - Assess for the presence of thrombus in the pathway (echodense material).
  - Flow in the conduit is interrogated from subcostal sagittal imaging and is low velocity and phasic.
  - Patency and size of the fenestration can be assessed by color Doppler from the apical views.
    - Measure the mean gradient across the fenestration by PW Doppler over several cardiac cycles from apical views (estimate of the transpulmonary gradient).

- Obstruction/narrowing in bidirectional Glenn/Hemi-Fontan procedure, as described previously.
- Obstruction in the pulmonary venous pathway because of improper baffle creation in the lateral tunnel or compression of the PVs by the extracardiac conduit.
  - Identify drainage and connection of all four PVs by 2D imaging color Doppler and spectral Doppler (SSN short axis, subcostal coronal, parasternal short axis views).
- Similar to post-Norwood and post-BDG echo assessments, it is important to assess AVVR, neo-AV insufficiency, ventricular function, presence of systemic venovenous collaterals, and aortic-to-pulmonary collaterals.

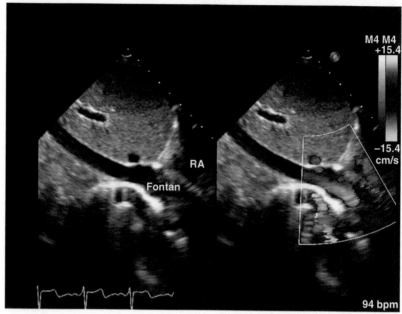

Figure 10-21. Hybrid palliation of HLHS. High left parasternal window profiling the struts of the ductal stent. Flow across the stent is noted in systole from the PA to the aorta.

Suggested Reading

1. Bevilacqua M, Sanders SP, Van Praagh S, et al. Double-inlet single left ventricle: echocardiographic anatomy with emphasis on the morphology of the atrioventricular valves and ventricular septal defect. *J Am Coll Cardiol.* 1991;18:559-568.
   It discusses the echocardiographic anatomy of DILV with special attention to the morphology, size, and function of the AVVs and VSD and their relationship to PS, aortic stenosis, and AAO.

2. Orie JD, Anderson C, Ettedgui JA, et al. Echocardiographic morphologic correlations in tricuspid atresia. *J Am Coll Cardiol.* 1995;26:750-758.
   It describes how TA in most cases is secondary to the absence of an RA-RV junction along with the associated findings in TA.

3. Fraisse A, Colan SD, Jonas RA, et al. Accuracy of echocardiography for detection of aortic arch obstruction after Stage I Norwood procedure. *Am Heart J.* 1998;135 (2 Pt 1):230-236.
   This study evaluates the accuracy of echo in the diagnosis of AAO after a stage I Norwood procedure, identifies echocardiographic predictors of arch obstruction, and examines the time course of its development. It shows that echo is a highly specific but poorly sensitive modality in detecting AAO after a stage I Norwood procedure. Early cardiac catheterization with possible intervention should be considered in patients with moderate or severe RV dysfunction, moderate or severe TR, or an abnormal abdominal Doppler flow pattern during that period.

4. Jacobs ML, Mayer Jr JE. Congenital Heart Surgery Nomenclature and Database Project: single ventricle. *Ann Thorac Surg.* 2000;69(Suppl 4):S197-S204.
   The STS-Congenital Heart Surgery Database Committee and the European Association for Cardiothoracic Surgery have proposed a classification that is relevant to surgical therapy.

5. Cook AC, Anderson RH. The anatomy of hearts with double inlet ventricle. *Cardiol Young.* 2006;16(Suppl 1): 22-26.

6. Munoz-Castellanos L, Espinola-Zavaleta N, Keirns C. Anatomoechocardiographic correlation double inlet left ventricle. *J Am Soc Echocardiogr.* 2005;18(3):237-243.
   Anatomoechocardiographic correlation between the morphologic features of equivalent anatomic specimens and the echocardiographic images of patients to provide a means of interpreting the image correctly and making a more precise diagnosis of the cardiac defect.

7. Cardis BM, Fyfe DA, Ketchum D, et al. Echocardiographic features and complications of the modified Norwood operation using the right ventricle to pulmonary artery conduit. *J Am Soc Echocardiogr.* 2005;18(6):660-665.

8. Galantowicz M, Cheatham JP. Lessons learned from the development of a new hybrid strategy for the management of hypoplastic left heart syndrome. *Pediatr Cardiol.* 2005;26:90-99.

9. Jacobs ML, Anderson RH. Nomenclature of the functionally univentricular heart. *Cardiol Young.* 2006;16(Suppl 1):3-8.
   It provides an anatomic distinction between the functionally univentricular heart or the functional SV and the hearts with an SV chamber.

10. Khairy P, Poirier N, Mercier LA. Univentricular heart. *Circulation.* 2007;115(6):800-812.
    An overview of the nomenclature and classification of the univentricular heart, epidemiology and pathological subtypes, genetic factors, physiology, clinical features, diagnostic assessment, therapy, and postoperative sequelae. The focus is on information of interest and relevance to the adult cardiologist and cardiac sonographer.

Right Heart Anomalies

11

Maggie L. Likes and Mark B. Lewin

Basic Principles

Right Ventricle
- There are three portions of a normally formed morphologic right ventricle (RV): inlet (supports the tricuspid valve [TV]), body (trabecular portion), and outlet (infundibulum or conal region).[1]
- The tripartite RV is loosely crescent shaped rather than conical shaped like the left ventricle (LV).
- Coarse muscular trabeculations and numerous small papillary muscles with attachments to both the septal and free walls further help to define a normal morphologic RV[2] (Fig. 11-1).

Right Heart
- Normally, the TV annulus is displaced slightly more apical than the mitral valve (MV) annulus.
- Embryologic aberrations can cause a wide variety of anomalies of the right heart including abnormalities of the TV and pulmonary valve (pulmV).

Ebstein's Anomaly

Background
- Ebstein's anomaly (or malformation) is characterized by an increased downward (apical) displacement of the TV annulus caused by failure of delamination of the posterior and septal leaflets.[3]
- There is subsequent variable thinning of the wall of the "atrialized" RV (aRV) along with redundancy and tethering of the anterior leaflet of the TV.
- The clinical manifestations of Ebstein's anomaly depend largely on the degree of severity of the TV displacement and the resultant physiologic effects.
- Right ventricular function becomes impaired and the abnormal TV becomes regurgitant, resulting in decreased forward flow through the pulmV.
- The combined right atrium (RA) and aRV becomes dilated with resultant right-to-left shunt across the interatrial septum (IAS).
- Clinically, infants with severe Ebstein's anomaly will present with extreme cyanosis, cardiomegaly, and heart failure.
- Most patients with Ebstein's anomaly will have other associated cardiac lesions. The most common associated lesion is an atrial septal communication, usually a patent foramen ovale (PFO), or secundum atrial septal defect (ASD). Other associated lesions include pulmV stenosis or atresia, ventricular septal defect (VSD), tetralogy of Fallot (TOF), left ventricular noncompaction (LVN), coarctation of the aorta (Ao), as well as other left-sided heart lesions. In congenitally corrected transposition of the great arteries (cc-TGA), the systemic left-sided TV may have some degree of Ebstein's anomaly[3-5] (Fig. 11-2).

Overview of Echocardiographic Approach
- The majority of clinically important information will be acquired with transthoracic two-dimensional (2D) imaging. The remaining physiologic data can be obtained with spectral and color Doppler.
- The goal of imaging is to define the anatomy associated with Ebstein's anomaly and to describe the severity of the lesion.
- Ebstein's anomaly can be diagnosed prenatally with fetal echocardiography (echo) (Table 11-1).

Anatomic Imaging
Acquisition
- Transthoracic echo (TTE) in the neonate is the diagnostic gold standard and defines the severity of Ebstein's anomaly.
- Parasternal long axis and short axis (PLAX and PSAX), subcostal long axis and short axis

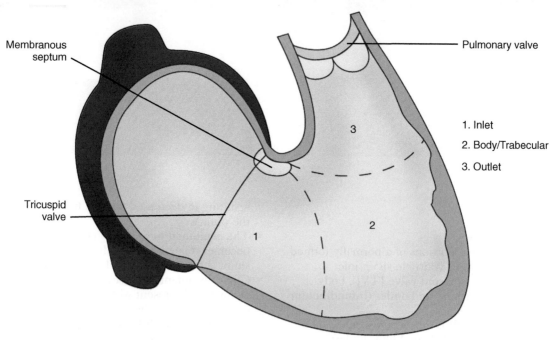

Figure 11-1. Schematic of a tripartite right ventricle (RV): inlet (1), body or trabecular portion (2), and outlet (3). Oriented toward the right ventricular aspect of the interventricular septum with the free wall of the RV removed. The inlet portion borders the tricuspid valve (TV), whereas the outlet portion borders the pulmonary valve (pulmV). The body contains the muscular or trabecular portion of the RV.

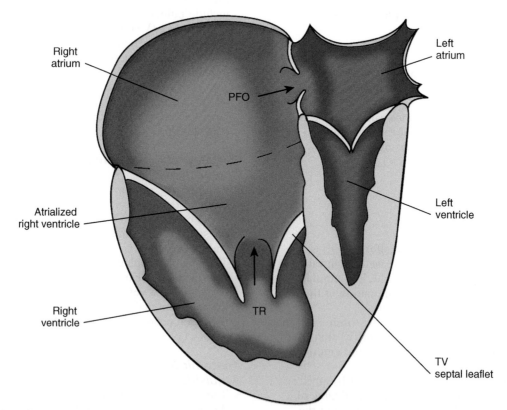

Figure 11-2. Schematic of Ebstein's anomaly in an apical four-chamber (A4C) view. Note the apically displaced TV septal leaflet, enlargement of the right atrium (RA) with the atrialized portion of the RV (aRV). There is usually tricuspid regurgitation (TR) as well as a right-to-left shunt across a patent foramen ovale (PFO). *(From Otto CM. Textbook of Clinical Echocardiography, 4th ed. Philadelphia: Saunders/Elsevier, 2009.)*

TABLE 11-1 EBSTEIN'S ANOMALY ECHOCARDIOGRAPHIC APPROACH

	Details	Acquisition	Image Planes	Analysis	Comments/Tips
Anatomic Imaging					
TV	Septal leaflet displacement	TTE, fetal	A4C, fetal 4C	Measure from MV hinge point to TV septal leaflet hinge point	Normal < 0.8 cm/m^2 Ebstein's > 0.8 cm/m^2
	Septal leaflet attachments	TTE	PLAX, PSAX, A4C, SC	Free edges and chordal attachments Hinge point as above	
	Anterior leaflet	TTE	PLAX, PSAX, A4C, SC	Hinge point seen from A4C, chordal attachments, and free edges from others	Anterior leaflet is often large and redundant, can cause RVOTO
	Posterior leaflet	TTE	SC sagittal	Hinge point, free edges, and chordal attachments	May be apically displaced
	Annulus Z score	TTE	A4C	Measure from anterior TV leaflet hinge point to the septal surface	Measurement of the "true" TV annulus
RA	Dilatation	TTE, fetal	A4C, fetal 4C, PSAX, SC	Degree of dilatation, often profound	
IAS	PFO, ASD	TTE, fetal	SC coronal, PSAX, fetal 4C	Size of ASD if present	
Great Ormond Street ratio	Severity score	TTE	A4C in diastole	(RA + aRV)/(RV + LA + LV)	Grade 1 < 0.5, Grade 2 = 0.5–0.99 Grade 3 = 1–1.49, Grade 4 > 1.5
PDA	Presence	TTE	SSN, "ductal"	Measure size of PDA if present	
Associated lesions	Rule out	TTE	All views	Look for associated cardiac lesions	PS/PA, VSD, TOF, LVN CoA, other left heart lesions, cc-TGA
Physiologic Data					
IAS	Shunt flow	Color, PW Doppler	SC, PSAX, fetal 4C	Determine direction and velocity of shunting across IAS	Often is right-to-left shunting
TR/TS	Severity	Color, CW Doppler	A4C, PLAX/SAX SC	Determine severity of TR/TS, estimated pressure gradient	May have to decrease Nyquist limit to capture low-velocity TR
PulmV	PS/PI	Color, PW Doppler, CW Doppler	PLAX/SAX, SC anterior apical	Note any forward flow across pulmV as well as PI or PS	Take note of the "circular" shunt Rule out RVOTO with large anterior TV leaflet
Ventricular function	RV and LV	2D, M-mode	A4C, PSAX	Note size and wall motion of RV	LV function may be impaired due to large RV or LVN

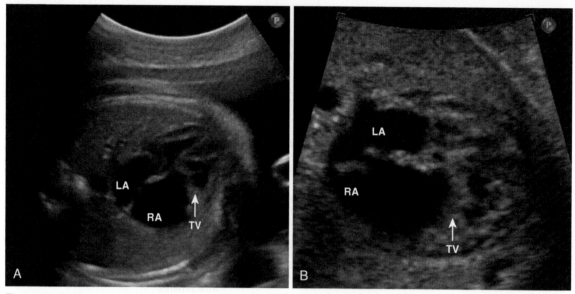

Figure 11-3. Fetal images of Ebstein's anomaly. **A,** Fetal 4C view of Ebstein's anomaly. Note apically displaced TV, dilated RA as well as slightly enlarged cardiothoracic ratio. **B,** Magnification of fetal 4C view of the same patient.

(SCLAX and SCSAX), and apical four-chamber (A4C) views are the most useful imaging planes to visualize the RA, IAS, TV, RV, and pulmV.

- Transesophageal echo (TEE) is used intraoperatively to assess the adequacy of the surgical repair.
- In the adult patient with Ebstein's anomaly, TTE is usually adequate to visualize the right heart. However, TEE may be required if the TV leaflets are difficult to visualize with TTE.
- In fetal echo, the TV abnormality is best seen in the 4C view. The cardiothoracic ratio is also useful to demonstrate the extreme cardiomegaly seen with Ebstein's anomaly (Fig. 11-3).

Analysis

- The septal TV leaflet (and the posterior/inferior leaflet in severe forms) is apically displaced relative to the anterior leaflet of the MV. A displacement more than 0.8 cm/m^2 is diagnostic of Ebstein's anomaly. The A4C view best demonstrates the displacement and allows for measurement[6] (Fig. 11-4).
- The profound right atrial dilation characteristic of Ebstein's anomaly may best be seen in the A4C view, parasternal short axis view, and the subcostal view.
- Define the anatomy of the TV anterior, septal, and posterior leaflets (including attachments, tethering, dysplasia, and redundancy). The TV is best visualized from parasternal long

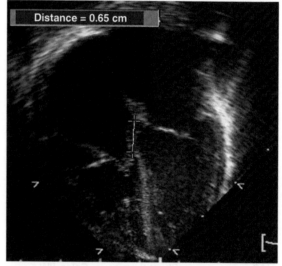

Figure 11-4. A4C view. The measurement of the TV apical displacement is shown from the mitral valve hinge point to the septal leaflet of the TV hinge point. Normal displacement is considered less than 0.8 cm/m^2. Ebstein's anomaly is defined by displacement greater than 0.8 cm/m^2. This patient's displacement of 0.65 cm is 3.6 cm/m^2 and diagnostic for Ebstein's anomaly.

axis and short axis, A4C, and subcostal views.[5] Using an anatomic classification described by Carpentier et al.,[7] a type A, B, C, or D category may be designated (Table 11-2). This classification can be helpful to the surgeon when considering whether to repair the TV[6] (Fig. 11-5).

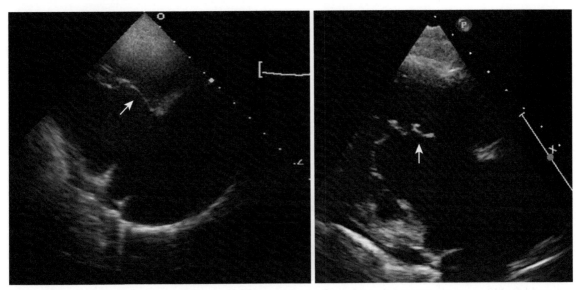

Figure 11-5. Parasternal long axis (PLAX) view angled toward the TV. The large and redundant anterior TV leaflet is seen well in this view in two different patients with Ebstein's anomaly. The *arrows* depict the anterior TV leaflet.

TABLE 11-2	ANATOMIC CLASSIFICATION
Type A	Septal and posterior leaflet adherance without functional RV restriction of volume
Type B	Atrialized RV with normal anterior leaflet hinge point
Type C	Anterior leaflet stenosis
Type D	RV entirely atrialized except for a small infundibulum

Data from Carpentier A, Chauvaud S, Mace L, et al. A new reconstructed operation for Ebstein's anomaly of the tricuspid valve. *J Thorac Cardiovasc Surg.* 2006;132: 1285–1290.

- Three-dimensional (3D) TTE may be useful to further define leaflet attachments and tethering.[8]
- The echocardiographic assessment of severity can be measured using the Great Ormond Street (GOS) ratio described by Celermajer et al.[9] The ratio is obtained from the A4C view in end-diastole. It is the ratio of the area of the RA plus the area of the aRV compared with the area of the functional RV plus the left atrial and left ventricular areas (RA + aRV)/(RV + LA + LV). The increasing grade of severity is grade 1, ratio less than 0.5; grade 2, ratio 0.5 to 0.99; grade 3, ratio 1 to 1.49; grade 4, ratio greater than 1.5. Grades 3 and 4 have an increased risk of mortality[9] (Fig. 11-6).
- Other important anatomic features to define include the normalized dimension of the TV annulus via Z score (usually at the level of the anterior leaflet proximal hinge points, where the true tricuspid annulus is located), the size of the ASD (if present), the presence or absence of a patent ductus arteriosus (PDA), and other associated cardiac anomalies (discussed previously).[10]

Pitfalls
- It is sometimes difficult to distinguish isolated TV dysplasia from true Ebstein's anomaly. In TV dysplasia, the functional right ventricular chamber is usually larger and the TV orifice is directed to the apex of the RV. In Ebstein's anomaly, the functional RV is usually smaller and the TV orifice is directed to the right ventricular outflow tract (RVOT).
- Right ventricular dysplasia can cause significant right atrial and right ventricular enlargement that can mimic Ebstein's anomaly. In right ventricular dysplasia, however, there will not be an apical displacement of the septal leaflet of the TV.[11]

Physiologic Data
Acquisition
- After a thorough description of the anatomy of Ebstein's anomaly has been achieved, the physiologic characteristics of the lesion should be delineated.
- The use of pulsed wave (PW) Doppler, continuous wave (CW) Doppler, and color Doppler is of paramount importance to define the direction of blood flow through the heart: either forward flow through the RV and out the pulmV or reverse flow across the IAS to

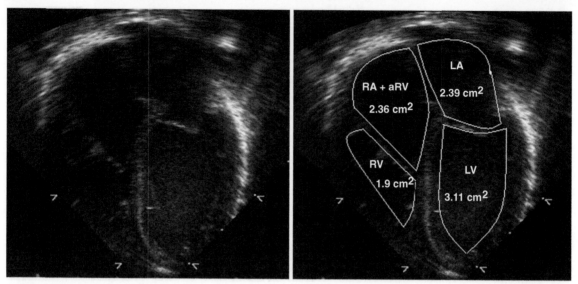

Figure 11-6. A4C view without and with the Great Ormond Street (GOS) ratio measurements. The ratio is the area of the RA + aRV divided by the area of the RV + LA + left ventricle. Severity is graded from 1 to 4 with 4 being the most severe. Grade 1 is a ratio less than 0.5; grade 4 is a ratio more than 1.5. In this patient, the GOS ratio is 0.32, which is a grade 1 on the severity scale. Clinically, this patient has been followed serially and has not required any interventions to date.

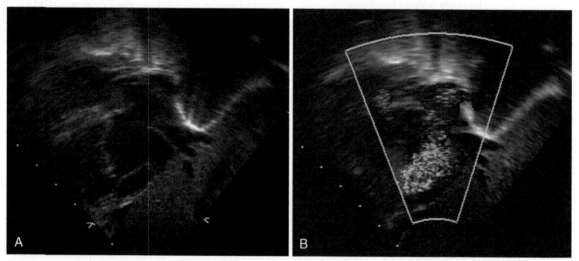

Figure 11-7. Subcostal (SC) view of an atrial septal defect (ASD) in a patient with severe Ebstein's anomaly. **A,** Two-dimensional (2D) image demonstrating a dilated RA and a large atrial communication. **B,** Color flow Doppler demonstrating right-to-left flow across the interatrial septum (IAS).

the LV, out the aortic valve (AV) and then across the PDA.
- Parasternal, subcostal, and apical views are important to visualize IAS flow and valvular stenosis or regurgitation. The suprasternal notch (SSN) views along with the "ductal" view will help to define PDA flow (if present).

Analysis
- Focusing on the IAS from either the subcostal or parasternal view, use color Doppler along with PW Doppler to demonstrate the direction and velocity of shunting across the ASD. There is usually right-to-left atrial-level shunting in hemodynamically significant Ebstein's anomaly (Fig. 11-7).

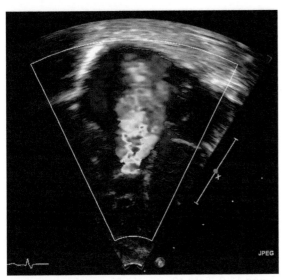

Figure 11-8. A4C view with color Doppler across the TV in a patient with Ebstein's anomaly. Note the severe TR that originates at the coaptation point of the apically displaced TV leaflets.

- From the A4C view as well as the parasternal and subcostal views, use color Doppler to demonstrate the severity of TV regurgitation (TR) and/or stenosis (TS). Use CW Doppler of the tricuspid regurgitant jet to estimate functional right ventricular pressure (Fig. 11-8).
- Investigate the pulmV with color Doppler, PW Doppler, and CW Doppler for forward flow, insufficiency, and stenosis from the parasternal short axis and long axis views as well as the subcostal views. This may be seen from an anteriorly directed apical view as well. Take special care to note pulmonary insufficiency (PI) in the setting of tricuspid regurgitation (TR), right-to-left atrial-level shunting, and left-to-right ductal shunting (the so-called circular shunt). Also pay special attention to the RVOT, as a large, redundant anterior leaflet of the TV can cause RV outflow tract obstruction (RVOTO). Some patients may exhibit "functional" pulmonary stenosis (PS) in which the valve leaflets fail to open in the setting of reduced right ventricular output and accompanying elevated pulmonary artery pressure (PAP) of the newborn. Pulmonary regurgitation can be a tip-off that the pulmonary valve will in fact eventually open when the PAP incrementally decreases.
- Right and left ventricular function should be evaluated. Pay attention to the size and wall motion of the RV. Measure left ventricular shortening fraction with M-mode

measurements from the parasternal short axis view at the level of the papillary muscles.
- TEE can be helpful in the setting of surgical repair of Ebstein's anomaly (TV repair/replacement or RV exclusion). The preoperative assessment should be used to confirm the anatomy found on TTE and further define the TV attachments if needed. Postoperatively, it is important to assess the TV repair (residual TR or TS) or the right ventricular exclusion patch fenestration depending on the surgical repair or palliation. Evaluate the IAS, ventricular function, MV pulmV function, and the PDA (if applicable) as well.

Pitfalls
- TR may be difficult to visualize if there are low-velocity jets. Remember to lower the Nyquist limit to investigate the TV fully. There may also be regurgitant jets through fenestrations of the anterior leaflet.[5]

Alternate Approaches
- Usually a complete diagnosis can be made based on echocardiographic data alone in Ebstein's anomaly.
- On rare occasions, if there are anatomic questions unable to be answered by echo (TTE or TEE), other imaging modalities can be considered including MRI or cardiac catheterization. Catheterization is particularly important if hemodynamic data are required.

KEY POINTS

- Ebstein's anomaly is characterized by an increased apical displacement of the TV annulus caused by failure of delamination of the posterior and septal leaflets.
- The TV is often regurgitant into the atrialized portion of the RV, causing severe right atrial enlargement and right-to-left flow across an ASD.
- The clinical manifestations of Ebstein's anomaly depend largely on the severity of the TV displacement and the resultant physiologic effects. Infants with severe Ebstein's anomaly will present with extreme cyanosis, cardiomegaly, and heart failure.
- The echocardiogram is crucial for accurate diagnosis and prognostic interpretation of disease severity.
- Key features on the echocardiogram include anatomy of the TV leaflets, degree of TR and/or stenosis, degree of right atrial enlargement, shunting across the IAS, PDA flow, ventricular function, and other associated cardiac lesions.

Pulmonary Atresia with Intact Ventricular Septum

Background

- Pulmonary atresia with intact ventricular septum (PA/IVS) is a rare and unique clinical entity in which the pulmV is atretic or imperforate and there is no interventricular communication.
- This combination of cardiac lesions leads to a spectrum of clinical disease.
- On the severe end of the spectrum, the pulmV is imperforate and the RV is severely hypoplastic. The TV is often dysplastic and hypoplastic as well. Due to the lack of egress of antegrade right ventricular blood flow, the right ventricular pressure is often suprasystemic. There is a higher incidence of coronary sinusoids from the RV in this scenario.
- RV-dependent coronary circulation (RVDCC) occurs in a small proportion of patients with PA/IVS. There may be stenosis that develops within the coronary artery system as well as ostial stenosis or atresia at the aortic cusp.[5] As a result, the normal perfusion from oxygenated blood through the coronary arteries cannot take place. Instead, the perfusion to the myocardium becomes partially supplied by deoxygenated blood from the RV through coronary fistulous connections from persistent sinusoids. The presence of RVDCC has important clinical implications discussed further below.
- On the less severe end of the spectrum, patients can have pulmV atresia with a large or even dilated RV. These patients are less likely to have coronary sinusoids and more likely to have severe TR.
- Patients will initially require an intervention, either catheter based or surgical, to establish pulmonary blood flow (PBF). Depending on the severity of the lesion, including the presence or absence of RVDCC, the patient may eventually have a two-ventricle repair or a staged 1.5-ventricle or single-ventricle (SV) palliation.[12–14]

Overview of Echocardiographic Approach

TTE plays an integral role in defining the anatomy and clinical severity of patients with pulmonary atresia with IVS (Table 11-3).

- PA/IVS can be diagnosed prenatally with fetal echo (Fig. 11-9).
- The goal of echo is to delineate the severity of right ventricular hypoplasia and related anatomy to help elucidate the physiology.

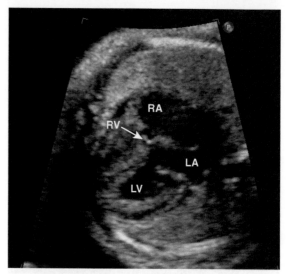

Figure 11-9. Fetal 4C view of a 26-week fetus with pulmonary atresia with intact ventricular septum (IVS) with a severely hypoplastic RV and TV.

- In this lesion in particular, echo plays a complementary role to invasive diagnostic and interventional cardiac catheterization. One major complication of severe PA/IVS, RVDCC, cannot be identified with echo alone. The presence of RVDCC eliminates the possibility of a two-ventricle repair or a 1.5-ventricle palliation via opening the pulmV either surgically or interventionally and decompressing the RV.

Anatomic Imaging
Acquisition

- TTE in the neonate is the first step in imaging to making the diagnosis of PA/IVS.
- The initial 2D imaging should include defining the severity of right ventricular hypoplasia, measuring the TV Z score, evaluating the atretic pulmV and RVOT anatomy, identifying the main pulmonary artery (MPA) and branch pulmonary arteries, and identifying other associated lesions including a PFO and PDA.
- Parasternal, apical, and subcostal views will be the most helpful planes with which to begin to define the anatomy of PA/IVS.

Analysis

- As stated previously, the RV can be severely hypoplastic to severely dilated. The A4C view is a good place to start to get a sense of the size of the RV as well as the size of the inflow

TABLE 11-3   PULMONARY ATRESIA WITH IVS—ECHOCARDIOGRAPHIC APPROACH

	Details	Acquisition	Image Planes	Analysis	Comments/Tips
Anatomic Imaging					
RV	Hypoplasia	TTE, fetal	Apical, parasternal, SC	Degree of hypoplasia or dilatation, evaluate function	Determine whether it is tripartite
TV	Annulus Z score	TTE, fetal	Apical, PLAX	Measure annulus from hinge points of the TV leaflets	Measure in two planes
RVOT	Anatomy	TTE	PLAX, PSAX, SC	Presence of an RVOT and degree of hypoplasia	Note proximity to atretic pulmV
PulmV	Leaflets, annulus	TTE, fetal	PLAX, PSAX, en-face view	Thickened and fused valve leaflets	High PSAX for en-face view
MPA, branch PAs	Sizes, confluence	TTE, fetal	SSN, PSAX	Diameter of MPA and branch PAs, confluence of PAs	Report Z scores
Associated lesions	Presence	TTE, fetal	All views	PFO or ASD, PDA	Left heart lesions rare
Physiologic Data					
PV	Atresia	Color	PLAX, PSAX, SC	Antegrade blood flow or insufficiency is not atretic pulmV	Lower Nyquist limit
TV	Regurgitation	Color, CW Doppler	Apical, PSLAX	Degree of TR and peak TR velocity	Dilated RV likely to have significant TR
Coronary arteries	Origins and course	2D, color Doppler	PSAX	Demonstrate direction of proximal coronary blood flow	If there is RVDCC, normal coronary flow may not be present
Coronary sinusoids	Presence	Color Doppler	Apical, parasternal, SC	If present, does not indicate RVDCC without catheterization	Lower Nyquist limit
Ventricular function	RV and LV	2D, M-mode	Apical, PSAX	Look for regional wall motion abnormalities	
PFO or ASD	Shunt	Color, PW Doppler	SC, PSAX, fetal 4C	Determine direction and velocity of shunting across IAS	Shunt is usually right to left
PDA	Shunt	Color, PW Doppler	SSN, "ductal"	Demonstrate direction and velocity	PA/IVS is a "ductal dependent" lesion, flow should be left to right

portion. By using multiple imaging plane sweeps (parasternal, subcostal), determine whether the RV is tripartite (inflow, body, and outflow) (Fig. 11-10).

- The majority of patients who have hypoplasia of the RV will also have hypoplasia of the TV.[14] Measure the annulus of the TV from the apical and parasternal long axis planes (with Z score). The Z score of the TV and the degree of right ventricular hypoplasia will influence the type of clinical management; single ventricle versus two-ventricle palliation or repair[13] (Fig. 11-11).
- Evaluate the RVOT from PLAX, PSAX, and SC views. Determine whether there is a well-formed infundibulum, a moderately hypoplastic RVOT that tapers down but ends in close proximity to the atretic pulmV or a severely hypoplastic RVOT (muscular pulmonary atresia) that terminates remotely from the pulmV. These details are important to the interventionalist if consideration is being given to opening the pulmV with radiofrequency perforation and balloon valvuloplasty.
- Image the pulmV and describe the appearance of the valve leaflets. Determine if there are thickened and fused leaflets with a well-formed pulmonary annulus. Measure the diameter of the pulmV annulus. An en face

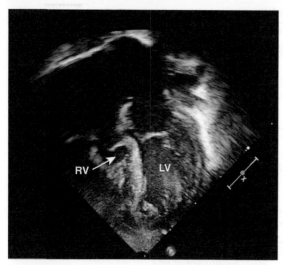

Figure 11-10. Apical view. Note the severely hypoplastic RV. A small inlet portion of the RV is seen in this image.

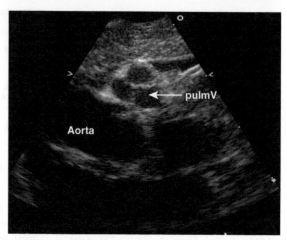

Figure 11-12. High parasternal view with transducer rotated away from the aortic valve to bring the pulmV into an "en face" view. This is an image of an atretic pulmV. There are three cusps to the valve seen with slightly thickened leaflets. The leaflets were completely fused.

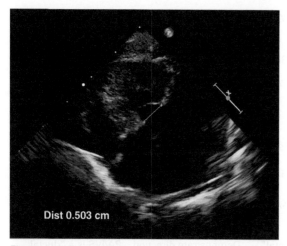

Figure 11-11. PLAX view angled down toward the TV. The TV annulus measures 0.5 cm in this patient, which is a Z score of −3.5.

view of the pulmV can be obtained in a high parasternal short axis view by rotating the transducer away from the aortic valve until the pulmV comes into view (Fig. 11-12).

- Image the MPA segment as well as the presence or absence of confluent branch PAs. Measure the diameter of the MPA and branch PAs with the Z score. The SSN and PSAX view may be the most helpful.
- Identify other associated cardiac lesions including a PFO or an ASD and a PDA. It is extremely uncommon to have left-sided cardiac lesions (like coarctation of the aorta) and PA/IVS. There may rarely be left ventricular outflow tract obstruction seen

due to bowing of the interventricular septum from a suprasystemic RV.

Pitfalls
- If the RV is severely dilated, there will likely be significant TR when evaluated with color Doppler. Obtain focused images of the TV leaflets and attachments paying attention to leaflet function and coaptation.

Physiologic Data
Acquisition
- After the anatomy has been carefully described with thorough 2D imaging, the physiologic data gathered with color Doppler and spectral Doppler will further delineate the severity of PA/IVS.

Analysis
- The first step is to determine whether the pulmV is functionally or completely atretic. Use color Doppler across the pulmV with a low Nyquist limit to evaluate for any evidence of antegrade PBF or PI (Fig. 11-13).
- Evaluate the degree of TR with color Doppler. A dilated RV will likely have significant TR, whereas a hypoplastic TV and RV may have very little TR. If present, use CW Doppler to obtain a peak TR velocity to estimate right ventricular pressure (including an estimate of right atrial pressure).
- In the PSAX view, identify the origins and proximal course of the right and left coronary arteries with 2D imaging and color Doppler. Attempt to demonstrate the direction of

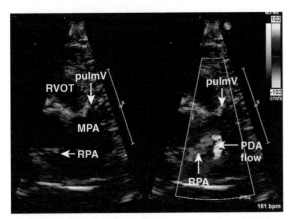

Figure 11-13. Parasternal short axis (PSAX) view angled up to the pulmV with a side-by-side comparison with 2D imaging and color Doppler. There is a thick and atretic pulmV without any antegrade blood flow. There is left-to-right ductal blood flow seen entering the main pulmonary artery (MPA). The right PA (RPA) is seen being filled by ductal blood flow.

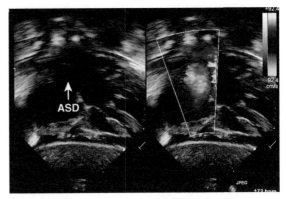

Figure 11-14. SC view of the IAS in a patient with PA/IVS. Note that a large ASD is present. This patient underwent a balloon atrial septostomy shortly after birth. On color Doppler interrogation, laminar right-to-left flow across the ASD is seen.

proximal coronary blood flow. Take note that if there is RVDCC, there may not be normal proximal coronary blood flow in one or both of the coronary arteries.

- Attempt to demonstrate coronary sinusoids. With the Nyquist limit turned very low, it is sometimes possible to capture the flow of coronary sinusoids over the right ventricular myocardium. If they are present, if does not necessarily indicate RVDCC. A cardiac catheterization must be performed with a right ventricular injection. However, patients with tricuspid annulus Z scores greater than −2.5 are less likely to have coronary sinusoids and RVDCC by catheterizations.[16]
- Assess right and left ventricular function, paying attention to regional wall motion abnormalities.
- Evaluate the direction of flow across the IAS using color Doppler. There is a right-to-left shunt in patients with PA/IVS. Take note of color turbulence at the defect indicating a possible restrictive IAS. Use PW Doppler to interrogate the peak velocity across the defect. Also note whether there is one or multiple defects (Fig. 11-14).
- Patients with PA/IVS are dependent on a PDA for PBF. Use color Doppler and spectral Doppler to interrogate the PDA. The flow should be left to right.

Pitfalls

- With the large amount of left-to-right flow across a PDA, there may not be any antegrade PBF seen even if the pulmV is only

functionally atretic. Take special care to look for PI for a clue that the valve may in fact open.

Alternate Approaches

- Cardiac catheterization is used as a diagnostic tool to identify RVDCC. Catheterization also is used interventionally to open the pulmV when there is a formed RVOT and valve plate that will lend itself to either crossing through a small opening or via radiofrequency perforation and balloon valvuloplasty. This procedure may be attempted once RVDCC is excluded.

Key Points
• PA/IVS is a rare and unique clinical entity in which the pulmV is atretic or imperforate and there is no interventricular communication.
• There is a spectrum of disease severity seen ranging from a severely hypoplastic RV and TV to a dilated RV and regurgitant TV.
• In this lesion in particular, echo plays a complementary role to invasive diagnostic and possibly interventional cardiac catheterization because one major but rare complication, RVDCC, cannot be diagnosed with echo alone.
• Goals of 2D imaging should include defining the severity of right ventricular hypoplasia, measuring the TV Z score, evaluating the atretic pulmV and RVOT anatomy, identifying the MPA and branch PAs, and identifying other associated lesions including a PFO and PDA.
• Use color Doppler across the pulmV with a low Nyquist limit to evaluate for any evidence of antegrade PBF or PI.

Pulmonary Stenosis

Background

- PS encompasses valvar PS as well as subvalvar and supravalvar PS[17] (Fig. 11-15).
- A normal pulmV is trileaflet and opens/coapts well.
- Most causes of native pulmV stenosis are congenital. Isolated pulmV stenosis can occur due to three typical valve types: doming pulmV (most commonly fusion of valve leaflets), dysplastic pulmV (thickened leaflets with poor mobility), or an abnormal number of cusps (unicuspid, bicuspid, quadricuspid). The latter form of pulmV stenosis is usually seen in conjunction with other forms of congenital heart disease (CHD) rather than in isolation.
- PulmV stenosis is also seen with several genetic syndromes or disorders including Noonan syndrome, Alagille syndrome, Williams syndrome, and congenital rubella.
- Stenosis may occur below the pulmV (subvalvar) in association with other CHD such as TOF or as a result of the development of infundibular muscle bundle hypertrophy (double-chamber RV [DCRV]) because of concomitant VSD jet lesions and right ventricular hypertension. Other rare causes of RVOT obstruction include hypertrophic cardiomyopathy or an infiltrative process such as Pompe disease.[16]
- Stenosis above the pulmV (supravalvar) may occur in association with the mentioned genetic disorders as well as in isolation.
- Most patients with PS are asymptomatic, even with moderate to severe stenosis. Mild PS does not tend to progress outside of the neonatal period and may improve over time.
- Those patients with moderate to severe disease with or without symptoms may benefit from catheter-based or surgical valve opening based on well-documented recommendations by the American College of Cardiology and the American Heart Association (ACC/AHA).[17]
- The dysplastic type of pulmV stenosis usually is not amenable to catheter-based valvuloplasty and requires surgical intervention.
- Clinical consequences of PS include right ventricular hypertrophy (RVH), increased right ventricular systolic and diastolic pressures, and eventual right-to-left shunting across a PFO if one is present. The degree of RVH and upstream effects is related to the severity of the stenosis.
- Neonates with critical PS are at the severe end of the spectrum for this disease process. They present with cyanosis from right-to-left atrial-level shunting and have PDA-dependent PBF with suprasystemic right ventricular pressure.

Overview of Echocardiographic Approach

- PS can be diagnosed with fetal echo as well as TTE (Fig. 11-16).
- The echocardiographer should attempt to demonstrate the morphology of the pulmV, the degree of stenosis, the degree of RVH, evaluate for TR and atrial-level shunting.
- The precise data obtained by echo will largely dictate the clinical management to follow (Table 11-4).

Anatomic Imaging
Acquisition

- TTE of the neonate or child is usually the mainstay for the initial diagnosis and grading of severity.

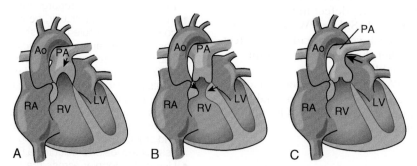

Figure 11-15. Three anatomic types of pulmonary stenosis (PS). **A,** Valvar PS. **B,** Subvalvar PS. **C,** Supravalvar PS. Note that there can be a combination of these lesions as well. (*From Park MK. Pediatric Cardiology for Practitioners, 4th ed. St. Louis, MO: Mosby; 2002; Figure 13-1.*)

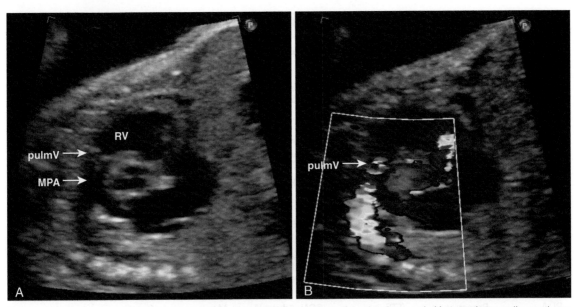

Figure 11-16. Images of fetal pulmV stenosis. This is a 27-week fetus found to have pulmV stenosis as well as at least moderate TV regurgitation and right atrial dilation. **A,** 2D image of a thickened and hypoplastic pulmV (4 mm; Z score −3.2). The main PA (MPA) and branch PAs were normal size. **B,** Color Doppler across the pulmV with flow turbulence at the valve. The peak velocity obtained was 3.2 m/s.

- The pulmV is best visualized in the PSAX and PLAX views. It may also been seen in the apical view angled anteriorly as well as via SC imaging planes.
- TEE is not required to diagnose and evaluate PS in children. TEE is used intraoperatively to assess subvalvar resection, pulmonary valvotomy, or supravalvar stenosis repair.

Analysis
- The first step is to evaluate the pulmV morphology with 2D imaging. Identify whether the valve is doming with fusion of the leaflet cusps, is dysplastic with thickened and poorly mobile leaflets, or has an abnormal number of cusps. The pulmV function and leaflet morphology are best visualized in the parasternal and subcostal views. Measure the valve annulus in systole (including calculation of valve dimension Z score) (Fig. 11-17). Stenotic pulmV can be hypoplastic as can be seen in critical neonatal PS. To identify the number of cusps, the valve must be seen in an en face view. This is best accomplished in a higher parasternal view with slight rotation of the transducer away from the aortic valve until the pulmV comes into view (Fig. 11-18).
- The next step is to evaluate the subvalvar region for evidence of RVOT narrowing or infundibular muscle hypertrophy. There can be a ridge of tissue causing obstruction toward the proximal end of the infundibulum seen best in the PSAX view. There may also be muscle bundle hypertrophy or accessory muscle bundles that can divide the right ventricular body into proximal and distal chambers (DCRV). This is best seen in the subcostal anterior oblique view (the same view that is used to evaluate the infundibular area in TOF).
- Assess the degree of RVH and systolic function in the A4C view as well as PLAX and SC views. The amount of hypertrophy is relative to the degree of PS.
- Evaluate the IAS for a PFO or ASD. Measure the diameter. This is best seen in the standard atrial septal views (subcostal, PSAX, right parasternal).
- Assess for supravalvar PS. Measure the diameter of the MPA and the area of narrowing seen due to either a discrete ridge of tissue or a narrowed vessel. Measure both branch PAs. The MPA and branches are best visualized from PSAX/PLAX as well as SSN and high left parasternal views.
- Assess for the presence of a PDA. If present, measure the diameter of the ampulla. The PDA is best seen in the high left parasternal view.

TABLE 11-4 PULMONARY STENOSIS—ECHOCARDIOGRAPHIC APPROACH

	Details	Acquisition	Image Planes	Analysis	Comments/Tips
Anatomic Imaging					
PulmV	Morphology	TTE, fetal	PSAX/LAX, SC fetal outflow	Measure PV annulus (Z score) Describe valve anatomy	High parasternal for en-face view of pulmV
RVOT	Subvalvar stenosis	TTE	SC anterior oblique PSAX	Look for muscle bundle hypertrophy and DCRV also	Rule out associated VSDs if DCRV seen
RV	Hypertrophy	TTE	A4C, PSAX, PLAX	Describe severity of RVH	Degree of hypertrophy related to severity of stenosis
IAS	PFO, ASD	TTE, fetal	SC, PSAX, right PS, fetal 4C	Size of ASD if present	
MPA, branch PAs	Supravalvar stenosis	TTE	PSAX/PLAX, SSN, high left parasternal	Diameter of MPA and branch PAs, diameter of MPA narrowing	May be discrete ridge of tissue vs. hypoplastic vessel
PDA	Presence	TTE	SSN, "ductal"	Measure size of PDA if present	
Physiologic Data					
PulmV	Qualitative	Color Doppler	PSAX/LAX, SC fetal outflow	Note where flow turbulence initiates (below, at, above pulmV)	Maximize Nyquist limit Assess for PI
PulmV	Quantitative	CW Doppler, PW Doppler	PSAX/LAX, SC	CW Doppler across valve, use highest value, PW Doppler below, at, above valve	Trace envelope to calculate the mean gradient
TV	Regurgitation	TTE, fetal	A4C, PSAX, PLAX, fetal 4C	CW Doppler to estimated RV pressure with adding RA pressure	
IAS	Shunt flow	Color, PW Doppler	SC, PSAX, fetal 4C	Determine direction of shunting across atrial septum	Usually is left to right but can be right to left with severe PS
PDA	Shunt flow	Color, PW Doppler	SSN, "ductal"	Demonstrate direction and velocity	Can have PDA dependence with critical PS
RV	Function	2D	A4C, PSLAX	Qualitative systolic function assessment	Assess IVS position for evidence of high RV pressure

- Measure the TV annulus (with calculation of Z score) and note the morphology of the TV. In cases of severe PS, the TV may be hypoplastic and/or dysplastic.[19]

Pitfalls

- In the adult patient with poor subcostal windows, parasternal views along with color Doppler information are relied on more heavily. It can be difficult to obtain clear 2D imaging of subvalvar PS, but color Doppler information from parasternal long axis and short axis should assist with the diagnosis.[5]

- Poststenotic dilation of the MPA is often seen with pulmV stenosis from a doming-type pulmV. This is not seen with subvalvar stenosis. The degree of poststenotic dilation is not related to the degree of stenosis (Fig. 11-19).

- In the rare instance that a DCRV is present, be sure to look for associated VSDs.

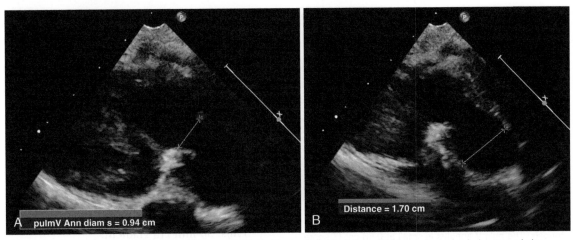

Figure 11-17. PLAX view angled toward the pulmV. **A,** Measurement of the pulmV annulus revealed a normal-size valve at 9.4 mm (Z score 0.17). **B,** This valve was found to be dysplastic and stenotic with moderate poststenotic dilation noted measuring 1.7 cm.

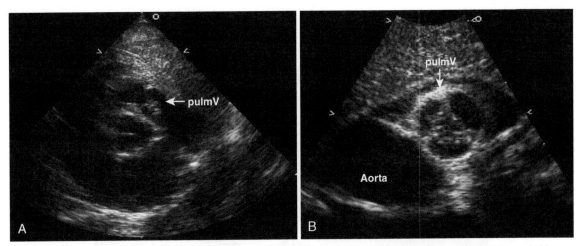

Figure 11-18. PSAX view. **A,** A thickened and dysplastic pulmV is identified (*arrow*). **B,** En face view of this pulmV obtained by sliding slightly superiorly and rotating the probe away from the aortic valve. Three cusps with thickened leaflets are seen.

Physiologic Data
Acquisition
- The quantitative assessment of the severity of PS is based on the systolic pressure gradient across the area of stenosis.
- Use color Doppler across the RVOT and pulmV with the Nyquist limit at its maximum to get a sense for where the flow turbulence begins (below, at, or above the valve).
- Using CW Doppler and the modified Bernoulli equation, the peak velocity across the site of stenosis can be acquired. Trace the full envelope to calculate the mean pressure gradient (Fig. 11-20).

- It is also important to use PW Doppler to measure the peak velocity below the valve, at the valve, and above the valve to determine the level of obstruction (or the relative contribution of multiple sites of stenosis) (Figs. 11-21 and 11-22).
- The highest velocity from multiple different planes should be used. In children, the Doppler angle will be the most accurate from SC or PSAX views. In adults without subcostal views, the best angle of interrogation will usually be on the PSAX view.
- Assess for the degree of PI while using color Doppler.

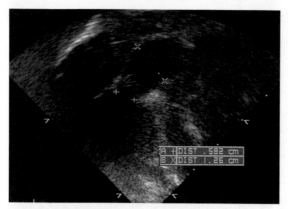

Figure 11-19. Apical view angled anteriorly to visualize the pulmV in an infant with moderate to severe pulmV stenosis. The pulmV annulus is small at 0.58 cm (Z score −2.27), and there is poststenotic dilation measuring at 1.26 cm.

- If the pulmV is interrogated intraoperatively with TEE, a transgastric view or a midesophageal view will align the Doppler angle the most accurately.

Analysis
- In 2006, the AHA and ACC defined grades of severity of PS based on systolic peak velocity or maximal instantaneous pressure gradients (MIPGs).[18] Grading is as follows:
  - Severe PS: peak systolic velocity greater than 4 m/s, 64-mm Hg gradient.
  - Moderate PS: peak systolic velocity, 3 to 4 m/s, 36- to 64-mm Hg gradient.
  - Mild PS: peak systolic velocity less than 3 m/s, 36-mm Hg gradient.
- Both the peak and mean systolic pressure gradients should be reported. In general, the peak-to-peak gradient measured in the cardiac

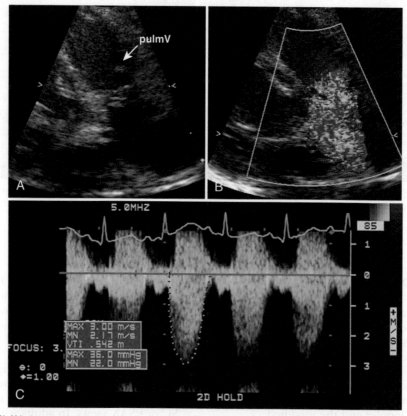

Figure 11-20. PLAX view angled toward the pulmV. **A,** 2D image of a thickened pulmV. **B,** Color Doppler across the pulmV with flow turbulence starting at the level of the valve. **C,** Continuous wave (CW) Doppler across the pulmV reveals a peak velocity of 3 m/s (maximal instantaneous pressure gradient [MIPG] of 36 mm Hg; 22-mm Hg mean gradient). This is considered mild to moderate pulmV stenosis.

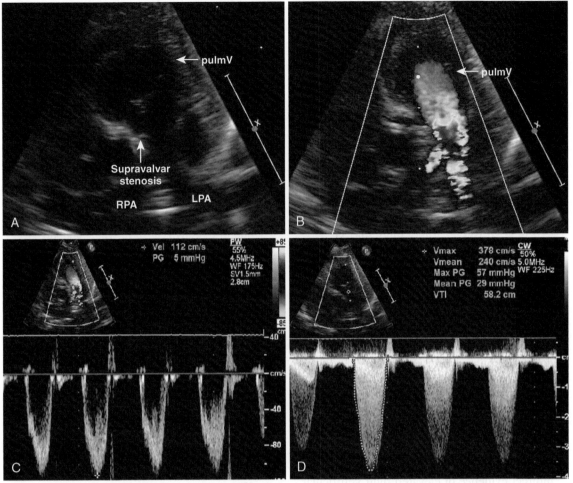

Figure 11-21. PLAX view angled toward the pulmV in a patient with supravalvar PS and hypoplastic PAs. **A,** 2D image of supravalvar PS (*arrow*). The pulmV annulus is normal size (7 mm, Z score –1.2), whereas the MPA is small (5 mm, Z score –2.6) as well as the right PA (RPA) (3 mm, Z score –2.2). The left PA (LPA) measures 4 mm (Z score –1.1). **B,** Color Doppler across the pulmV into the MPA and branch PAs. The color turbulence starts above the pulmV (*arrow*) at the level of MPA narrowing. **C,** Pulsed wave (PW) Doppler at the pulmV shows no increased velocity (peak velocity 1.1 m/s). **D,** CW Doppler through the pulmV and MPA. There is a peak velocity of 3.78 m/s (MIPG of 57 mm Hg) across the area.

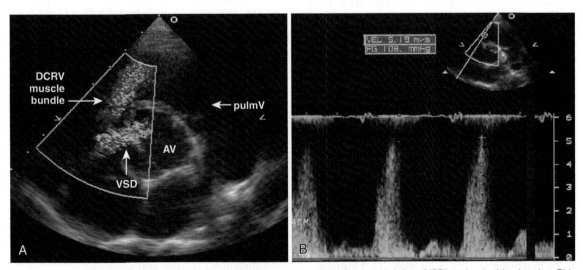

Figure 11-22. PSAX view in a patient with a perimembranous ventricular septal defect (VSD) and a double-chamber RV. **A,** There is a level of obstruction to flow caused by muscle bundles in the RV well below the level of the pulmV. **B,** PW Doppler in the RV just distal to the muscle bundle and proximal to the pulmV reveals a peak velocity of 5.19 m/s (MIPG of 108 mm Hg).

catheterization laboratory is lower than the Doppler-derived MIPG. Some would argue that the mean Doppler gradient measured correlates better with the catheterization measured peak-to peak gradient.[20]

- If TR is present, measure the CW Doppler pressure gradient to estimate right ventricular pressure (plus right atrial pressure).
- Demonstrate the atrial-level shunting with color Doppler and PW Doppler if there is a PFO or ASD present. The direction of blood flow should be left to right except in cases of severe or critical PS where there may be right-to-left shunting across the IAS from decreased right ventricular compliance or right ventricular outflow obstruction.
- If present, demonstrate the direction of flow across a PDA. Use PW Doppler to estimate the peak systolic velocity. This, along with knowledge of systemic systolic blood pressure, will allow for calculation of the downstream (poststenosis) PAP. In combination with the CW Doppler velocity across the region of stenosis, a calculation can then be performed to estimate right ventricular systolic pressure.
- Qualitatively assess the right ventricular function. Also note the interventricular septal position. A flattened interventricular septum is indirect evidence of elevated right ventricular pressure.[21]
- After intervention on the pulmV (either catheter based or surgically), the residual stenosis gradient should be assessed as well as evidence of PI. In a rare case, subvalvar (infundibular) stenosis can develop after the valvar PS is relieved (the "suicide" RV). This obstruction is dynamic in nature. The Doppler profile will be consistent with a dynamic rather than a fixed obstruction.

Pitfalls

- Accurate Doppler estimation of any peak velocity or pressure gradient is dependent on appropriate angle of interrogation. Attempt to align the Doppler signal with the jet of PS to maximize velocity measured.
- With multiple levels of obstruction, the modified Bernoulli equation ($\Delta P = 4v^2$) is not accurate to assess the distal obstruction. The proximal velocity must be taken in account. $\Delta P = 4(v_2^2 - v_1^2)$.

Alternate Approaches

- In most cases of PS, echo with 2D, Doppler, and color Doppler information can accurately define the anatomic reasons for and severity of the stenosis.

- On rare occasions, other imaging modalities, such as MRI or computed tomography (CT), can be beneficial.
- Cardiac catheterization is usually not required for diagnostic purposes but reserved for interventions for PS.

KEY POINTS

- Most causes of native pulmV stenosis are congenital. Isolated pulmV stenosis can occur due to three typical valve types: doming pulmV (most common, fusion of valve leaflets), dysplastic pulmV (thickened leaflets with poor mobility), or an abnormal number of cusps (unicuspid, bicuspid, quadricuspid).
- Obstruction below the pulmV (subvalvar) or above the valve (supravalvar) may be seen in isolation or in conjunction with pulmV stenosis.
- Echo is the primary tool used to define the anatomic reasons for PS as well as define the degree of severity. No further diagnostic tools should be required if the echocardiogram is complete and precisely executed.
- Using 2D imaging, fully demonstrate the anatomy and size of the pulmV as well as subvalvar or supravalvar narrowing if present. Other important features to define with 2D imaging are the presence of an ASD or PDA, the appearance of the TV, and the qualitative assessment of right ventricular function.
- Using spectral and color Doppler, the quantitative assessment of the severity of the obstruction can be analyzed. The direction of flow across an ASD and PDA (if present) and the degree of TR with an estimate of right ventricular pressure should also be assessed.
- AHA and ACC (2006) grades of severity of PS:
  - Severe PS: peak systolic velocity greater than 4 m/s, 64-mm Hg gradient.
  - Moderate PS: peak systolic velocity 3 to 4 m/s, 36- to 64-mm Hg gradient.
  - Mild PS: peak systolic velocity less than 3 m/s, 36-mm Hg gradient.

Branch Pulmonary Artery Stenosis

Background

- As with valvar PS, branch PA stenosis has a wide variation in its clinical presentation, subsequent course, and sequelae.
- In infants, physiologic branch PA stenosis often presents as a short systolic murmur in an asymptomatic neonate. On echocardiographic

investigation, the branch PAs are found to be slightly smaller than normal with mild flow turbulence through the right and left PAs (usually <2 m/s). The stenosis is usually bilateral and tends to regress without the need for any intervention by about 3 months of age.[22]

- Other forms of branch PA stenosis can be unilateral or bilateral and are often found in conjunction with other CHD (e.g., TOF, pulmonary atresia with VSD, other cyanotic heart defects), genetic syndromes (Williams, Noonan, Alagille), or acquired after cardiac surgery (e.g., after the LeCompte maneuver in an arterial switch operation for dextro transposition of the great arteries [d-TGA] repair, unifocalization of major aortopulmonary collaterals).
- Moderate to severe branch PA stenosis can cause similar physiologic consequences as pulmV stenosis. These include elevated right ventricular pressure, right ventricular dysfunction, TR, elevated right atrial pressures, and right-to-left atrial-level shunting if a PFO or ASD is present.
- Moderate to severe branch PA stenosis may be amenable to intervention in the cardiac catheterization lab including angioplasty and/or stent placement. Surgical options exist as well; however, with distal branch PA stenosis it is often difficult to achieve an adequate result with surgery.

Overview of Echocardiographic Approach

- Careful 2D and Doppler evaluation of the branch PAs will reveal most clinically important information with a few exceptions (see the following Pitfalls section).
- Similar to pulmV stenosis, the echocardiographer should attempt to demonstrate the 2D narrowing with measurements of the branch PAs, the degree of stenosis with Doppler, the degree of RVH, and the interventricular septal position and evaluate for TR and atrial-level shunting (Table 11-5).

Anatomic imaging
Acquisition

- The branch PAs are well visualized from the PSAX and PLAX views. The SSN views and the high left parasternal views are also helpful but may be more challenging in the adult patient.
- With 2D imaging, measure the diameter of the branch PAs and any discrete narrowing seen. Measure the MPA as well (Fig. 11-23).
- Along with performing a complete anatomic 2D evaluation, pay particular attention to associations with branch PA stenosis including pulmV abnormalities/stenosis and other CHD (especially conotruncal defects).

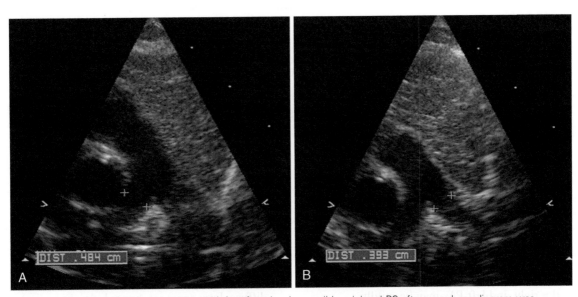

Figure 11-23. PSAX view in a 1-month-old infant found to have mild peripheral PS after an echocardiogram was performed for a murmur evaluation. **A,** The right PA measures 4.8 mm. **B,** The left PA measures 3.9 mm.

TABLE 11-5 BRANCH PULMONARY ARTERY STENOSIS—ECHOCARDIOGRAPHIC APPROACH

	Details	Acquisition	Image Planes	Analysis	Comments/Tips
Anatomic Imaging					
Branch PAs	Measurements	TTE, 2D	PSAX/PLAX, SSN, high left parasternal	Diameter on 2D, discrete narrowing	Report Z score
MPA	Measurements	TTE, 2D	PSAX/PLAX, SC	Diameter on 2D	Report Z score
PulmV	Morphology	TTE, 2D	PSAX/LAX, SC	pulmV annulus Z score, valve anatomy	High parasternal for en-face view of pulmV
RV	Hypertrophy	TTE, 2D	A4C, PSAX, PLAX	Describe severity of RVH	Degree of hypertrophy related to severity of stenosis
IAS	PFO, ASD	TTE, 2D	SC, PSAX, right PS	Size of ASD if present	
PDA	Presence	TTE, 2D	SSN, "ductal"	Measure size of PDA if present	
Associated lesions	Rule out	TTE, 2D	All views	Look for associated cardiac lesions	PS/pulmonary atresia with VSD, TOF, other cyanotic CHD
Physiologic Data					
MPA and branches	Qualitative	Color Doppler	PSAX/LAX, SC, SSN, high left parasternal	Note where flow turbulence initiates	Maximize Nyquist limit Assess for flow reversal and PI
Branch PAs	Quantitative	CW and PW Doppler	PSAX/LAX, SSN, high left parasternal	PW Doppler in branch PAs	Attempt to maximize Doppler angle to minimize error
RVOT, pulmV, MPA	Quantitative	CW and PW Doppler	PSAX/PLAX, SC	Measure velocity proximal to PAs	Use regular Bernoulli equation with proximal obstruction
TV	Regurgitation	CW Doppler	A4C, PSAX, PLAX	CW Doppler to estimate RV pressure with adding RA pressure	
IAS	Shunt flow	Color, PW Doppler	SC, PSAX, fetal 4C	Direction of atrial septal flow	Usually is left to right but can be right to left with severe branch PS
PDA	Shunt flow	Color, PW Doppler	SSN, "ductal"	Demonstrate direction and velocity	
RV	Function	2D	A4C, PSLAX	Qualitative systolic function assessment	Assess IVS position for evidence of high RV pressure

Analysis

- Report the Z scores of the 2D measurements of the right PA, left PA, MPA, and pulmV annulus. In physiologic branch PA stenosis, the right and left PAs may be mildly hypoplastic (on the order of 4 mm in the full-term infant), but the MPA and pulmV are typically normal.[22]
- Determine whether there is a discrete ostial stenosis to one or both branch PAs versus diffuse long-segment hypoplasia (Fig. 11-24).

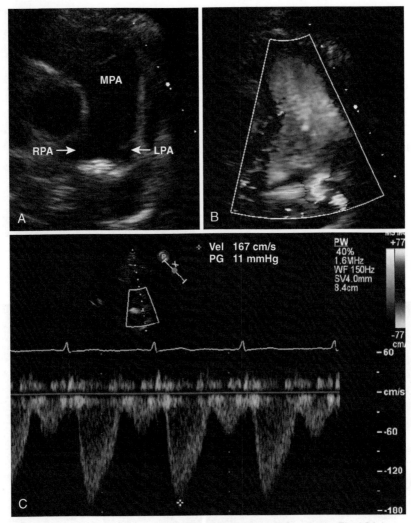

Figure 11-24. PSAX view. **A,** 2D image in an infant with unilateral branch PA stenosis. The LPA has a discrete stenosis at its origin. **B,** Color Doppler demonstrating flow turbulence originating at the branch point of the LPA. Flow through the MPA and RPA is laminar. **C,** Spectral Doppler of the LPA showing mild branch PS (peak velocity 1.67 m/s).

- The branch PA abnormalities associated with specific cardiac lesions are discussed in their respective chapters.
- Assess for signs of severe stenosis. Look for evidence of elevated right ventricular pressure (IVS position), RVH, and RV systolic function.

Pitfalls

- In cases of unilateral branch PA stenosis, there is decreased blood flow through the stenotic vessel and increased flow through the opposite vessel. The nonstenotic vessel may appear larger on 2D measurements, and the RV may or may not have evidence of elevated pressure.
- Postsurgical imaging of branch PAs is discussed in their respective chapters (i.e.,

imaging the branch PAs in their atypical orientation after a LeCompte maneuver for d-TGA) (Fig. 11-25).

Physiologic Data
Acquisition

- After 2D imaging, data are gathered; spectral and color Doppler information should be obtained to quantify the degree of stenosis.
- Color Doppler across the MPA and branch PAs will identify the site(s) of flow turbulence. Also take note of flow reversal, where the flow reversal begins, and the degree of PI. Be sure to maximize the Nyquist limit (Fig. 11-26).

Figure 11-25. Color Doppler image demonstrating branch PA stenosis in a patient with dextro transposition of the great arteries who underwent an arterial switch operation. The PA anatomy is often difficult to visualize due to the anteroposterior orientation of the branch PAs straddling the aorta. In this image, flow turbulence is seen at the LPA and RPA.

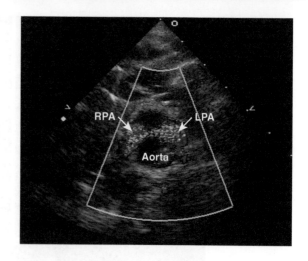

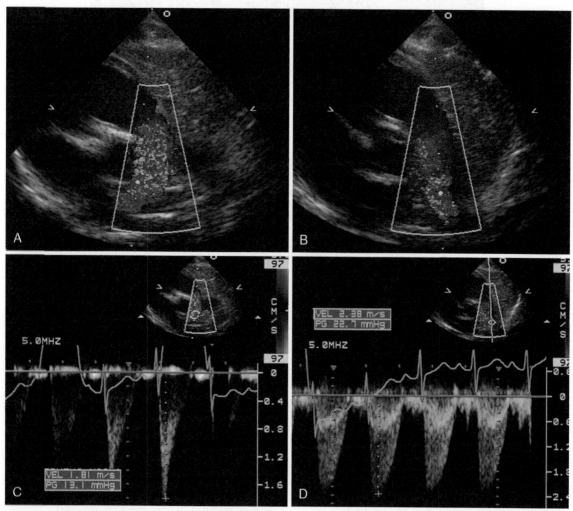

Figure 11-26. PSAX images in an infant with bilateral branch PA stenosis. This is the same patient as in Figure 11-23. **A,** Color Doppler demonstrating flow turbulence in the RPA. **B,** Color Doppler demonstrating flow turbulence in the LPA. **C,** Spectral Doppler of the RPA showing stenosis (peak velocity 1.81 m/s). **D,** Spectral Doppler of the LPA showing stenosis (peak velocity 2.38 m/s).

Analysis

- Unlike pulmV stenosis, there is not a specific severity grading scale for branch PA stenosis. There are anatomic issues that can complicate the interpretation of Doppler-derived velocity information (see the following Pitfalls section).
- PW Doppler profiles should be obtained in each branch PA, MPA, and pulmV. A CW Doppler profile can be obtained as well, although it may not give specific information as to the site of the obstruction. If the branch PA stenosis is being followed at serial clinic visits, it is important to measure the velocity in similar locations and views with similar echo settings at each visit so that a reasonable comparison can be made over time. It is also important to align the Doppler angle with the stenotic jet to minimize error.
- If TR is present, measure the CW Doppler pressure gradient to estimate RV pressure (plus right atrial pressure).
- Demonstrate the atrial-level shunting with color Doppler and PW Doppler if there is a PFO or ASD present. The direction of blood flow should be left to right except in cases of severe branch PS in which there may be right-to-left shunting across the IAS.
- If present, demonstrate the direction of flow across a PDA. Use PW Doppler to estimate the peak systolic velocity.
- Qualitatively assess the right ventricular function. Also note the interventricular septal position. A flattened interventricular septum is indirect evidence of elevated right ventricular pressure.[21]

Pitfalls

- In unilateral branch PA stenosis, there can be increased blood flow through the opposite branch PA with an increased flow velocity recorded with PW Doppler and turbulence seen on color Doppler interrogation. The stenotic vessel will have decreased blood flow. For this reason, the velocity across this vessel may not be an accurate predictor of the severity of stenosis.
- Doppler-measured velocity in branch PAs has been shown to overestimate the catheterization lab measured peak-to-peak gradient across the stenosis. This is another reason to be cautious when assigning a degree of severity to branch PA stenosis.[23]
- Similar to pulmV stenosis, with multiple levels of obstruction (i.e., pulmV and branch PA stenosis), the modified Bernoulli equation

($\Delta P = 4v^2$) is inaccurate in assessing branch PA obstruction. The proximal velocity must be taken in account. $\Delta P = 4(v_2^2 - v_1^2)$.

Alternate Approaches

- In cases of unilateral branch PA stenosis, a lung perfusion study will help to clarify the percentage of blood flow going to each lung field. This information may assist the clinician in assessing the severity of stenosis.
- Occasionally the branch PAs are difficult to visualize well by echo. In these cases, MRI or CT could be considered to augment echo information.
- Catheterization is usually reserved for intervention on branch PA stenosis. Once the stenosis is deemed severe enough (based on clinical symptoms, echo, lung perfusion scan, and/or MRI information), the pressure gradient can be assessed invasively before possible intervention.[24,25]

KEY POINTS

- In infants, physiologic branch PA stenosis often presents as a short systolic murmur in an asymptomatic neonate. The branch PAs are found to be slightly smaller than normal with mild flow turbulence through the right and LPAs (usually <2 m/s). Stenosis tends to regress by about 3 months of age without the need for intervention.
- Other forms of branch PA stenosis can be unilateral or bilateral and are often found in conjunction with other CHD or genetic syndromes or acquired after cardiac surgery.
- The branch PAs are well visualized from the PSAX, PLAX, SSN, and high left parasternal views.
- Obtain 2D measurements (with Z score) of each branch PA, MPA, and pulmV annulus.
- Color Doppler across the MPA and branch PAs will identify the site(s) of flow turbulence as well as flow reversal and the degree of PI.
- PW Doppler profiles should be obtained in each branch PA, MPA, and pulmV, although this tends to overestimate invasive peak-to-peak gradient measurements. Be careful to define proximal stenosis in addition to branch PA stenosis.
- Assess for evidence of elevated right ventricular pressures.
- In unilateral branch PA stenosis, there can be a blood flow differential between stenotic and nonstenotic PA branches that will affect the color Doppler and Doppler velocity measurement interpretation.

References

1. Allen HD, Driscoll DJ, Shaddy RE, Feltes TF, ed. *Moss and Adams' Heart Disease in Infants, Children, and Adolescents: Including the Fetus and Young Adults.* 2007.
2. Keane JF, Lock JE, Flyer DC. *Nadas' Pediatric Cardiology.* 2nd ed. Philadelphia: Saunders/Elsevier; 2006.
3. Attenhofer Jost CH, Connolly HM, Dearani JA, et al. Ebstein's anomaly. *Circulation.* 2007;115:277-285.
4. Silverman NH, Gerlis LM, Horowitz ES, et al. Pathologic elucidation of the echocardiographic features of Ebstein's malformation of the morphologically tricuspid valve in discordant atrioventricular connections. *Am J Cardiol.* 1995;76:1277-1283.
5. Lai WW, Mertens LL, Cohen MS, Geva T, eds. *Echocardiography in Pediatric and Congenital Heart Disease: From Fetus to Adult.* Oxford, UK: Wiley-Blackwell; 2009.
6. Paranon S, Acar P. Ebstein's anomaly of the tricuspid valve: from fetus to adult: congenital heart disease. *Heart.* 2008;94:237-243.
7. Carpentier A, Chauvaud S, Mace L, et al. A new reconstructive operation for Ebstein's anomaly of the tricuspid valve. *J Thorac Cardiovasc Surg.* 1988;96:92-101.
8. Patel V, Nanda NC, Rajdev S, et al. Live/real time three-dimensional transthoracic echocardiographic assessment of Ebstein's anomaly. *Echocardiography.* 2005;22:847-854.
9. Celermajer DS, Cullen S, Sullivan ID, et al. Outcome in neonates with Ebstein's anomaly. *J Am Coll Cardiol.* 1992;19:1041-1046.
10. Celermajer DS, Bull C, Till JA, et al. Ebstein's anomaly: presentation and outcome from fetus to adult. *J Am Coll Cardiol.* 1994;23:170-176.
11. Ammash NM, Warnes CA, Connolly HM, et al. Mimics of Ebstein's anomaly. *Am Heart J.* 1997;134:508-513.
12. Steinberger J, Berry JM, Bass JL, et al. Results of a right ventricular outflow patch for pulmonary atresia with intact ventricular septum. *Circulation.* 1992;86(5 Suppl):167-175.
13. Odim J, Laks H, Plunkett MD, Tung TC. Successful management of patients with pulmonary atresia with intact ventricular septum using a three tier grading system for right ventricular hypoplasia. *Ann Thorac Surg.* 2006;81:678-684.
14. Hanley FL, Sade RM, Blackstone EH, et al. Outcomes in neonatal pulmonary atresia with intact ventricular septum. A multiinstitutional study. *J Thorac Cardiovasc Surg.* 1993;105:406-423.
15. Satou GM, Perry SB, Gauvreau K, Geva T. Echocardiographic predictors of coronary artery pathology in pulmonary atresia with intact ventricular septum. *Am J Cardiol.* 2000;85(11):1319-1324.
16. Park MK. *Pediatric Cardiology for Practitioners.* 4th ed. St. Louis, MO: Mosby; 2002.
17. Baumgartner H, Hung J, Bermejo J, et al. Echocardiographic assessment of valve stenosis: EAE/ASE recommendations for clinical practice. *J Am Soc Echocardiogr.* 2009;22:1-23.
18. Developed in Collaboration With the Society of Cardiovascular Anesthesiologists, Endorsed by the Society for Cardiovascular Angiography and Interventions and the Society of Thoracic Surgeons, Writing Committee Meers, et al. ACC/AHA 2006 Guidelines for the Management of Patients With Valvular Heart Disease: A Report of the American College of Cardiology/American Heart Association Task Force on Practice Guidelines (Writing Committee to Revise the 1998 Guidelines for the Management of Patients With Valvular Heart Disease). *Circulation.* 2006;114:e84-e231.
19. Kovalchin JP, Forbes TJ, Nihill MR, Geva T. Echocardiographic determinants of clinical course in infants with critical and severe pulmonary valve stenosis. *J Am Coll Cardiol.* 1997;29(5):1095-1101.
20. Silvilairat S, Cabalka AK, Cetta F, et al. Echocardiographic assessment of isolated pulmonary valve stenosis: which outpatient Doppler gradient has the most clinical validity? *J Am Soc Echocardiogr.* 2005;18:1137-1142.
21. King ME, Braun H, Goldblatt A, et al. Interventricular septal configuration as a predictor of right ventricular systolic hypertension in children: a cross-sectional echocardiographic study. *Circulation.* 1983;68(1):68-75.
22. Rodriguez RJ, Riggs TW. Physiologic peripheral pulmonic stenosis in infancy. *Am J Cardiol.* 1990;66:1478-1481.
23. Frank DU, Minich LL, Shaddy RE, Tani LY. Is Doppler an accurate predictor of catheterization gradients for postoperative branch pulmonary stenosis? *J Am Soc Echocardiogr.* 2002;15(10 Pt 2):1140-1144.
24. Rocchini AP, Kveselis D, Dick M, et al. Use of balloon angioplasty to treat peripheral pulmonary stenosis. *Am J Cardiol.* 1984;54:1069-1073.
25. Suda K, Matsumura M, Hayashi H, Nishimura K. Comparison of efficacy of medium-sized cutting balloons versus standard balloons for dilation of peripheral pulmonary stenosis. *Am J Cardiol.* 2006;97:1060-1063.

Suggested Reading

1. Attenhofer Jost CH, Connolly HM, Dearani JA, et al. Ebstein's anomaly. *Circulation.* 2007;115:277-285.
2. Paranon S, Acar P. Ebstein's anomaly of the tricuspid valve: from fetus to adult: congenital heart disease. *Heart.* 2008;94:237-243.
3. Reemtsen BL, Fagan BT, Wells WJ, Starnes VA. Current surgical therapy for Ebstein anomaly in neonates. *J Thorac Cardiovasc Surg.* 2006;132(6):1285-1290.
4. Powell AJ, Mayer JE, Lang P, Lock JE. Outcome in infants with pulmonary atresia, intact ventricular septum, and right ventricle-dependent coronary circulation. *Am J Cardiol.* 2000;86(11):1272-1274.
5. Odim J, Laks H, Plunkett MD, Tung TC. Successful management of patients with pulmonary atresia with intact ventricular septum using a three tier grading system for right ventricular hypoplasia. *Ann Thorac Surg.* 2006;81:678-684.
6. ACC/AHA 2006 Guidelines for the Management of Patients With Valvular Heart Disease: A Report of the American College of Cardiology/American Heart Association Task Force on Practice Guidelines (Writing Committee to Revise the 1998 Guidelines for the Management of Patients With Valvular Heart Disease). *Circulation.* 2006;114:e84-e231.
7. Silvilairat S, Cabalka AK, Cetta F, et al. Echocardiographic assessment of isolated pulmonary valve stenosis: which outpatient Doppler gradient has the most clinical validity? *J Am Soc Echocardiogr.* 2005;18:1137-1142.
8. Frank DU, Minich LL, Shaddy RE, Tani LY. Is Doppler an accurate predictor of catheterization gradients for postoperative branch pulmonary stenosis? *J Am Soc Echocardiogr.* 2002;15(10 Pt 2):1140-1144.

Left Heart Anomalies

12

Brian D. Soriano and David S. Owens

Background

- Left heart anomalies include lesions of the mitral valve (MV), left ventricular outflow tract (LVOT), aortic valve (AV), coronary arteries, and aorta (Ao). Within each of these structures there is a wide spectrum of both congenital and acquired diseases.
- Certain genetic lesions are associated with left heart lesions (Table 12-1).

Overview of Echocardiographic Approach

- Any abnormality that is detected by echocardiography (echo) should trigger the detailed evaluation of structures both upstream and downstream of the lesion. For example, if coarctation of the aorta is diagnosed, both the AV and MV should be carefully evaluated to rule out associated functional or structural abnormalities (Box 12-1).
- Evaluation of lesions by two-dimensional (2D) echo should be performed via all available acoustic windows because subtle diagnostic or anatomic clues can be gleaned. A single en face view of the MV, for example, would not be able to determine whether there are problems with the submitral apparatus or whether there are signs of supramitral obstruction.
  - Fine-tune 2D images to maximize resolution. Use the highest frequency transducer that windows will permit. Eliminate unnecessarily wide views by narrowing the 2D sector angle or by zooming into a region of interest. Consider changing line density if higher frame rates take priority over spatial resolution.
- Doppler imaging is critical to evaluate the hemodynamic impact of the anomaly. The regions immediately adjacent to an identified anomaly should be carefully performed to determine whether problems exist in series. Color Doppler complements spectral Doppler and can help visualize the location and degree of stenosis or regurgitation and the presence or absence of turbulence.
  - Nyquist limits are inversely related to transducer frequency; if color Doppler maps or pulsed wave (PW) Doppler scales are limited, consider switching to a lower frequency setting or switch to a lower frequency transducer.
  - A good-quality color Doppler map is best predicted by the quality of the 2D image and the acoustic windows. If the acoustic window or the 2D image is poor, the color Doppler maps are unlikely to be useful.
  - A surprisingly good spectral Doppler tracing, however, can frequently be obtained even if 2D images are suboptimal.
  - If necessary, intravenous contrast can enhance spectral Doppler images.

Left Atrial Anomalies

Cor Triatriatum
- Can be either obstructive or widely patent.
- Typically seen as an "extra" atrial septum that partially divides the left atrium (LA) into a pulmonary venous chamber and the true left atrial chamber.

Anatomic and Physiologic Imaging
- The true left atrial chamber can be identified by locating the left atrial appendage orifice.
- The pulmonary venous chamber would not include the appendage orifice.

TABLE 12-1   SYNDROMES AND DISEASES ASSOCIATED WITH LEFT HEART LESIONS

Left Heart Disease	Association
Coarctation of the aorta	Turner syndrome
	Bicuspid AV
	Unicuspid AV
Supravalvular aortic stenosis	Williams syndrome
Dilated aorta	Bicuspid AV
	Marfan syndrome
	Loeys-Dietz syndrome
	Ehlers-Danlos syndrome
	Shprintzen-Goldberg syndrome
	Turner Syndrome
Simultaneous left heart obstructions: mitral stenosis, aortic stenosis, coarctation	Shone syndrome
	Hypoplastic left heart syndrome

This list is intended to summarize more commonly associated syndromes and is not all-inclusive.

- PW Doppler and color Doppler should be used to determine whether any restriction across the cor membrane is present. Mean gradients greater that 3 mm Hg should be considered abnormal.

KEY POINTS

- Cor triatriatum is a rare intra-atrial septation that requires careful anatomic and physiologic interrogation when suspected.
- When cor triatriatum occurs in the right atrium (cor triatriatum dextrum), it must be differentiated from prominent Eustacean and Thebesian valves.

Aortic Valve Anomalies

Congenital Anomalies
Bicuspid Aortic Valve
- Most common left-sided lesion.
- Typically fusion of the intercoronary commissure is present.
- The entire length of the commissure does not necessarily have to be fused; partial fusion can be present.
  - Less common anatomic variants include unicuspid (Fig. 12-1) and quadricuspid AVs (Fig. 12-2).

BOX 12-1 Suggested Echocardiographic Approach for Left Heart Lesions

Left Heart Obstruction
- Detailed evaluation of anatomy by 2D from multiple windows
- PW Doppler evaluation both upstream and downstream of region
- Spectral Doppler and color Doppler map of the region
- Evaluate for left ventricular hypertrophy or dysfunction
- Evaluate for the presence or absence of pulmonary hypertension

AV Regurgitation
- Detailed 2D views of valvular and subvalvular regions
- Evaluate lesion with PW Doppler across the LVOT and supravalvular area, CW Doppler across region, and color Doppler
- Evaluate LV: size, function, and mass

MV Regurgitation
- Detailed 2D views of valve, chordae, and papillary muscles
- Color Doppler of regurgitant jet
- Evaluate left atrial size
- Evaluate for the presence or absence of pulmonary hypertension

Coronary Artery Lesions
- Evaluate right and left ventricular function
- If acoustic windows allow, the origins of coronary arteries must be evaluated
  - Use low Nyquist color Doppler (≤40 cm/s) to fill the imaged vessels

- In truncus arteriosus, individuals are born with a single semilunar valve, which can be quadricuspid.

Acquired Aortic Valve Disease
- Rheumatic aortic stenosis (AS) and regurgitation.
- Postinterventional regurgitation.
- AV prolapse.
  - Usually associated with ventricular septal defects (VSDs), especially with subpulmonary (supracristal) defects.

Anatomic Imaging
- Leaflet thickness, position, and mobility are best evaluated in the parasternal long axis and short axis. M-mode cursors can evaluate motion with good temporal resolution. With modern-day ultrasound carts, however, temporal resolution of the 2D images is almost as fine.

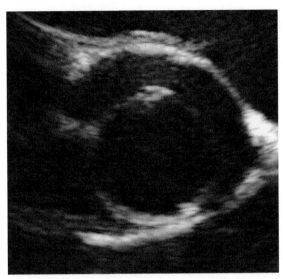

Figure 12-1. En face view of a unicuspid aortic valve (AV).

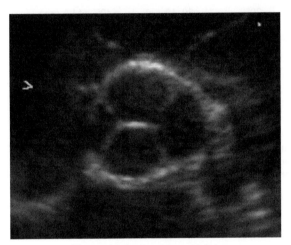

Figure 12-2. Quadricuspid AV.

- In adults, estimations of AV area can determined by using the continuity equation or, less frequently, by 2D planimetry.
  - Valve areas are less frequently measured in pediatric patients due to the relative lack of precision in smaller patients as well as the low frequency of low-output AS for which the AV area would be diagnostically useful.
  - Three-dimensional imaging of the AV can assist in evaluating both morphology and depth of the cusps.

Physiologic Data

- PW Doppler and continuous wave (CW) Doppler of the subaortic and supravalvular regions should be obtained to determine whether any additional obstruction exists (Fig. 12-3).
- Peak velocity and mean gradients can be obtained from the apical windows. The mean gradient from this view best correlates with peak-to-peak estimations by catheterization.
- Overestimation of pressure gradients can occur when velocities are obtained in the suprasternal notch (SSN) or high parasternal views. Pressure recovery phenomena may account for these discrepancies.
- Severity of AS can be underestimated when there is left ventricular systolic dysfunction.
- The degree of aortic regurgitation (AR) can be determined using both color Doppler and spectral Doppler.
  - PW Doppler of the ascending and descending aorta should be obtained to evaluate the volume of regurgitation.
  - Pressure half-time.
- Guidelines for assessing valve stenosis and regurgitation are outlined in Table 12-2.

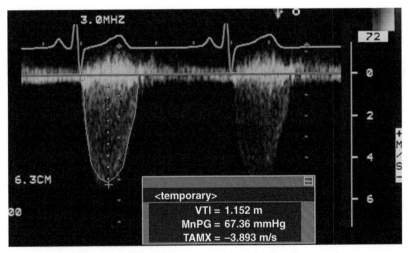

Figure 12-3. Spectral Doppler tracing of subaortic stenosis.

TABLE 12-2   ECHOCARDIOGRAPHIC ASSESSMENT OF THE SEVERITY OF VALVE DISEASE IN ADULTS

Valve Disease	Indicator (unit of measure)	Severity		
		Mild	Moderate	Severe
Aortic stenosis	Jet velocity (m/s)*	<3.0	3.0–4.0	>4.0
	Mean gradient† (mm Hg)*	<25	25–40	>40
	Valve area (cm²)	>1.5	1.0–1.5	<1.0
	Valve area index (cm²/m²)			<0.6
Mitral stenosis	Mean gradient† (mm Hg)*	<5	5–10	>10
	PASP (mm Hg)*	<30	30–50	>50
	Valve area (cm²)	>1.5	1.0–1.5	<1.0
Aortic regurgitation	Jet width (% of LVOT)*	<25	25–65	>65
	Vena contracta (cm)	<0.3	0.3–0.6	>0.6
	Regurgitant volume (mL/beat)	<30	30–59	≥60
	Regurgitant fraction (%)	<30	30–49	≥50
	ROA (cm²)	<0.1	0.1–0.29	≥0.3
	LV size*			Enlarged
Mitral regurgitation	Jet area (% of LA area)	<20% LA area	20–40	>40% of LA area or wall-impinging jet
	Vena contracta (cm)	<0.3	0.3–0.69	>0.7
	Regurgitant volume (mL/beat)	<30	30–59	≥60
	Regurgitant fraction (%)	<30	30–49	≥50
	ROA (cm²)	<0.2	0.2–0.39	≥0.4
	LA size*			Enlarged
	LV size*			Enlarged

*These measures are commonly used in pediatric patients, though they do not have robust outcomes data associated with them and therefore some values may vary in pediatric patient (i.e., mean gradient > 50 mm Hg is generally considered severe AS).
†Valve gradients are flow dependent and should be interpreted in the context of the cardiac output shunts or forward flow across the valve.
Modified from the ACC/AHA Guidelines for the Management of Patients with Valvular Heart Disease, *Circulation.* 2006;114 e84-e231. Data from American Heart Association.

KEY POINTS

- Congenital AV disease is usually due to abnormalities in the number of valve leaflets and may result in AS and/or regurgitation.
- Assessment of valvular AS requires the integration of both 2D and Doppler data; when the valve appears to open well despite high transvalvular velocities, subaortic or supravalvular stenosis should be suspected.
- Congenital AV disease may be associated with an underlying connective disease disorder, and coarctation of the aorta and ascending aortic aneurysm are not uncommon associated findings.

Mitral Valve Anomalies

Congenital Anomalies
- MS variants include
  - Supramitral ring (Figs. 12-4 and 12-5).
  - Commissure fusion.
  - Parachute valve (Figs. 12-6–12-8).
- Mitral arcade.
- Hypoplastic annulus.
- MV prolapse.
- Cleft MV.
  - Can be isolated (Figs. 12-9 and 12-10).
  - Is also present in other congenital diseases such as complete atrioventricular canal defects (see Chapter 6, Atrioventricular Septal Defect: Echocardiographic Assessment).

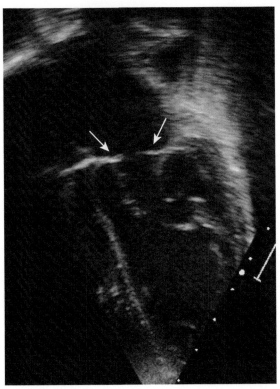

Figure 12-4. Apical view of a supramitral ring *(arrows)* in diastole. The mitral valve (MV) leaflets are tethered by the ring, leading to restricted mobility and a small orifice.

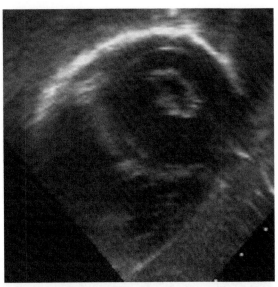

Figure 12-6. En face view of a parachute MV.

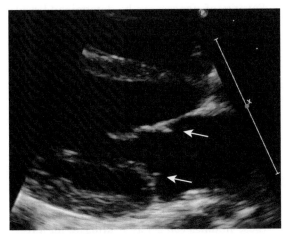

Figure 12-5. Parasternal long axis view of the supramitral ring *(arrows)*.

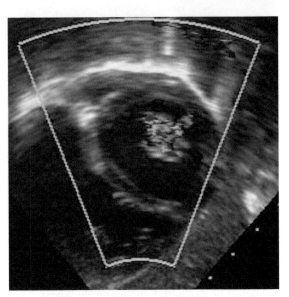

Figure 12-7. Color map of the same MV showing the aliased and turbulent flow as it enters the left ventricle.

Acquired Anomalies

- Rheumatic disease.
- Regurgitation from ischemic disease.
- Autoimmune diseases.
- Traumatic injury.

Anatomic Imaging

- Annular dimensions are recorded and should be compared with established normal data to determine whether the valve is considered to be an adequate size.
- Both congenital and acquired anomalies can involve different levels of the MV: supravalvular, MV leaflets, chordal arrangements and attachments, and papillary muscles. Characteristics of each structure

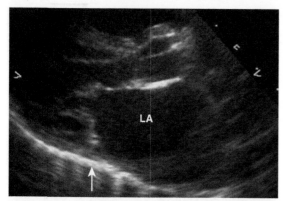

Figure 12-8. Parasternal long axis view of a parachute MV (*arrow*) in diastole. The leaflets are thickened and restricted.

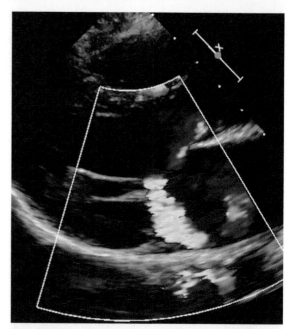

Figure 12-10. Color map of mitral regurgitation (MR) through an isolated cleft. The jet is directed posteriorly.

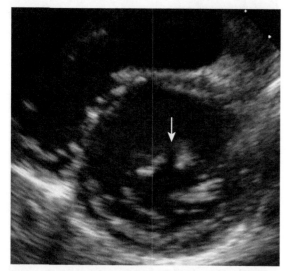

Figure 12-9. Isolated cleft MV. As opposed to a cleft MV (*arrow*) in septum primum atrial septal defects or in atrioventricular canal defects, the length of this cleft is oriented toward the left ventricular outflow tract (LVOT) instead of the crux of the heart.

should be evaluated, including thickness, mobility, and geometry.
- If there is suspicion of an abnormal MV, all levels of the valve's apparatus from base to apex should be imaged from a parasternal short axis view. Each aspect of the MV apparatus (leaflets, chords, and papillary muscles) can be evaluated.
- 2D and M-mode imaging can be used to assess valve motion.
- In MV prolapse, the leaflets should be evaluated from both the parasternal long axis and apical views.
- In chronic rheumatic heart disease, both MS and mitral regurgitation (MR) can be present. Valve leaflets can appear thickened with

restricted mobility, and the annulus can be dilated. Valve prolapse can also be associated with rheumatic disease.

Physiologic Data
- Severity of stenosis can be determined based on several techniques.
  - Pressure half-time.
  - Planimetry.
  - Mean gradient.
  - Transmitral jet width (Fig. 12-11).
- Severity of regurgitation is determined by
  - Vena contracta width.
  - Regurgitant color jet area within the LA.
  - Density of spectral Doppler regurgitation signals.
  - Presence or absence of flow reversal in the pulmonary veins.
- Estimations of pulmonary artery (PA) pressures should also be obtained because these findings can act as a surrogate for left atrial hypertension.

KEY POINTS
• Congenital MV disorders can be isolated or associated with other congenital disorders.
• Complete assessment of MV disease requires the integration of both 2D and Doppler data.

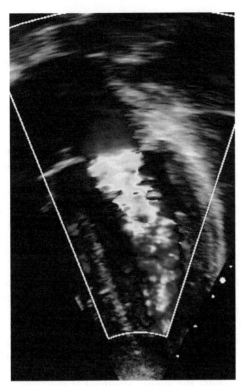

Figure 12-11. Color map showing aliasing at the level of the ring itself.

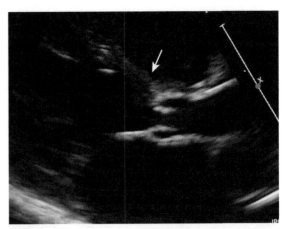

Figure 12-13. The conal or outlet septum (*arrow*) is deviated posteriorly into the LVOT. In this instance, both subaortic and valvular aortic stenosis is present.

BOX 12-2 Known Associations with Subaortic Stenosis
Complete atrioventricular canal defects Double-outlet right ventricle Rastelli repair (LV-to-Ao baffle) VSDs (repaired or unrepaired) Shone syndrome

Subaortic Stenosis

- Discrete subaortic stenosis is typically caused by a membrane or fibrous ridge extending from the ventricular septum. It can often be circumferential, with attachments to either the AV or the MV leaflets (Fig. 12-12).
- Complex congenital heart disease (CHD) such as VSD and malaligned conal septa can create subaortic obstruction (Fig. 12-13).
  - Patients with certain diseases that have been surgically "repaired" are at higher risk of subaortic obstruction (Box 12-2).
- Tunnel-like subaortic stenosis implies that instead of a discrete stenosis, a large portion of the LVOT is narrowed and tubular, with a cross-sectional area small enough to create a significant pressure gradient between the left ventricle (LV) and aorta (Fig. 12-14).

Anatomic Imaging

- 2D parasternal long axis and short axis views provide good views for evaluating the LVOT and obtaining dimensions.
- Apical windows provide additional information on subaortic lesions

Physiologic Data

- Similar to AS, serial PW Doppler assessments through the LVOT and proximal ascending

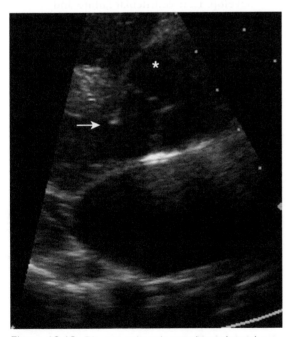

Figure 12-12. Discrete subaortic membrane (*arrow*). Note the mild distortion of the right coronary cusp and the displaced hinge point (*asterisk*), indicating that it prolapses slightly.

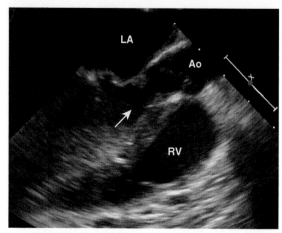

Figure 12-14. Transesophageal echocardiogram of tunnel-like subaortic stenosis in a repaired complete atrioventricular canal defect patient. In addition to the narrowed outflow tract, there is an additional fibrous ring located underneath the AV (*arrow*).

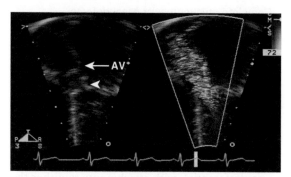

Figure 12-15. Apical 2D and color Doppler views of a subaortic membrane (*arrowhead*) and the AV located just above it.

aorta are important for determining which levels are obstructed. Use a low-frequency transducer to provide the highest Nyquist limit for both spectral Doppler and color Doppler (Fig. 12-15).

KEY POINTS

- Subaortic membranes may be difficult to visualize by transthoracic echo (TTE), and identification of subaortic stenosis may require a high index of suspicion. Early closure of the AV may be present.
- Transesophageal echo (TEE) generally offers better visualization of the subaortic anatomy and should be considered when there are high transvalvular velocities but normal AV leaflet excursion.

Aortic Diseases (Aortopathies)

Coarctation of the Aorta

- Coarctation is a congenital disease in which any part of the aorta can be hypoplastic or stenotic.
- The most typical location is at the isthmus, which is just distal to the origin of the left subclavian artery (Figs. 12-16 and 12-17).
- In some cases, the aortic arch may be diffusely hypoplastic (Fig. 12-18), creating obstruction along the length of the aortic arch.
- Interrupted aortic arch can be considered the extreme form of coarctation in which there is no continuity between part of the aortic arch and the descending aorta. In newborns, blood to the descending aorta is supplied by a patent ductus arteriosus (PDA).
- In rare cases, other segments of the aorta can be involved, including the descending aorta and abdominal aorta.
- The presence and significance of collateral vessels are directly proportional to the severity of the coarctation and the age of the patient.
  - In infants, critical coarctation can occur where the severe afterload of the coarctation develops when the ductus arteriosus closes, and there is not enough time for adequate collateral vessels to develop. Left ventricular failure and cardiogenic shock ensue.

Anatomic Imaging

- The presence or absence of a PDA, along with its flow patterns, should be carefully evaluated.
- Whereas SSN imaging is the typical location, part of the aorta can be masked by the trachea or mainstem bronchus.
- In infants and young children, the manubrium is not completely ossified and is used as an alternative window. If severe coarctation is present and the patient is dependent on a PDA to avoid shock, an interrupted aortic arch should be ruled out.
- Imaging the aorta in both the long axis and short axis views should also be performed.
- In coarctations that have been surgically repaired with patch angioplasty, aneurysmal dilation of the aorta is a long-term complication that may not be well seen with TTE.

Physiologic Data

- In discrete coarctations, the modified Bernoulli equation will overestimate peak-to-peak systolic pressure gradients measured by a blood pressure cuff or catheterization.

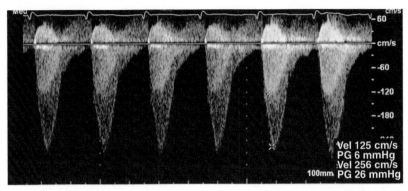

Figure 12-16. CW spectral Doppler pattern of the isthmus region shown in Figure 12-18. Notice the double envelope that represents the transverse arch (velocity 125 cm/s) and the posterior shelf (velocity 256 cm/s).

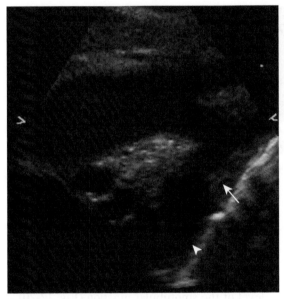

Figure 12-17. Narrowed aortic isthmus (*arrow*) and normal-sized descending aorta (*arrowhead*).

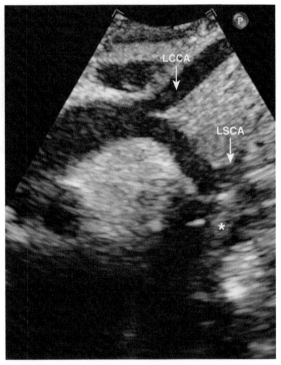

Figure 12-18. The distal transverse arch, located between the left common carotid artery (LCCA) and the subclavian artery (LSCA) is diffusely small. A posterior shelf, indicated by the *asterisk* and the echobright horizontal line to its left, is the narrowest part of the isthmus.

- Corrected velocities can be obtained by an expansion of the Bernoulli equation: $4 \times (V_2^2 - V_1^2)$.
- In patients with tubular hypoplasia of the aortic arch and in patients with multiple levels of obstruction, estimation of blood pressure gradients by spectral Doppler will be less accurate.
- Spectral Doppler evaluation includes all regions of the aorta, including the ascending proximal arch, distal arch, isthmus, descending, and abdominal (Fig. 12-19) regions.
    - Alternate imaging should be carefully considered in this population because echo does not always visualize the important areas of the aorta in every patient.

- Computed tomography (CT) angiography and magnetic resonance (MR) angiography will provide the best noninvasive visualization, will define collateral vessels, and will better define the presence or absence of aneurysms.
    - CT angiography and MR angiography can better define and evaluate aneurysms throughout the thoracic aorta, particularly in the descending aorta in the area of previous repair.

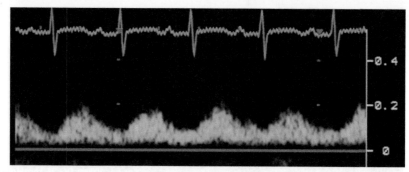

Figure 12-19. Abdominal aorta Doppler in severe coarctation. Pulsatility and peak velocities are severely blunted.

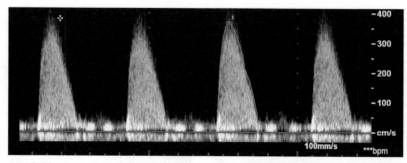

Figure 12-20. Spectral Doppler example of supravalvular AS from a suprasternal notch view.

- The American College of Cardiology/ American Heart Association Adult Congenital Heart Disease Guidelines recommend MR/CT evaluation of the coarctation repair site at least once every 5 years.
- Cardiac catheterization should be considered when additional hemodynamic data are required or if there is a potential for an intervention.

KEY POINTS

- When coarctation of the aorta is present, patency of the ductus arteriosus should be evaluated, particularly in the neonatal period; patients with severe coarctation may be dependent on a PDA for hemodynamic stability.
- The simplified Bernoulli equation may not be a reliable means of assessing coarctation gradients, and the expanded equation is often needed.
- Complementary imaging techniques (e.g., CT and MR angiography) may be needed for full evaluation of coarctation anatomy, aneurysm formation, and collateral flow.

Supravalvular Aortic Stenoses

Congenital
- Supravalvular AS is a condition in which narrowing of the aorta typically occurs at the level of the sinotubular junction (Fig. 12-20).

Acquired Stenosis
- Rarely, supravalvular stenosis can occur either as an early or as a late complication of cardiac or aorta surgical procedures. It is also a complication of profound lipid abnormalities such as homozygous hyperlipidemia.

Anatomic imaging
- 2D parasternal long axis and short axis views provide the best views for evaluating supravalvular stenosis and obtaining dimensions.
- As with other aortic diseases, CT/MR angiography may provide better imaging of the proximal aorta.

Physiologic Data
- Similar to AS, serial PW Doppler assessments through the LVOT and proximal ascending aorta are important to determine which levels are obstructed. Use a low-frequency

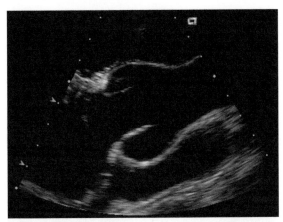

Figure 12-21. Example of a dilated aortic root without effacement of the sinotubular junction.

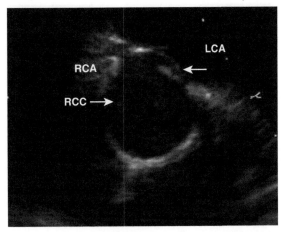

Figure 12-23. Anomalous left coronary artery (LCA) from the right coronary cusp (RCC).

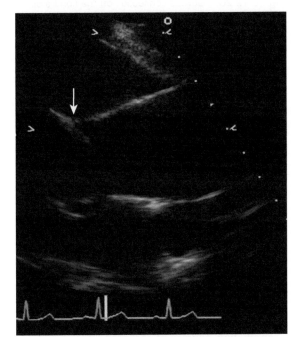

Figure 12-22. Dilation of the ascending aorta. The aortic root (arrow) is not as affected and part of the sinotubular junction is effaced.

transducer to provide the highest Nyquist limit for both spectral Doppler and color Doppler.
- There may be a "Coanda effect" of entrainment of blood toward the right subclavian artery that may be seen on Doppler and can manifest as a slightly higher blood pressure in the right arm.

KEY POINT
• Supravalvular AS should be suspected when there are high transvalvular velocities, normal AV leaflet opening, and a small sinotubular junction diameter.

Dilated Aorta

- Can be associated with connective tissue diseases (see Table 12-1).
- Is associated with congenital diseases such as bicuspid AV or as a consequence of systemic hypertension (Figs. 12-21 and 12-22).

Congenital Coronary Artery Anomalies

- Unusual coronary artery patterns that do not appear to have functional significance include
  - Single coronary artery origins that give rise to the left coronary artery (LCA) and right coronary artery (RCA).
  - Circumflex artery from the RCA.
- Anomalous origin from the opposite sinus (Fig. 12-23).
  - Associated with sudden death.
  - Some authorities postulate that a patient with the anomalous origin of the LCA from the right sinus of Valsalva is at greater risk of sudden death (see Fig. 12-23) compared with a patient with an anomalous RCA from the left sinus.
- Anomalous origin from the PA (Figs. 12-24 and 12-25).

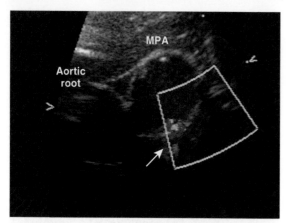

Figure 12-24. Color Doppler of the anomalous LCA connection *(arrow)*. Flow courses from the coronary artery into the main pulmonary artery (MPA).

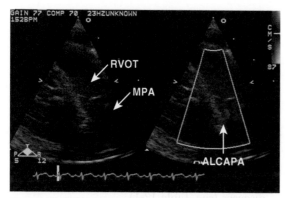

Figure 12-25. Parasternal long axis view of the anomalous connection, located at the inferior aspect of the MPA. Flow from the coronary artery courses retrograde.

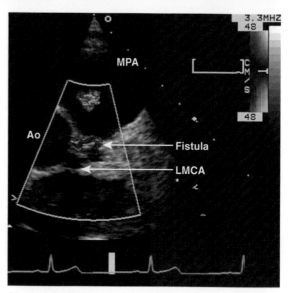

Figure 12-26. Fistulous connection off the nondilated LMCA. Despite the color Doppler map, the terminal connection of this fistula could not be located.

- Can be either the LCA (anomalous origin of the LCA from the PA) or the RCA (anomalous origin of the RCA from the PA), usually originating off the main PA (MPA).
- In infancy, can present with cardiogenic shock and ventricular dysfunction.
- In older children and adults, collateral circulation from the normally connected coronary artery will have developed.
- Coronary artery fistulae.
  - Also known as coronary-cameral fistulas, these lesions are present when flow from a coronary artery is shunted to an adjacent chamber, typically the MPA or atrium (Fig. 12-26). Most are clinically silent, but some are associated with ischemic symptoms or signs of volume overload.

Anatomic Imaging
- Identification and direct visualization of the origins are critical.
  - Proximal coronary artery vessels are more easily imaged than origins, but their presence may not be used to imply that the origin is normal.
  - Use both still frame and cine (moving) images to determine location.
  - In young pediatric patients, anomalous coronary artery origins can be reliably diagnosed by echo.
  - In older patients such as adolescents and adults, visualization of the origins can be limited by windows.
- Color Doppler can assist in defining anomalous courses of coronary arteries and locating fistulae. Low Nyquist settings (≤40 cm/s) should be used to ensure that adequate signals are detected.

Physiologic Data
- Hemodynamically significant fistulous connections can be supported by the presence of coronary artery, atrial, or ventricular dilation. Identification of ventricular dysfunction can also serve as a surrogate.
- Spectral Doppler evaluation of coronary arteries is limited due to the lack of data defining normal and abnormal flow patterns and motion of the aortic root.

Alternate Imaging

- Electrocardiography-gated coronary CT angiography can be used to identify anatomy and fistulous connections.
- Cardiac MR imaging (MRI) spatial resolution is not as fine as CT, but can be used to determine shunt volumes and chamber volumes.
- Cardiac catheterization is often needed to define the course and treatment options for coronary fistulae.

Alternate Approaches to Echo in Left Heart Anomalies

- Supplemental modalities can be considered if transthoracic windows are poor and echo cannot answer the clinical questions.
  - TEE can be used for intracardiac, and most ascending and descending aorta evaluation. The aortic arch and part of the ascending aorta are not well visualized, however.
  - Cardiac MRI can be used if additional physiologic data are required such as determination of regurgitant volumes, ventricular volumes, and myocardial viability. Anatomic imaging can also be accomplished, but the spatial resolution will not always be as good as that with TEE or CT.
  - Cardiac CT can be used with good spatial resolution, but blood flow and pressure gradients cannot be estimated.
- Positron emission tomography/CT can evaluate flows, but use of this modality is not as widespread.
  - The relative strengths and weaknesses of supplemental modalities are outlined in Table 12-3.
- In all cases, structures immediately upstream and downstream of any identified lesion can also be abnormal and should be evaluated carefully.

KEY POINTS

- Coronary artery anomalies are an important cause of sudden cardiac death in young people, particularly when the coronary artery trasverses between the PA and the aorta.
- When imaging quality allows, coronary artery ostia can be well visualized echocardiographically; visualization of the bifurcation of the left anterior descending and the left circumflex arteries is needed to exclude anomalous takeoffs.
- Coronary angiography will provide additional assessment of coronary anatomy and arterial course and should be performed whenever coronary anomalies are suspected.

TABLE 12-3 RELATIVE ADVANTAGES AND DISADVANTAGES OF ALTERNATIVE IMAGING MODALITIES

	Echocardiography	MRI	CT
Spatial resolution	+++	++	+++
Temporal Resolution	++++	+++	+
Physiology/blood flow	++++	+++	+
Pericardium visualization	++	++++	+++

+, Poor; ++, fair; +++, better; ++++, best.

Suggested Reading

1. Rheumatic Fever and Rheumatic Heart Disease. Report of a WHO Expert Consultation. WHO Technical Report Series. 2001. http://www.who.int/cardiovascular_diseases/resources/trs923/en/.
   Web article from the World Health Organization that provides a detailed description of rheumatic fever diagnosis and clinical findings.
2. Aboulhosn J, Child JS. Left ventricular outflow obstruction: subaortic stenosis, bicuspid aortic valve, supravalvar aortic stenosis, and coarctation of the aorta. *Circulation.* 2006;114:2412-2422.
3. Basso C, Maron BJ, Corrado D, Thiene G. Clinical profile of congenital coronary artery anomalies with origin from the wrong aortic sinus leading to sudden death in young competitive athletes. *J Am Coll Cardiol.* 2000;35:1493-1501.
   Good series on a rare coronary anomaly.
4. Baumgartner H, Hung J, Bermejo J, et al. Echocardiographic assessment of valve stenosis: EAE/ASE recommendations for clinical practice. *J Am Soc Echocardiogr.* 2009;22:1-23; quiz 101-102.
   Detailed, up-to-date review of valve stenosis.
5. Frommelt PC, Frommelt MA. Congenital coronary artery anomalies. *Pediatr Clin North Am.* 2004;51:1273-1288.
   Authors have a number of articles and presentations that cover this subject and can be considered to be among the leading authorities.

6. Gibbs JL. Ultrasound and coarctation of the aorta. *Br Heart J*. Aug 1990;64(2):109-110.

7. Kurtz CE, Otto CM. Aortic stenosis: clinical aspects of diagnosis and management, with 10 illustrative case reports from a 25-year experience. *Medicine (Baltimore)*. 2010;89:349-379.

8. Lancellotti P, Tribouilloy C, Hagendorff A, et al. European Association of Echocardiography recommendations for the assessment of valvular regurgitation. Part 1: aortic and pulmonary regurgitation (native valve disease). *Eur J Echocardiogr*. 2010;11:223-244.

9. Lancellotti P, Moura L, Pierard LA, et al. European Association of Echocardiography recommendations for the assessment of valvular regurgitation. Part 2: mitral and tricuspid regurgitation (native valve disease). *Eur J Echocardiogr*. 2010;11:307-332.

10. Shaddy RE, Snider AR, Silverman NH, Lutin W. Pulsed Doppler findings in patients with coarctation of the aorta. *Circulation*. 1986;73(1):82-88.
Important article that describes the subtleties of spectral Doppler patterns.

11. Tani LY, Veasy LG, Minich LL, Shaddy RE. Rheumatic fever in children younger than 5 years: is the presentation different? *Pediatrics*. 2003;112(5):1065-1068.

12. Zoghbi WA, Enriquez-Sarano M, Foster E, et al. Recommendations for evaluation of the severity of native valvular regurgitation with two-dimensional and Doppler echocardiography. *J Am Soc Echocardiogr*. 2003;16:777-802.
Another article that describes the multiple techniques and the various limitations of regurgitation severity assessment. The tables alone are worth the time for review.

Myocardial Pathology

David S. Owens and Mariska Kemna

13

HYPERTROPHIC CARDIOMYOPATHY

Background

- Hypertrophic cardiomyopathy (HCM) is characterized by pathologic thickening of the left ventricle (LV) due to sarcomeric gene mutations.
- HCM commonly involves asymmetrical hypertrophy of the anterior septum, but can manifest as concentric hypertrophy or hypertrophy of other segments (Figs. 13-1 through 13-3).
- Resting left ventricular outflow tract obstruction (LVOTO) due to systolic anterior motion of the mitral apparatus is present in about one third of HCM patients; another one third has provocable obstruction.
- The presence of LVOTO is neither necessary nor sufficient to diagnose HCM.
- A diagnosis of HCM is suggested by wall thickness greater than 1.5 cm in adults or a Z score indexed to body surface area of more than 2 in children (in the absence of other causes for hypertrophy).
- Structural or valvular abnormalities that increase left ventricular afterload (e.g., aortic stenosis, coarctation of the aorta) need to be excluded before a diagnosis of HCM can be made.
- Other conditions that mimic HCM include hypertensive heart disease, infiltrative disorders (e.g., amyloidosis), and glycogen storage disorders (e.g., Fabry disease, Danon disease, *PRKAG2* mutations).
- In infants, 30% to 50% of cases of an HCM-like phenotype can be attributed to metabolic or syndromal disorders (e.g., Noonan syndrome). Infants born to diabetic mothers can have transient biventricular hypertrophy.
- Physiologic adaptation to exercise can lead to mild to moderate ventricular hypertrophy, which can mimic HCM. Features distinguishing "athlete's heart" from HCM are shown in Table 13-1.
- Massive left ventricular hypertrophy (LVH)—wall thickness greater than 30 mm in adults or a Z score for body surface area greater than +15 in children—is a risk factor for sudden death in HCM patients.

Echocardiographic Approach
(Table 13-2)

Anatomic Imaging
- Step 1: Assess the magnitude and extent of LVH.
  - Whenever possible, wall thickness measurements should be confirmed in more than one imaging plane (see Fig. 13-1).
  - Short axis view imaging of the LV at multiple levels usually provides the best means of assessing wall thickness and overall hypertrophy.
  - The right ventricular moderator band and papillary muscle insertions should not be included in wall thickness measurements. The parasternal long axis view is most susceptible to mismeasurement.
  - Apical windows may be more suited to estimating LV wall thickness of the inferior septum and lateral wall, common regions of dropout on short axis view imaging.
  - Use of contrast agents can improve endocardial border detection in patients with suspected midcavitary or apical hypertrophy.
- Step 2: Quantify systolic function.
  - HCM patients often have an increase in circumferential shortening, but a decrease in longitudinal shortening.
  - Hyperdynamic systolic function is also commonly seen in hypertensive heart disease or situations of decreased afterload.

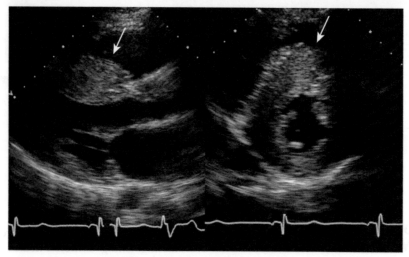

Figure 13-1. Parasternal long axis and short axis two-dimensional images of a patient with classic reverse curvature hypertrophic cardiomyopathy (HCM) and primary involvement of the basal anterior septum. Measurement of maximal wall thickness is performed at the greatest diameter, excluding right ventricular band insertion.

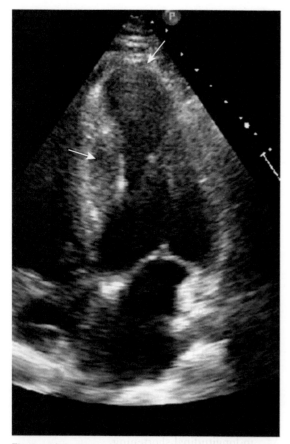

Figure 13-2. Apical four-chamber (4C) view of a patient with mid-ventricular HCM demonstrating mid-ventricular and papillary muscle hypertrophy and secondary apical aneurysm formation due to midventricular obstruction.

TABLE 13-1	FEATURES DISTINGUISHING "ATHLETE'S HEART" FROM HCM IN ADULTS*	
Feature	**Athlete's Heart**	**HCM**
Maximal wall thickness	≤16 mm	≥13 mm
Pattern of LVH	Predominantly concentric	Concentric or asymmetrical
LV cavity dimension	Often > 55 mm (in endurance athletes)	Usually < 45 mm
Diastolic function	Normal	Normal or abnormal
Gender	Male > female	Male = female
Family history of HCM or SCD	No	Yes or no
Delayed enhancement (MRI)	No	Yes or no
Exercise capacity	Above normal	Normal to below normal
Response to deconditioning	LVH regression	No change in LVH

*Intended for adults or adult-sized teenagers. Corresponding Z scores can be calculated for children but have not been validated.

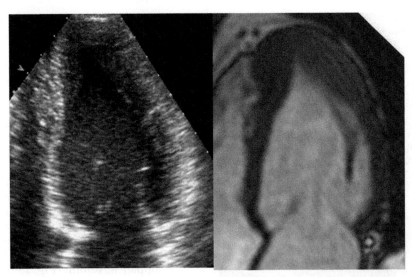

Figure 13-3. Apical 4C echocardiographic (*left*) and cardiac magnetic resonance imaging (MRI) (*right*) views of a patient with apical HCM. Cardiac MRI can provide a good depiction of apical thickness and function when echocardiographic imaging is inadequate.

TABLE 13-2   ECHOCARDIOGRAPHIC FEATURES OF CARDIOMYOPATHIES

	HCM	DCM	LVN	RCM
LV size	Normal	Increased	Normal to increased	Normal
LV ejection fraction	Increased	Decreased	Normal to decreased	Normal to decreased
LV wall thickness	Increased	Normal	Normal	Normal to increased
LV diastolic function	Decreased	Decreased	Normal to decreased	Markedly decreased
LV filling pressures	Increased	Increased	Normal to increased	Markedly increased
LA size	Increased	Increased	Normal to increased	Markedly increased
PA pressures	Normal to increased	Normal to increased	Normal	Increased

- A small subset (~5%) of HCM patients have declining LV systolic function due to progressive fibrosis.
- Step 3: Assess mitral leaflet motion for possible systolic anterior motion (SAM).
  - SAM is best viewed in either the parasternal or apical long axis windows (Fig. 13-4).
  - M-mode depiction of mitral leaflet motion is essential for determining the timing of SAM and the duration of mitral-septal contract (Fig. 13-5).
  - The presence of LVOTO in the absence of SAM suggests fixed subaortic stenosis, and additional causes of obstruction should be sought.
  - Early closure of the aortic valve (AV) on M-mode echocardiography (echo) is a nonspecific finding that may be present with either fixed or dynamic LVOTO.

- Step 4: If significant SAM is present, assess mitral leaflets and subvalvular anatomy.
  - HCM can be associated with abnormalities in papillary muscle anatomy.
  - Features that predispose to LVOTO include elongated mitral leaflets, chordal slack, direct insertion of the papillary muscle into the mitral leaflets, septal chordal attachments, and anteriorly or apically displaced papillary muscles.

Physiologic Data
- Step 1: Assess the presence and severity of intracardiac obstruction.
  - Obstruction can occur at either the midventricular or left ventricular outflow tract (LVOT) level.
  - Midventricular obstruction predisposes to apical aneurysm formation and scarring;

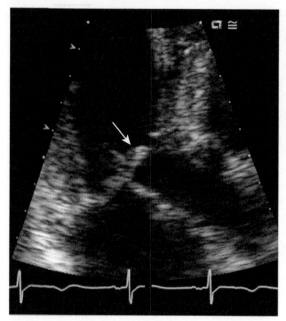

Figure 13-4. Apical long axis view of a patient with outflow tract obstruction due to systolic anterior motion of the mitral valve (MV) leaflets.

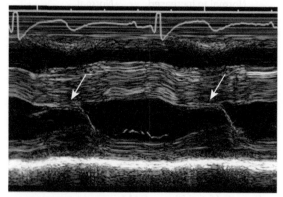

Figure 13-5. M-mode at the level of the MV tips showing septal hypertrophy and systolic anterior motion of the mitral apparatus in a patient with HCM.

contrast agents should be considered if the apex is not well visualized.
- Changes in left ventricular geometry can alter intracardiac flow patterns, dragging the mitral leaflets anteriorly into the LVOT.
- Anterior movement of the tips of the mitral leaflets may result in a loss of coaptation and posteriorly directed mitral regurgitation (MR).
- This LVOTO is a complex, dynamic process that is affected by LV contractility, loading conditions, and both mitral leaflet and subvalvular anatomy.

- Step 2: Measure the velocity of blood flow down the length of the LV using pulsed wave (PW) Doppler.
  - Marching the PW Doppler sample from apex to base allows localization of the site of obstruction.
  - Anterior displacement of the mitral leaflets causes associated MR to originate more anteriorly, and thus care must be taken to differentiate LVOT flow from regurgitation flow.
  - Resting LVOT velocities greater than 5 m/s are uncommon and should be confirmed by finding a separate, even higher velocity (>7 m/s) mitral regurgitant jet.
  - Dynamic obstruction may produce a characteristic dagger-shaped, late-peaking Doppler waveform (Fig. 13-6A); however, complete LVOTO may produce a characteristic "lobster claw" appearance (Fig. 13-6B).
- Step 3: Assess changes in LVOT velocity with provocation in adults and older children.
  - Perform in patients with known or suspected HCM without resting LVOTO.
  - Provocation can unmask resting LVOT gradients; patients with provocable LVOTO are more likely to have exercise-induced obstruction.
  - Common provocative factors include Valsalva maneuver, pharmacologic agents (amyl nitrate or isoproterenol), and exercise.
- Step 4: Assess MR.
  - MR can be difficult to quantify because of its timing (originating in mid to late systole) and eccentricity, making proximal isovelocity surface area (PISA) calculations less reliable.
  - If the mitral regurgitant jet is not posteriorly directed, other etiologies for the MR should be suspected.
- Step 5: Assess diastolic function.
  - Assessment of diastolic function in HCM patients is challenging due to asymmetrical hypertrophy and changes in calcium kinetics.
  - Because of the asymmetrical hypertrophy, mitral annular relaxation velocities should be sampled from the septal, lateral, anterior, and inferior aspects of the annulus, with an average velocity used to assess global diastolic function.
  - The ratio of mitral inflow velocity deceleration (E wave) to early mitral annular relaxation (E′) velocity is not as robust a predictor of filling pressure as in other conditions.

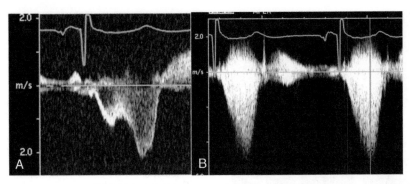

Figure 13-6. Complete LVOTO may result in a "lobster claw" appearance of the pulsed wave (PW) Doppler (**A**); more commonly, a characteristic dagger-shaped, late-peaking continuous wave (CW) Doppler signal is seen (**B**).

- Abnormalities in diastolic relaxation can precede the development of hypertrophy in patients carrying otherwise subclinical sarcomeric gene mutations (Fig. 13-7).
- Step 6: Assess consequences of HCM.
  - Assess left atrial enlargement.
  - Assess pulmonary artery pressures (PAPs).
  - Assess right ventricular function and hypertrophy.

Alternate Approaches

- Exercise echo is particularly useful in evaluating patients with suspected exercise-induced LVOTO.
- Cardiac magnetic resonance imaging (MRI) is useful for determining maximal wall thickness, and the use of delayed gadolinium enhancement can provide assessment of the extent of fibrosis.
- Consider the use of contrast agents for better visualization of the left ventricular apex in patients with midcavitary obstruction.
- 3D TEE can aid in the assessment of subvalvular architecture and the location of intracardiac obstruction.

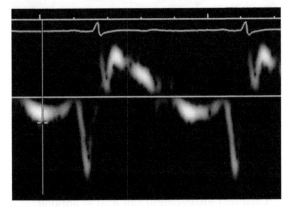

Figure 13-7. Septal mitral annular tissue Doppler sample in a carrier of a known HCM gene mutation before the development of left ventricular hypertrophy (LVH). In this patient, the myocardial early relaxation velocity is markedly decreased.

DILATED CARDIOMYOPATHY

Background

- Dilated cardiomyopathy (DCM) is characterized by spherical enlargement of the LV with reduction in global systolic function. Four-chamber enlargement and dysfunction are often present (Fig. 13-8).
- Echo is an essential component of diagnosing and managing patients with DCM.
- DCM is often classified as ischemic (due to coronary artery disease) or nonischemic, based on the presence or absence of myocardial ischemia or infarction. Potential causes of DCM are listed in Table 13-3.
- Most cases of primary DCM in children are idiopathic, but a positive family history is present in 30% of cases, suggesting a genetic component.

KEY POINTS

- HCM can present with asymmetric hypertrophy of any cardiac segment, and may also manifest as concentric hypertrophy.
- The presence of LVOTO is neither necessary nor sufficient to diagnose HCM.
- When LVOTO is present, care must be taken to differentiate the LVOT Doppler signal from MR.
- Abnormalities in mitral valve and papillary muscle anatomy are common in HCM and can predispose to LVOTO.

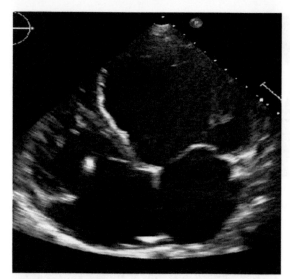

Figure 13-8. Apical 4C image of a dilated cardiomyopathy (DCM) showing globular 4C enlargement.

TABLE 13-3   CONGENITAL AND ACQUIRED CAUSES OF DCM PRESENTING IN CHILDREN AND ADULTS

Children	Adults
Congenital	**Congenital**
Familial/genetic	Familial/genetic
Neuromuscular disorders	Neuromuscular
Inborn errors of metabolism	**Acquired**
Left-sided stenotic lesions	Ischemic causes
Coronary anomalies (e.g., ALCAPA)	Myocarditis
Malformation syndromes	Infectious (viral, HIV)
Acquired	Medications (anthracyclines)
Myocarditis	Toxins (alcohol, stimulants)
Infectious (viral, HIV)	Infiltrative disorders (amyloid, sarcoid)
Medications (anthracyclines)	Peripartum
Tachycardia mediated	Stress-induced (takotsubo)
High output (chronic anemia, shunts)	Thyroid disorders
Idiopathic	Tachycardia mediated
	High output (chronic anemia, shunts)
	Idiopathic

- Anomalous origin of the left coronary artery from the pulmonary artery (ALCAPA) can present with DCM in the first weeks of life due to decreasing PAP and resultant myocardial ischemia.
- Chamber enlargement can lead to annular dilation and leaflet tethering of the semilunar valves, causing secondary (functional) valve regurgitation.
- In contrast, a primary valvular cardiomyopathy (CM) should be suspected when significant aortic regurgitation (AR) is present in the setting of DCM.
- Diastolic dysfunction is commonly present in patients with impaired systolic function, with increase in LV filling pressures.
- Important sequelae of DCM include atrial enlargement, pulmonary hypertension, ventricular aneurysm formation, and intracardiac thrombosis.

Echocardiographic Approach
(See Table 13-2)

Anatomic Imaging
- Step 1: Assess LV size and anatomy.
  - A single left ventricular dimension, standardly taken from the parasternal long axis or short axis views at the level of the MV tips, using M-mode or 2D measurements, is a reasonable first estimate of left ventricular chamber size.

- Left ventricular volume measurements give more accurate assessments of cavity size and can be estimated using 2D formulae or 3D methods.
- Left ventricular dimensions and volumes should be indexed to body surface area in children and in adults when body size is particularly large or small.
- Stress-induced (takotsubo) CM demonstrates a characteristic pattern of apical ballooning.
- Step 2: Assess left ventricular systolic function.
  - Assessment of left ventricular function should focus on both global and regional wall motion; regional wall motion abnormalities (RWMAs) suggest the presence of coronary artery disease (Fig. 13-9).
  - Global systolic function is estimated using either fractional shortening or ejection fraction (EF) calculations.
  - Volumetric methods for estimating EF are more robust than those based on 2D measures, which make assumptions of chamber geometry.
  - The presence of RWMAs can suggest fibrosis, previous myocardial infarction, or regions of hibernating myocardium.
  - Use of intravenous contrast agent can improve wall motion assessment through improved endocardial border definition.

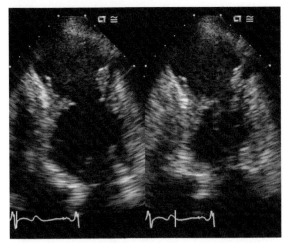

Figure 13-9.   Apical 4C images in diastole (*left*) and systole (*right*) of a patient with DCM and apical aneurysm secondary to Danon disease (i.e., *LAMP2* gene mutation).

- Patients with left ventricular dysfunction and alterations in ventricular conduction may demonstrate dyssynchronous ventricular contraction, wherein wall segments contact at slightly different times.
- Another good measure of global left ventricular contractility includes mitral regurgitant *dP/dt* (rate of change in pressure over time).
- Step 3: Evaluate the presence of aneurysms and intracardiac thrombi.
  - In patients with previous transmural myocardial infarctions or fibrosis, aneurysms can develop, most commonly seen in the left ventricular apex.
  - In patients with aneurysms or reduced systolic function, intracardiac thrombi can develop, especially in regions of aneurysm formation (Fig. 13-10).
  - Scanning for apical aneurysms is best performed using a slow anterior-to-posterior sweep with 4- to 8-s digital capture.
  - If aneurysms or thrombi are suspected but image quality is suboptimal, consider the use of intravenous contrast.
- Step 4: Evaluate valve anatomy.
  - Ventricular chamber enlargement can distort the geometry of the MV and tricuspid valve (TV), resulting in annular dilation and leaflet tethering (Fig. 13-11).
  - Severe annular dilation can result in failure of leaflet coaptation, which suggests the presence of severe regurgitation.
  - AR is not an expected sequela of DCM, and a primary valvular CM should be suspected when significant AR is present.

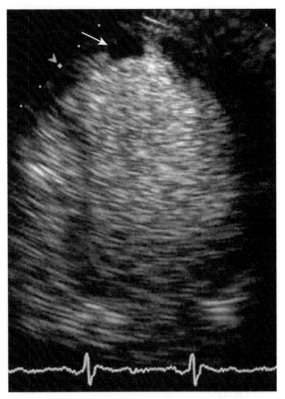

Figure 13-10. Contrast-enhanced apical 4C image showing a thrombus (*arrow*) within the left ventricular apex of a patient with apical akinesis.

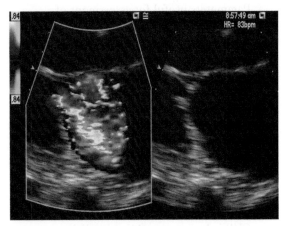

Figure 13-11. Zoomed parasternal long axis view of a patient with DCM and severe functional mitral regurgitation (MR) due to mitral annular dilation and limited coaptation of the mitral leaflets.

- Step 5: Exclude anatomic causes for DCM.
  - If intrinsic abnormalities of MV or TV anatomy are detected, a primary valvular etiology for the DCM should be considered.
  - Severe left-sided obstructive lesions, including AV stenosis and coarctation (see Chapter 12), can occasionally result in DCM and should also be excluded.

- ALCAPA (see Chapter 12, Left Heart Anomalies) may present as DCM within the first few weeks of life. Retrograde flow within the left main coronary artery is best detected using PW Doppler from the parasternal long axis or short axis view.

Physiologic Data
- Step 1: Assess valvular function.
  - Standard methods for assessing valvular function, using continuous wave (CW) Doppler, PW Doppler, and color Doppler, are appropriate.
  - Quantification of valvular regurgitation, using the PISA or flow volume at two sites method, is particular useful in DCM.
  - Functional MR or tricuspid regurgitation (TR) can improve or worsen with changes in patient's volume status.
- Step 2: Assess left ventricular diastolic function (Fig. 13-12).
  - Patients with significant systolic dysfunction will also have alterations in diastolic function. Estimation of left ventricular filling pressures is particularly useful in the management of patients with DCM.
  - When RWMAs are present, mitral annular velocities should be sampled from the most unaffected regions.
  - Parameters useful for assessment of diastolic function include transmitral flow velocities, the transmitral E/A ratio, the E-wave deceleration time, the isovolumic relaxation time (IVRT), tissue Doppler E′ velocities and the E/E′ ratio, and pulmonary vein flow patterns.
  - Diastolic filling patterns may change with changes in the patient's volume status.
- Step 3: Assess central venous pressure (CVP) and PA systolic pressure (PASP).
  - Patients with DCM are prone to the development of congestive heart failure, manifesting as elevations in CVP or PAP.
  - CVP is best assessed by visualizing the response of the inferior vena cava (IVC) to a deep, quick inspiration or sniff.
    - The IVC is best visualized through subcostal window.
    - A dilated IVC and/or less than 50% collapse of the IVC to sniff suggests elevation in CVP.
  - PASP can be estimated using the tricuspid regurgitant jet velocity, the modified Bernoulli equation, and estimates of CVP.

- PASP ≈ right ventricular systolic pressure = CVP + 4 × (peak TR jet velocity)^2.

Alternate Approaches

- Dobutamine stress echo can be useful for assessing myocardial viability in patients with RWMAs and reduced systolic function.
- Strain and strain rate echocardiographic imaging can be adjunctive in the assessment of global and regional systolic function.
- 3D transthoracic echo may provide more reliable volumetric assessments of the EF, but may be time-consuming for standard use.
- Several methods for quantifying left ventricular dyssynchrony using strain rate and 3D imaging are available, but the best predictors of a response to cardiac resynchronization therapy have not been established.
- Cardiac MRI can provide global and regional assessments of left ventricular function, and the use of delayed gadolinium enhancement can define the location and extent of scarring and viability.

KEY POINTS

- DCM is characterized by spherical enlargement of the LV with reduction in global systolic function; causes of DCM are varied.
- Echocardiographic assessment of systolic and diastolic function plays a key role in the diagnosis and management of patients with DCM.
- When significant regurgitation of the semilunar valves is present, careful interrogation of the valves is required to distinguish a primary valvular etiology from secondary functional regurgitation.
- When systolic function is severely decreased or aneurysms are present, it is important to exclude thrombus formation within the ventricle.

LEFT VENTRICULAR NONCOMPACTION

Background

- Left ventricular noncompaction (LVN) is a rare disorder characterized by alteration in myocardial wall development, resulting in a thinned compact myocardial layer, prominent left ventricular trabeculations, and deep intertrabecular recesses (Fig. 13-13).

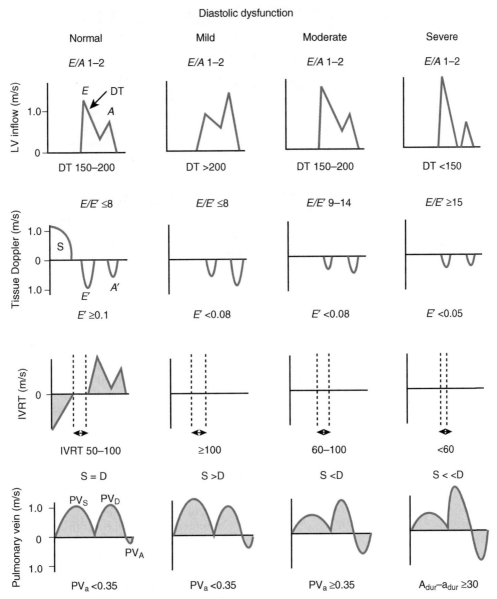

Figure 13-12. Assessment of diastolic function. Diagram comparing typical Doppler findings in patients with normal, mild, moderate, and severe diastolic dysfunction. *Top row:* Left ventricular inflow with early (E) and atrial (A) phases of diastolic filling. *Second row:* Tissue Doppler recorded at the septal side of the mitral annulus with the myocardial early (E') and atrial (A') velocities and the expected ratio of E/E'. *Third row:* Isovolumic relaxation time (IVRT). *Bottom row:* Pulmonary venous inflow pattern with systolic (S) and diastolic (D) antegrade flow and the pulmonary vein atrial (PVa) reversal of flow. *(From Otto C. Textbook of Clinical Echocardiography, 4th ed. Philadelphia: Saunders/Elsevier, 2009; Figure 7-28.)*

- Echo plays a critical role in identifying and diagnosing LVN.
- Several different sets of diagnostic criteria for LVN exist. Common echocardiographic findings include
  - More than three prominent trabeculations protruding from the left ventricular apex or midcavity (distinct from papillary muscles).
  - Greater than 2:1 ratio in thickness of noncompacted epicardial trabeculations to

thickness of compact endocardium, measured at end-systole.
  - Evidence of flow within the deep intertrabecular recesses.
- Although noncompaction can occur as an isolated finding (isolated LVN), it can also be seen in conjunction with other neuromuscular or congenital heart abnormalities.
- There is considerable genotypic and phenotypic overlap between LVN and dilated,

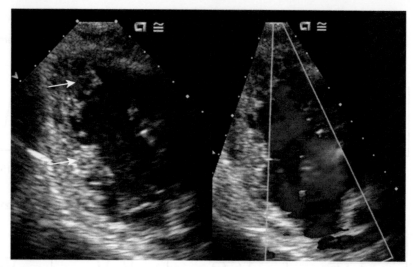

Figure 13-13. An apical 2C view showing left ventricular noncompaction characterized by prominent trabeculations along the inferior wall and apex. Color flow Doppler demonstrates flow within the intertrabecular recesses, differentiating this from HCM.

hypertrophic (particularly the apical variant), and restrictive cardiomyopathies.
- Patients with LVN often have progressive left ventricular systolic dysfunction and dilation.
- Additional clinical complications of LVN include atrial and ventricular tachyarrhythmias, sudden cardiac death, and thromboembolic complications including strokes, with the intertrabecular spaces likely serving as a nidus of thrombus formation.

Echocardiographic Approach
(See Table 13-2)

Anatomic Imaging
- Step 1: Assess left ventricular morphology and function.
  - Trabeculations are often best visualized from the apical windows and should be distinguished from the hypertrophy of the apical compact myocardium seen in HCM.
  - Use of intravenous contrast can help distinguish trabeculations (which are not generally visible with contrast) from compact myocardium.
  - Because DCM is common in LVN, standard assessment of left ventricular size and function is appropriate.
  - Trabecular microthrombosis is a common source of emboli in patients with LVN; screening for left ventricular thrombi, using contrast enhancement when appropriate, should be standard.

- Step 2: Screen for associated congenital abnormalities.
  - An array of congenital heart abnormalities have been described as being coincident with LVN, including coronary anomalies and coronary-cameral fistulae, atrial septal defects (ASDs), ventricular septal defects (VSDs), bicuspid AVs, and Ebstein's anomaly.
  - Coronary ostia can usually be identified in young patients from the parasternal short axis view, although this is more challenging in older individuals.
  - Screening for ASDs or VSDs is appropriate; consider use of saline solution contrast injections to screen for shunting.

Physiologic Imaging
- Step 1: Demonstration of flow in trabecular recesses.
  - Color Doppler should be used to demonstrate flow within the trabecular recesses, confirming that this layer is loosely organized. Because flow in the recesses is slow, adjustments to the color scale and Nyquist limits may be required.
  - If intertrabecular flow is not seen, alternative diagnoses should be considered.
- Step 2: Standard assessment of ventricular and valvular function (as described in the DCM section).

Alternate Approaches

- Cardiac MRI can be performed to help distinguish compact myocardium from trabeculation when the diagnosis of LVN is uncertain; separate MRI criteria for LVN have been proposed.

KEY POINTS

- LVN is caused by alteration in myocardial wall development, and results in a thinned compact myocardial layer, prominent left ventricular trabeculations, and deep intertrabecular recesses.
- LVN can mimic DCM and apical HCM echocardiographically.
- Demonstration of flow within the intertrabecular recesses distinguishes LVN from apical HCM.
- Thrombi formation within the intertrabecular recesses can be a source of strokes and other embolic events in patients with LVN.

RESTRICTIVE CARDIOMYOPATHY

Background

- Restrictive cardiomyopathy (RCM) is characterized by a nondilated LV with significant impairment in diastolic filling due primarily to abnormalities in myocardial compliance.
- Wall thickness in RCM can be normal or concentrically hypertrophied; left ventricular function is usually preserved but can be decreased in late-stage disease.
- Causes of RCM are varied and include infiltrative disorders (e.g., amyloidosis, sarcoidosis), storage disease (e.g., hemochromotosis, Fabry disease), endomyocardial fibrosis, hypereosinophilic syndrome, endomyocardial fibroelastosis, radiation exposure, or an underlying gene mutation. In children, RCM is most commonly idiopathic.
- RCM must be distinguished from constrictive pericarditis in which normal myocardium is constricted by a noncompliant pericardium, resulting in elevated filling pressures.
- Echo can suggest a diagnosis of RCM, but is not conclusive. RCM diagnosis is usually based on multimodality imaging, invasive hemodynamic testing, and possible pathologic examination of biopsy specimens.
- Myocardial tissue may appear echobright (e.g., a "starry sky" appearance with amyloidosis [Fig. 13-14]), or there may be a hyperechoic endocardial layer (e.g., in Fabry disease [Fig. 13-15]). These findings are suggestive, but not pathognomonic for RCM.
- Additional echocardiographic findings supporting a diagnosis of RCM include significant biatrial enlargement and elevated PAPs.
- Restrictive diastolic filling patterns can also be seen in patients with DCM and significant volume overload; these are not classified as RCM.

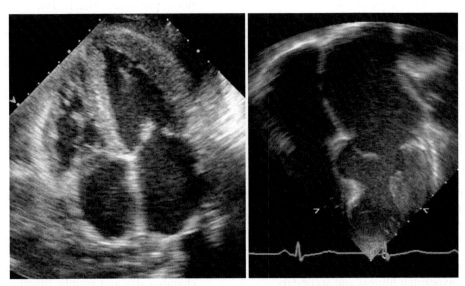

Figure 13-14. Apical 4C views of an adult with restrictive cardiomyopathy (RCM) (*left*) due to systemic amyloidosis demonstrating concentric LVH, a general increase in the echogenicity of the myocardium, severe biatrial enlargement, and mild thickening of the mitral leaflets. In children, RCM may give an "ice cream cone" appearance (*right*) with massive atrial enlargement with preserved ventricular size.

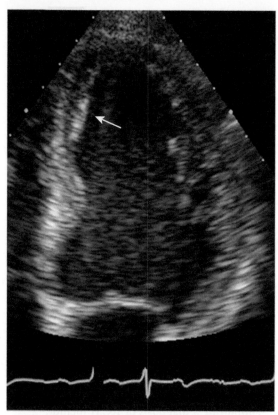

Figure 13-15. Apical 4C view of a patient with Fabry disease showing concentric LVH and increased echogenicity of the endocardium due to glycosphingolipid accumulation.

Echocardiographic Approach
(See Table 13-2)

Anatomic Imaging

- Step 1: Assess chamber morphology and function.
  - Standard assessment of left ventricular size and function is appropriate in patients with known or suspected RCM.
  - Although echocardiographic findings may vary in each condition, common features of RCM include a small or nondilated LV with preserved systolic function but significant elevation in left ventricular filling pressures.
  - Wall thickness is often concentrically hypertrophied but can be normal; when LVH is present, RCM must be distinguished from HCM.
  - Endomyocardial fibrosis and secondary thrombus formation can result in apical obliteration and markedly reduced left ventricular chamber volumes.

- Standard harmonic imaging may cause normal myocardium to appear echobright or hyperechoic. When RCM is suspected, additional imaging without harmonics should be performed.
- Concurrent right ventricular dysfunction may be present, with elevated central venous pressure.
- Significant biatrial enlargement is a common feature of RCM due to chronic elevation in right and left ventricular filling pressures.
- In children, an "ice-cream cone" appearance can be seen, created by grossly enlarged atria resting on top of relatively small ventricles (see Fig. 13-14).
- If pericardial thickening or echogenicity is appreciated, constrictive pericarditis should be considered.
- Step 2: Assess valvular anatomy and function.
  - Endomyocardial fibrosis can cause fibrosis of the atrioventricular subvalvular apparatuses, leading to leaflet tethering and regurgitation.
  - Amyloidosis can result in diffuse leaflet thickening.

Physiologic Data

- Step 1: Assess left ventricular diastolic filling and function.
  - Careful assessment of left ventricular diastolic filling and function is essential.
  - Over time, progressive restriction leads to slower diastolic relaxation, decreasing compliance, and increasing ventricular filling pressures (Fig. 13-16).
  - At the time of diagnosis, moderate to severe diastolic dysfunction is usually present, characterized by:
    - Elevated transmitral E-wave velocity with a rapid deceleration time.
    - Reduced tissue Doppler mitral annular E′ velocity.
    - Elevated E/E′ ratio.
    - Decreased IVRT.
    - Increased pulmonary vein A-wave amplitude and duration.
    - Pulmonary hypertension.
- Step 2: Differentiate RCM from constrictive pericarditis (Table 13-4).
  - In clinical practice, differentiating RCM and constrictive pericarditis is often challenging because both demonstrate elevated filling pressures with normal chamber size and systolic function.
  - Pericardial constriction may show signs of interventricular dependence, such as septal shifting with inspiration and discordant

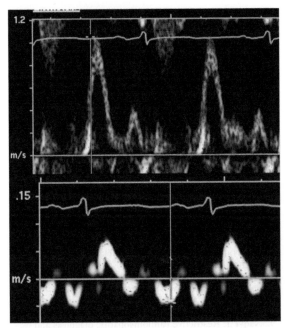

Figure 13-16. Left ventricular diastolic filling in a patient with RCM, with PW Doppler signal of transmitral inflow (*top*) and tissue Doppler imaging of the sepal mitral annulus (*bottom*). The mitral inflow E velocity is increased with a short deceleration time, whereas the aseptal annular E' velocity is reduced, yielding a significantly elevated E/E' ratio (>20).

respiratory variation in tricuspid and mitral inflow.
- Using a respirometer, PW Doppler sampling of mitral and tricuspid inflow should be performed.
- An M-mode of the left ventricular septum, obtained from a parasternal window, may show abrupt posterior motion of the septum during early diastole, suggesting a constrictive process.

- Associated features that favor a diagnosis of RCM over constrictive pericarditis include
  - PAPs greater than 60 mm Hg.
  - Severe biatrial enlargement.

Alternate Approaches

- A diagnosis of RCM should not be based on echocardiographic findings alone, and adjunctive data are needed.
- Cardiac MRI with gadolinium enhancement can be performed when infiltrative or storage disorders are suspected.
- Cardiac computed tomography scans can be performed to assess pericardial thickening or calcification.
- Invasive hemodynamic assessment may be necessary to differentiate RCM from constrictive pericarditis.
- Pathologic evidence of cardiac or extracardiac infiltration can support a diagnosis of RCM.

KEY POINTS

- The primary abnormality in RCM is decreased myocardial compliance and impaired diastolic relaxation, leading to severely increased diastolic filling pressures.
- RCM should be suspected when there is a normal to thick wall ventricle with elevated filling pressures and biatrial enlargement.
- RCM and constrictive pericarditis present with similar clinical findings and echocardiographic appearance, and multimodality investigation is often needed to confirm a diagnosis.

TABLE 13-4 ECHOCARDIOGRAPHIC PARAMETERS IN RCM AND CONSTRICTIVE PERICARDITIS

	RCM	Constrictive Pericarditis
LV size	Normal	Normal
LV systolic function	Normal	Normal
LV wall thickness	Normal to increased	Normal
LV filling pressures	Markedly increased	Increased
LA size	Markedly increased	Increased
PA pressures	Markedly increased	Increased
Pericardium	Normal	Echobright
Septal shifting with respiration	Absent	Present
Variability in MV inflow	Absent	Present
MV-TV inflow velocities	Concordant	Discordant

Suggested Reading

1. Woo A, Wigle ED, Rakowski H. Echocardiography in the evaluation and management of patients with hypertrophic cardiomyopathy. In: Otto CM, ed. *The Practice of Clinical Echocardiography*. Philadelphia: Elsevier/Saunders; 2007:653-709.
   This chapter provides an excellent overview of the use of echo in the clinical management of patients with HCM.

2. Nagueh SF, Mahmarian JJ. Noninvasive cardiac imaging in patients with hypertrophic cardiomyopathy. *J Am Coll Cardiol*. 2006;48(12):2410-2422.
   This review highlights the comparative utility of echo, nuclear spectroscopy, and cardiac MRI in the diagnosis and management of patients with HCM, including sections on the periprocedural evaluation of patients undergoing septal reduction therapies.

3. Ho CY, Sweitzer NK, McDonough B, et al. Assessment of diastolic function with Doppler tissue imaging to predict genotype in preclinical hypertrophic cardiomyopathy. *Circulation*. 2002;105(25): 2992-2997.
   Advances in gene technologies are allowing the identification of individuals who carry a sarcomeric gene mutation but who have yet to manifest LVH. This study suggests that the combination of low early relaxation tissue Doppler velocities and hyperdynamic systolic function may be able to identify individuals who carry such a genetic mutation.

4. Geske JB, Sorajja P, Nishimura RA, Ommen SR. Evaluation of left ventricular filling pressures by Doppler echocardiography in patients with hypertrophic cardiomyopathy: correlation with direct left atrial pressure measurement at cardiac catheterization. *Circulation*. 2007;116(23):2702-2708.
   Tissue Doppler imaging is widely used for the assessment of left ventricular filling pressures in patients with DCM. This study suggests that these methods are less reliable in patients with HCM due to the asymmetrical hypertrophy and the underlying genetic mutations that may affect intracellular calcium kinetics independent of changes in filling pressure.

5. St. John Sutton M. Doppler echocardiography in heart failure and cardiac resynchronization. In: Otto CM, ed. *The Practice of Clinical Echocardiography*. Philadelphia: Elsevier/Saunders; 2007:629-652.
   This chapter provides a detailed overview of the use of echo in the diagnosis and management of patients with heart failure, including both systolic and diastolic dysfunction, with a section on the potential use of echo in selecting patients for and optimizing resynchronization therapy.

6. Kirkpatrick JN, Vannan MA, Narula J, Lang RM. Echocardiography in heart failure: applications, utility, and new horizons. *J Am Coll Cardiol*. 2007;50(5):381-396.
   This review article summarizes the prognostic utility of echocardiographic findings in patients with heart failure and addresses some of the new technologies.

7. Frischknecht BS, Attenhofer Jost CH, Oechslin EN, et al. Validation of noncompaction criteria in dilated cardiomyopathy, and valvular and hypertensive heart disease. *J Am Soc Echocardiogr*. 2005;18(8):865-872.
   Several sets of criteria exist for the diagnosis of LVN. This study examines a proposed set of echocardiographic criteria and validates these criteria against several patient populations that can mimic LVN on noninvasive imaging.

8. Eidem BW. Noninvasive evaluation of left ventricular noncompaction: what's new in 2009? *Pediatr Cardiol*. 2009;30(5):682-689.
   This review article summarizes the latest echocardiographic approach to the diagnosis and management of patients with LVN, including the use of tissue Doppler, strain, and strain rate imaging for the detection of RWMAs.

9. Naqvi T. Restrictive cardiomyopathy: diagnosis and prognostic implications. In: Otto CM, ed. *The Practice of Clinical Echocardiography*. Philadelphia: Elsevier/ Saunders; 2007:679-711.
   This chapter provides an excellent summary of the echocardiographic findings and clinical management of patients with RCM, including the use of echo to help differentiate RCM from pericardial restriction.

10. Pieroni M, Chimenti C, De Cobelli F, et al. Fabry's disease cardiomyopathy: echocardiographic detection of endomyocardial glycosphingolipid compartmentalization. *J Am Coll Cardiol*. 2006;47(8):1663-1671.
    Fabry disease is caused by mutations in the α-galactosidase gene, resulting in the accumulation of glycosphingolipids within myocytes. This article suggests that a binary appearance of the endocardium on echo is a sensitive and specific finding for Fabry disease and is directly related to the glycosphingolipid deposition.

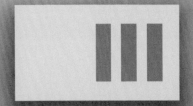

ACQUIRED HEART DISEASE IN THE CHILD

Kawasaki Disease: Echocardiographic Assessment

14

Jeffrey A. Conwell

KEY POINTS

- Kawasaki disease is an acute inflammatory illness that can cause dilation or aneurysms in the coronary arteries, occurring predominantly in children younger than the age of 5 years, but can occur in other age groups.
- Aneurysms of the coronary arteries are rarely seen before 10 days into the illness, and if there have been no aneurysms by 6 to 8 weeks after the acute illness, then aneurysms do not develop.
- Kawasaki disease results in diffuse inflammation, which can affect the myocardium, endocardium, pericardium, and valves. It is therefore important to assess for not only coronary involvement, but also myocarditis, valvulitis, and pericardial effusion.
- Echocardiographic assessment should focus on the coronary arteries, but because the illness occurs predominantly in young children, patients should also undergo a complete echocardiogram to evaluate for possible structural cardiac disease.
- Use the highest frequency transducer possible to image the coronary arteries and decrease the gain and dynamic range to improve the imaging.
- Coronary arteries should be measured from inner edge to inner edge and dimensions compared with reference values. Coronary arteries can be just diffusely dilated (ectasia) and not have aneurysms.

Background

Kawasaki disease is an acute febrile illness that has a systemic vasculitis and can involve the coronary arteries, causing dilation and/or aneurysmal dilation. Diagnosis is by history and clinical examination with supportive laboratory studies. The classic features of Kawasaki disease include fever for at least 5 days, changes in the extremities, rash, bilateral nonexudative conjunctivitis, erythema of the lips and oral mucosa, and cervical lymphadenopathy. Kawasaki disease most frequently occurs in children younger than 5 years of age and has a higher frequency in patients of Asian descent. The etiology of Kawasaki disease is unknown.

In the acute phase of the illness, patients may have pericarditis, myocarditis, and/or endocarditis. After resolution of the fever, there is a vasculitis that can affect the coronary arteries, resulting in ectasia, aneurysm, and/or thrombosis. If aneurysms occur, they tend to regress over time.

Echocardiography (echo) is used to monitor for coronary artery involvement with examinations recommended at the time of diagnosis, 2 weeks from diagnosis, and 6 to 8 weeks after diagnosis, but may be done more frequently if a patient is at high risk for the development of aneurysms (Box 14-1). If the echocardiogram is normal at 6 to 8 weeks, then further follow-up by echo is considered optional. Patients with positive echocardiographic findings will require ongoing follow-up studies.

Patients with a history of Kawasaki disease and coronary artery aneurysms are at an increased risk of early atherosclerosis. If the coronary arteries were only transiently dilated and no aneurysms were detected, this group of patients may be at increased risk of early atherosclerosis.

Overview of Echocardiographic Approach

Because Kawasaki disease can affect the coronary arterial system, echo provides an essential part of the evaluation of patients with Kawasaki disease. The initial echocardiogram should be a complete study to rule out any structural cardiac abnormalities, but also be focused to look at findings seen in Kawasaki disease. Careful examination of the coronary arteries is needed, and all major segments of the coronary arteries should be visualized, if possible. In addition, assessment of global ventricular function, presence of valvar regurgitation, and evaluation for pericardial effusion should be performed (Box 14-2).

BOX 14-1 Increased Risk of Aneurysms

Younger than 1 year of age
Male
Delayed treatment with intravenous
    immunoglobulin
Persistent fever after treatment
Worsening inflammation

**BOX 14-2 Initial Echocardiographic Assessment
in Kawasaki Disease**

Structural cardiac disease
Coronary artery abnormalities
    Image all coronary arteries:
        LMCA
        LAD
        Cx
        RCA
        PDA
Left ventricular dimensions and function
Wall motion abnormalities
Valve regurgitation
Presence of pericardial effusion
Aortic root dilation

BOX 14-3 Goals of Echocardiogram

Identify coronary artery abnormalities:
    Perivascular inflammation (brightness)
    Ectasia
    Aneurysm
    Location of abnormalities
    Severity of abnormalities
    Assess for coronary stenosis or thrombus
Identify valve abnormalities:
    Atrioventricular valve regurgitation
    Aortic valve regurgitation
    Aortic root dilation
Identify myocardial involvement:
    Global ventricular function
    Regional wall motion abnormalities
Identify pericardial involvement:
    Pericardial effusion

Anatomic Imaging

Anatomic imaging in patients with Kawasaki disease focuses on the coronary arteries (Fig. 14-1). However, a complete assessment of the patient needs to be done initially. A complete transthoracic echocardiogram with two-dimensional (2D), spectral, and color Doppler should be performed to assess for any structural cardiac disease. Areas of particular focus are global ventricular function and assessment for focal wall motion abnormalities, coronary artery abnormalities, valve regurgitation, and the presence of a pericardial effusion (Box 14-3).

Coronary abnormalities seen in patients with Kawasaki disease include perivascular brightness, a lack of distal tapering of the coronaries, diffuse dilation (typically referred to as ectasia [Fig. 14-2]), and aneurysmal dilation (Figs. 14-3 and 14-4) of the coronary arteries. Aneurysms are rarely seen before 10 days into the illness. Coronary scarring, calcification, and stenosis are typically seen in later phases of the illness. Thrombosis of the coronary arteries can occur at any time during the illness. Aneurysms can be classified as saccular with equal lateral and axial dimensions giving the appearance of a round bead, fusiform with proximal and distal tapering of the aneurysm giving a more tubelike appearance, or giant where the aneurysm measures more than 8 mm in size (Box 14-4).

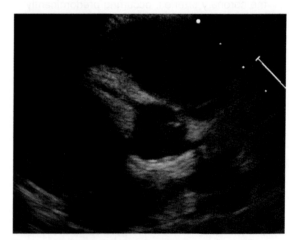

Figure 14-1. Normal coronary arteries in the parasternal short axis.

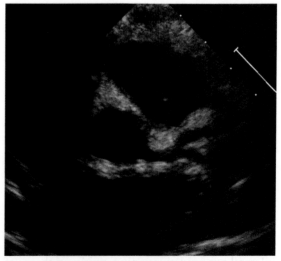

Figure 14-2. Diffuse dilation (ectasia) of the left main coronary artery (LMCA), left anterior descending artery (LAD), and circumflex coronary artery (Cx).

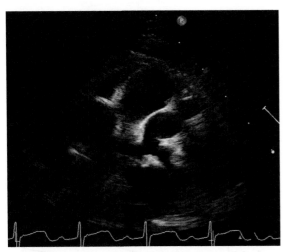

Figure 14-3. Saccular aneurysm of the LAD.

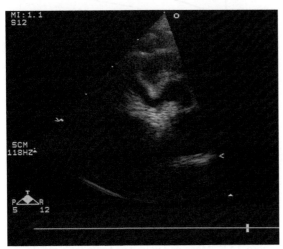

Figure 14-4. Aneurysm of the proximal right coronary artery (RCA).

Mitral valve (MV) regurgitation can be present in as many as 25% of patients with Kawasaki disease in the acute phase of the illness. Aortic regurgitation may also be seen, but is less common. Usually, any valve regurgitation that is present is not hemodynamically significant and frequently resolves. In the rare case of coronary occlusion resulting in papillary muscle ischemia/infarction, mitral regurgitation may persist.

A transient pericardial effusion may be present in the acute phase of the illness but is rarely hemodynamically significant.

Myocarditis can occur in Kawasaki disease and may result in decreased ventricular function and ventricular dilation in the acute phase. If coronary aneurysms have developed in patients, they are at risk of thrombosis, and regional wall motion abnormalities (RWMAs) may develop.

BOX 14-4 Coronary Abnormalities

Ectasia (dilation of coronary without aneurysm)
Lack of tapering
Perivascular brightness
Aneurysms:
    Saccular: equal lateral and axial dimensions
    Fusiform: symmetrical dilation with proximal
      and distal tapering
    Giant: measuring 8 mm or greater
    Aneurysm frequency: LAD > proximal RCA >
      LMCA > Cx > distal RCA > junction RCA
      and PDA

Mild dilation of the aortic root is commonly seen in patients with Kawasaki disease: the aortic root should be imaged and measured, and the measurement compared with normal values for body surface area (BSA).

Acquisition
Initial echocardiogram is used as a baseline and should be a complete study.

Step 1: Complete Transthoracic Echocardiogram
- Although the focus of the echocardiogram is looking for coronary artery abnormalities, patients should be assessed for structural cardiac disease.
- A complete echocardiogram should be performed including 2D imaging, pulsed wave (PW), and color Doppler.

Step 2: Assess Coronary Arteries
- Image all major coronary arteries (left main [LMCA], left anterior descending [LAD], circumflex [Cx], right coronary [RCA], and posterior descending [PDA]).
- Coronary arteries should be measured, and the values for the LMCA, LAD, and RCA should be compared with normal values (Figs. 14-5 and 14-6).
  - Avoid measuring near branch points because this may cause an overestimation of size.
- Coronary arteries may be diffusely dilated (ectasia) and may not appear to taper normally.
- Aneurysms may be present, and the number and location of aneurysms should be documented.
- If an aneurysm is present, make sure to evaluate for possible thrombus within the aneurysm or the presence of stenosis.
- Flow in the coronary arteries should be demonstrated; using color Doppler with a low Nyquist limit is helpful.

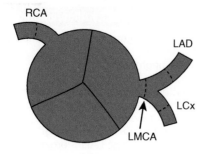

RCA - Right coronary artery
LAD - Left anterior descending
LMCA - Left main coronary artery
LCx - Circumflex

Figure 14-5. Coronary artery measurements.

- Use the highest frequency transducer possible.
- A slight clockwise rotation of the transducer in parasternal short axis views may help to visualize RCA and LMCA (see Fig. 14-1).
- Coronary artery visualization (Box 14-5).
  - In the parasternal long axis, a right-to-left sweep may demonstrate the LMCA, LAD, and Cx (Fig. 14-7).
  - The apical four-chamber (4C) view with anterior angulation will show the distal Cx in the anterior atrioventricular groove (Fig. 14-8).
  - The proximal RCA can be seen from an apical 4C view with anterior angulation in the anterior atrioventricular groove or from a subcostal coronal view (Fig. 14-9).
  - The middle RCA can be seen in cross section in the parasternal long axis angled toward the tricuspid valve (TV) and lateral atrioventricular groove.
  - The distal RCA and posterior descending coronary artery can be seen in the apical 4C view with posterior angulation in the posterior atrioventricular groove or from the subcostal frontal view with posterior angulation.

Step 3: Assess Valve Function
- All valves should be assessed for the presence and degree of regurgitation using both PW and color Doppler.
- MV regurgitation occurs in about 25% of patients with Kawasaki disease but is usually trivial to mild. TV regurgitation may also be present.
- Aortic valve (AV) regurgitation occurs less frequently than MV regurgitation and is usually trivial.

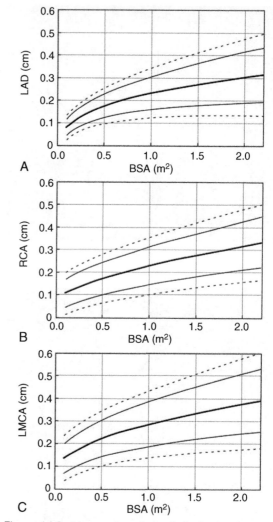

Figure 14-6. Mean and prediction limits for 2 and 3 standard deviations for size of the LAD (**A**), proximal RCA (**B**), and LMCA (**C**) according to body surface area for children 18 years old. LMCA Z scores should not be based on dimension at orifice and immediate vicinity; enlargement of LMCA secondary to Kawasaki disease usually is associated with ectasia of the LAD, Cx, or both. (From Newburger JW, Takahashi M, Gerber MA, et al. Diagnosis, treatment, and long-term management of Kawasaki disease: A statement for health professionals from the Committee on Rheumatic Fever, Endocarditis, and Kawasaki Disease, Council on Cardiovascular Disease in the Young. American Heart Association. *Pediatrics.* 2004;114:1708–1733.)

Step 4: Assess Ventricular Function
- Myocarditis may be present in the acute phase of the illness, and mildly depressed ventricular function may be noted.
- An assessment of global ventricular function should be performed and may be done by M-mode with calculation of a shortening fraction or apical imaging to calculate an ejection fraction.

BOX 14-5 Echocardiographic Views for Coronary Arteries

LMCA:
 Parasternal short axis at the AV level
 Parasternal long axis of the left ventricle (LV)
 Subcostal left ventricular long axis
LAD:
 Parasternal short axis at level of the AV
 Parasternal long axis of the LV
 Parasternal short axis of the LV
Left Cx:
 Parasternal short axis at level of AV
 Apical 4C
RCA, proximal:
 Parasternal short axis at the AV level
 Parasternal long axis of the LV
 Subcostal coronal projection of the RVOT
 Subcostal short axis at the level of the
  atrioventricular groove
RCA, middle segment:
 Parasternal long axis inferior tangential of the
  LV
 Apical 4C
 Subcostal left ventricular long axis
 Subcostal short axis at the level of the
  atrioventricular groove
RCA distal segment:
 Apical 4C
 Subcostal atrial long axis
PDA:
 Apical 4C
 Subcostal atrial long axis
 Parasternal long axis imaging of the posterior
  interventricular groove

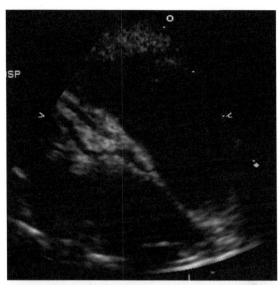

Figure 14-7. LAD seen in the parasternal long axis.

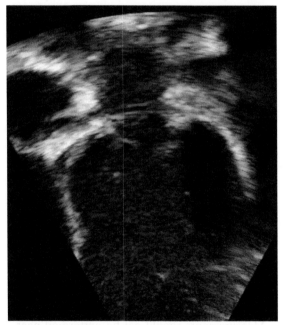

Figure 14-8. Cx seen from the apical four-chamber (4C) view with anterior angulation in the anterior atrioventricular groove.

- Patients with coronary abnormalities should be assessed for RWMAs that would suggest coronary ischemia or infarct. Views including parasternal long axis, parasternal short axis, and apical 4C and two-chamber are useful for imaging the 16 (or 17) standard myocardial segments useful in describing the location of wall motion abnormalities and determining the specific coronary artery distribution affected.

Step 5: Assess Aortic Root
- The aortic root should be imaged in the parasternal long axis view and measured during systole (per pediatric convention).
- Measurements should be compared with normal values for BSA (Z scores).

Step 6: Assess for Pericardial Effusion
- A transient pericardial effusion may be present in the acute phase of Kawasaki disease and is usually not hemodynamically significant.
- Size and location of the effusion should be noted.

Follow-up echocardiograms can be limited to evaluation of ventricular function and coronary arteries. If there is a history of valve regurgitation or other abnormalities, this should be reevaluated.

Pitfalls
- Using a low-frequency transducer may make imaging of coronary arteries difficult. It is best to use the highest frequency transducer possible.

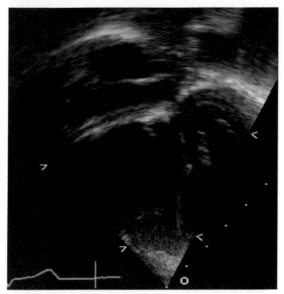

Figure 14-9. RCA seen from the apical 4C view with anterior angulation in the anterior atrioventricular groove.

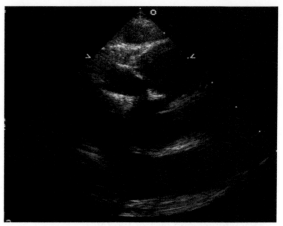

Figure 14-10. Giant aneurysm of the RCA.

- Optimize imaging by decreasing the gain and dynamic range (compression).
- If the patient has poor transthoracic images, transesophageal echo may need to be performed to assess the proximal LMCA and RCA.
- Recording images in a dynamic imaging format or digital cine format allows for better assessment of structures than a still-frame image.

Analysis

Coronary Artery Measurements
- Coronary arteries should be measured from inner edge to inner edge.
- Measurements should not be performed near branching points because this may overestimate the size of the coronary artery.
- Reference Z scores available for LMCA, LAD, and proximal RCA based on BSA (see Fig. 14-6).
- Coronary arteries are thought to be dilated if the measurement is a Z score greater than 2.5.
- Aneurysm size:
  - Small to medium, larger than 3 mm but smaller than 6 mm (coronary Z score +3 to +7, based on a "typical" BSA for a 5 year old).
  - Large: 6 mm or greater.
  - Giant: 8 mm or greater (Fig. 14-10).

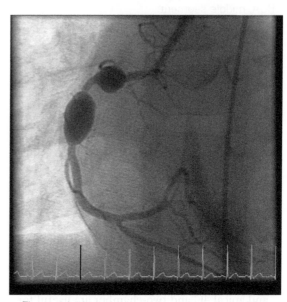

Figure 14-11. Angiogram of aneurysms in the RCA.

Alternate Approaches

- Dobutamine stress echo may be used to assess for segmental wall motion abnormalities.
- Magnetic resonance imaging/magnetic resonance angiography is an alternative method to image coronary arteries and assess for aneurysms, coronary occlusions, and coronary stenosis.
- Computed tomography has been demonstrated to be useful for imaging proximal aneurysms.
- Cardiac catheterization allows for assessment of both proximal and distal aneurysms along with assessing for coronary stenosis (Fig. 14-11).

- Transesophageal echo may allow assessment of the proximal RCA and LMCA in patients with limited echo windows.

Suggested Reading

1. Baer AZ, Rubin LG, Shapiro CA, Sood SK, Rajan S, Shapir Y, et al. Prevalence of coronary artery lesions on the initial echocardiogram in Kawasaki syndrome. *Arch Pediatr Adolesc Med*. 2006;160:686-690.
2. Crystal MA, Syan SK, Yeung RS, Dipchand AI, McCrindle BW. Echocardiographic and electrocardiographic trends in children with acute Kawasaki disease. *Can J Cardiol*. 2008;24:776-780.
3. Fukazawa R, Ogawa S. Long-term prognosis of patients with Kawasaki disease: at risk for future atherosclerosis? *J Nippon Med Sch*. 2009;76:124-133.
4. Gordon JB, Kahn AM, Burns JC. When children with Kawasaki disease grow up: myocardial and vascular complications in adulthood. *J Am Coll Cardiol*. 2009; 54:1911-1920.
5. Gupta-Malhotra M, Gruber D, Abraham SS, Roman MJ, Zabriskie JB, Hudgins LC, et al. Atherosclerosis in survivors of Kawasaki disease. *J Pediatr*. 2009;155: 572-577.
6. Heuclin T, Dubos F, Hue V, Godart F, Francart C, Vincent P, et al. Increased detection rate of Kawasaki disease using new diagnostic algorithm, including early use of echocardiography. *J Pediatr*. 2009;155:695, 9.e1.
7. JCS Joint Working Group. Guidelines for diagnosis and management of cardiovascular sequelae in Kawasaki disease (JCS 2008)–digest version. *Circ J*. 2010;74: 1989-2020.
8. Mavrogeni S, Papadopoulos G, Karanasios E, Cokkinos DV. How to image Kawasaki disease: a validation of different imaging techniques. *Int J Cardiol*. 2008;124: 27-31.
9. McCrindle BW, Li JS, Minich LL, Colan SD, Atz AM, Takahashi M, et al. Coronary artery involvement in children with Kawasaki disease: risk factors from analysis of serial normalized measurements. *Circulation*. 2007;116:174-179.
10. McMorrow Tuohy AM, Tani LY, Cetta F, Lewin MB, Eidem BW, Van Buren P, et al. How many echocardiograms are necessary for follow-up evaluation of patients with Kawasaki disease? *Am J Cardiol*. 2001; 88:328-330.
11. Minich LL, Tani LY, Pagotto LT, Young PC, Etheridge SP, Shaddy RE. Usefulness of echocardiography for detection of coronary artery thrombi in patients with Kawasaki disease. *Am J Cardiol*. 1998;82:1143, 6, A10.
12. Newburger JW, Takahashi M, Gerber MA, Gewitz MH, Tani LY, Burns JC, et al. Diagnosis, treatment, and long-term management of Kawasaki disease: a statement for health professionals from the Committee on Rheumatic Fever, Endocarditis, and Kawasaki Disease, Council on Cardiovascular Disease in the Young. American Heart Association. *Pediatrics*. 2004;114: 1708-1733.
13. Ren X, Banker R. Cardiac manifestation of mucocutaneous lymph node syndrome (Kawasaki disease). *J Am Coll Cardiol*. 2009 Jun 30;54(1):89.
14. Seve P, Stankovic K, Smail A, Durand DV, Marchand G, Broussolle C. Adult Kawasaki disease: report of two cases and literature review. *Semin Arthritis Rheum*. 2005;34:785-792.

Thromboembolic Phenomena and Vegetations

15

Peter J. Cawley and Brian D. Soriano

Background

Thrombi and vegetations may result in clinical symptoms when embolism occurs. Vegetations may result in clinical symptoms when significant valve destruction occurs or with systemic symptoms such as fever and malaise. Tumors may also present clinically due to embolism, but tumors are not covered in this section.

Thrombus
- Thrombus is predisposed to form in areas of the heart where there is low-velocity blood flow or flow stasis.
- The left atrium (LA) (especially the left atrial appendage [LAA] [Fig. 15-1]) is a common area of thrombus formation when associated with atrial arrhythmias or mitral stenosis.
- The left ventricle (LV) is a common area of thrombus formation when associated with left ventricular dysfunction (global or regional) (Fig. 15-2), aneurysm, or pseudoaneurysm (Fig. 15-3). The apex is a common area for thrombus formation.
- Thrombus formation within the right heart may occur in cases of severe right atrial enlargement (i.e., atriopulmonary Fontan) or right ventricular dysfunction. More commonly, thrombus formation occurs within veins and embolizes to the right heart. Thrombus may become trapped in the right atrium (RA) (Chiari network or Eustachian valve), in the right ventricle (RV) (tricuspid valve apparatus or right ventricular trabeculations), or pulmonary arteries (PAs) as it embolizes (Fig. 15-4).
- Thrombus formation may occur on intracardiac devices seen within the right heart such as pacing/defibrillator leads and central venous catheters. Thrombus formation can result on intracardiac walls of the right heart if a central venous catheter tip results in local trauma.
- Thrombus formation may occur in surgically placed conduits (Glenn shunt, Fontan shunt, RV-to-PA conduit). Thrombus can be difficult to visualize on echocardiography (echo) due to artifact from conduits or the lack of an ultrasound window. Magnetic resonance imaging (MRI) or computed tomography (CT) may be more helpful in this regard.
- Intracardiac shunting can result in venous thrombi embolizing to the arterial system. The most common shunts for which this may occur are a patent foramen ovale (PFO), atrial septal defects (ASDs), baffle/conduit leaks, and larger ventricular septal defects (VSDs) with right-to-left shunting such as Eisenmenger physiology.
- Thrombus can also occur on prosthetic valves. Clinical presentation may occur as a result of an embolic event or symptomatic valve dysfunction or may be directly visualized by echo in an asymptomatic patient.

Vegetations
- Vegetations are most commonly the result of bacterial or fungal infections.
- Noninfectious vegetations may also occur and are commonly referred to as marantic or nonbacterial thrombotic endocarditis (NBTE). NBTE usually occurs in the context of a malignancy or autoimmune disease (Fig. 15-5). A metastatic malignancy does not necessarily have to be present. Although blood cultures and an accurate determination of whether the patient was exposed to antibiotics at the time of blood sampling for culture are essential in identifying vegetations as infectious or noninfectious, there are some imaging characteristics of NBTE: vegetations tend to be less mobile, more sessile, and located toward the base of the leaflets. Because the base of the valve leaflets is more commonly affected, less severe valve regurgitation is noted. Anticoagulation should be considered in patients with NBTE.
- Mobility and location are important distinguishing features of a vegetation.

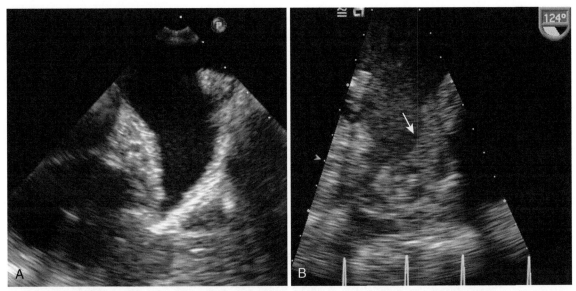

Figure 15-1. **A,** Narrow-sector transesophageal (TEE) image of the left atrial appendage (LAA) without any thrombus. **B,** Narrow-sector TEE image of the LAA with thrombus (*arrow*).

Vegetations have motion independent of a valve leaflet and are most commonly associated with the upstream surface of a valve leaflet (e.g., the right atrial side of the tricuspid valve [Fig. 15-6]) but have also been reported on the Eustachian valve, residual Chiari network, subvalvular apparatus, and chamber wall. Commonly, the vegetations are not rounded in appearance. Vegetations usually have low reflectance of ultrasound waves but over time may become more calcified (high reflectance). Visualization of vegetations in more than one ultrasound window decreases the likelihood of an ultrasound artifact.

- Vegetations can occur on intracardiac devices such as pacing/defibrillator leads and central venous catheters (Fig. 15-7).
- Destruction of the valve apparatus (annulus or leaflet) can result in a fistulous connection between adjacent cardiac chambers (e.g., aorta to RA) or valve regurgitation.
- Paravalvular abscesses may occur as a result of endocarditis and typically occur in the annular part of the valve apparatus. Abscesses may be echogenic or echolucent spaces near the valve annulus.
- Infections of bioprosthetic or prosthetic valves are more typically an annular disease, which can result in valve dehiscence or annular abscess (Fig. 15-8).
- Adequate sampling of blood for culture and obtaining blood cultures before the commencement of antibiotics are critical for the timely diagnosis of infectious endocarditis.

A more detailed discussion of the evaluation of endocarditis can be found in Chapter 14 of the *Echocardiography Review Guide* by C. M. Otto and R. G. Schwaegler.

Overview of Echocardiographic Approach

In many infants and young children, transthoracic acoustic windows are typically adequate enough that the structures of the heart are well visualized and there is little incremental benefit to transesophageal echo (TEE). TEE should be considered when transthoracic findings are equivocal or if specific structures of the heart are not well visualized. TEE may also be useful in guiding the surgical approach.

M-Mode
- Displaying cardiac motion over time in a "pencil-beam" portion of the heart can be very helpful diagnostically to demonstrate the rapid movements of a valve vegetation or thrombus.

Two-Dimensional
- Transthoracic echo (TTE) allows direct visualization of the cardiac chambers such as the left and right ventricles.
- The left ventricular apex is better visualized by TTE than TEE. Thus TTE is more sensitive for the detection of ventricular thrombi.

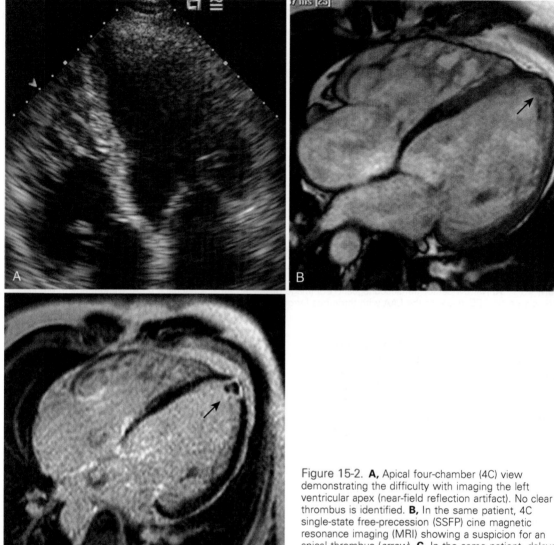

Figure 15-2. **A,** Apical four-chamber (4C) view demonstrating the difficulty with imaging the left ventricular apex (near-field reflection artifact). No clear thrombus is identified. **B,** In the same patient, 4C single-state free-precession (SSFP) cine magnetic resonance imaging (MRI) showing a suspicion for an apical thrombus (*arrow*). **C,** In the same patient, delayed contrast imaging demonstrating scar (white part of myocardium) in the apex with an apical thrombus (*arrow*).

- The LA and the LAA are better visualized by TEE than TTE. Thus TEE is more sensitive for the detection of atrial thrombi.
- TEE has a higher degree of sensitivity for detecting valve thrombosis.
- TTE can detect PFOs and ASDs, but TEE has a higher degree of sensitivity and specificity. The addition of saline microbubbles testing with two-dimensional (2D) imaging increases the sensitivity of detecting shunting.
- TTE can detect vegetations and paravalvular abscesses, but TEE has a higher degree of sensitivity and specificity (Figs. 15-9 and 15-10).

Color Doppler
- Doppler imaging is not useful for detecting the presence or absence of thrombus but is useful for detecting shunting when paradoxical embolization is clinically suspected.
- Useful for determining the presence of valve regurgitation and distinguishing between physiologic and pathologic valve regurgitation. Regurgitation or leaflet perforation may be a consequence of valve vegetations.
- Useful for distinguishing abnormal fistulous connections. A fistula may be a consequence of annular infections.

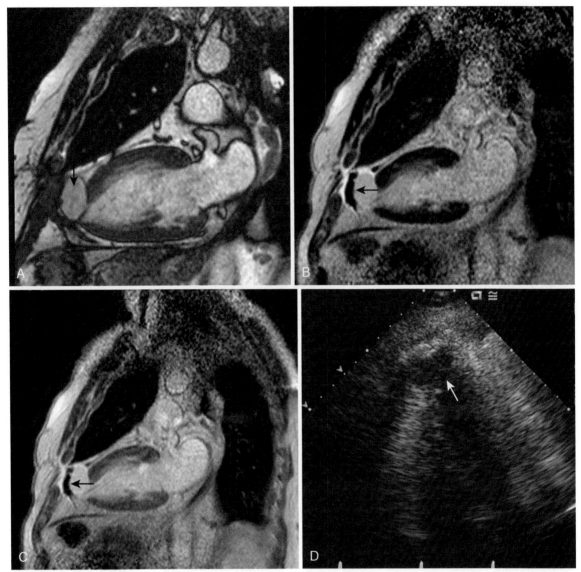

Figure 15-3. **A,** Vertical long axis (two-chamber [2C]) SSFP cine MRI demonstrating an apical pseudoaneurysm (*arrow*). **B,** In the same patient, delayed-enhancement imaging with a normal inversion time demonstrating the pseudoaneurysm. The *arrow* points to an area suspicious for thrombus but is best proved by prolonging the inversion time (**C**) and thus proving that thrombus did not take up the gadolinium contrast. **D,** Apical 4C transthoracic echocardiography (TTE) in the same patient demonstrates the apical pseudoaneurysm (*arrow*), but the echo images do not demonstrate the thrombus as clearly as the MRI, and it is harder to appreciate thrombus within pseudoaneurysm.

- Useful for determining flow disturbances, which are often the first echocardiographic signs of an abnormality that can then be further characterized by 2D imaging.
- Limited value for determining the severity of valve regurgitation.

Continuous Wave Doppler
- Useful for determining the severity of regurgitation.
- Useful for determining the location of fistulous connections by determining the peak velocity and the timing of the flow with the cardiac cycle.

Anatomic Imaging

Left Atrial Thrombus
Image Acquisition
- Use TEE.
- Decrease the image depth to maximize the entire LA. Scan the LA while repositioning the probe in the esophagus from superior to

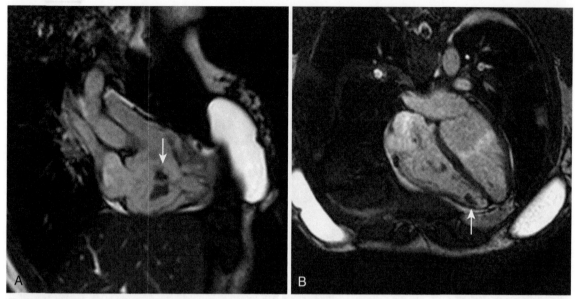

Figure 15-4. **A,** Right ventricular long axis SSFP cine MRI showing thrombus (*arrow*) entangled in the tricuspid subvalvular apparatus. **B,** In the same patient, a 4C SSFP cine demonstrating a thrombus (*arrow*) at the apex of the right ventricle.

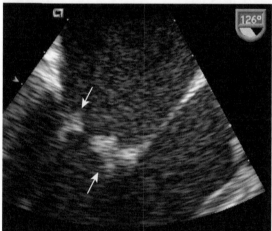

Figure 15-5. Narrow-sector TEE image (midesophageal long axis view) in a patient with nonbacterial thrombotic endocarditis secondary to lupus. These vegetations (*arrows*) tend to be more sessile and less mobile.

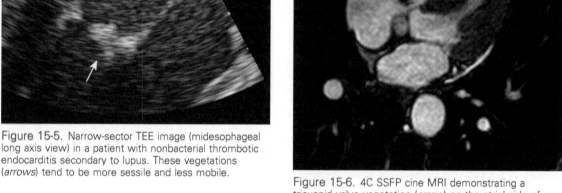

Figure 15-6. 4C SSFP cine MRI demonstrating a tricuspid valve vegetation (*arrow*) on the atrial side of the valve.

inferior and turning the probe left to right to capture the entire LA. Rotate the multiplane knob to scan the LA from 0 to 180 degrees.

- The exam must be individualized but commonly the LAA is best located by rotating the multiplane knob to between 60 and 100 degrees. Center the LAA in the imaging sector. Narrow the sector to maximize imaging resolution. Attempt to look into the LAA by avoiding the ridge of cardiac tissue between the left superior pulmonary vein (PV) and the LAA.

Pitfalls

- Spontaneous echocardiographic contrast is indicative of decreased flow areas and may be mistaken for cardiac thrombus.
- Reverberation artifact may be mistaken for a thrombus when the ridge of tissue between the left superior PV and the LAA is located between the source of the ultrasound beam and the LAA.

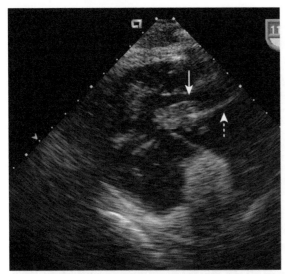

Figure 15-7. Transgastric right ventricular inflow view on TEE demonstrates a large mass (*solid arrow*) attached to a right-sided pacing/defibrillator lead (*dashed arrow*) as it crosses the tricuspid valve.

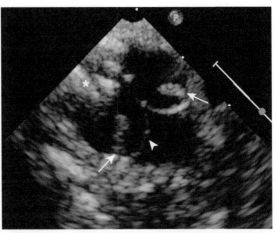

Figure 15-9. Diastolic TEE image (multiplane at 129 degrees) of a bioprosthetic pulmonary valve demonstrating normal valve leaflets (*arrowhead*) with thick, mobile densities adherent to the hinge points of the valve cuffs (*arrows*). The distal end of the conduit is partially obscured by a right pulmonary artery stent (*asterisk*).

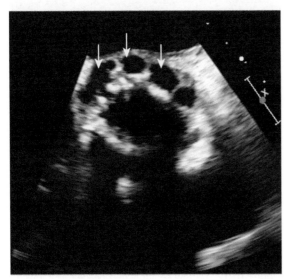

Figure 15-8. Narrow-sector TEE image of a bioprosthetic aortic valve in short axis. Note the echolucent spaces (*arrows*) along the annulus in this patient with an annular abscess.

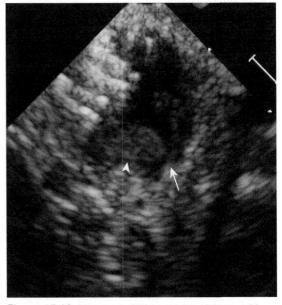

Figure 15-10. Short axis TEE image (multiplane at 90 degrees) of a bioprosthetic valve. The valve leaflets remain thin (*arrow*) but a prominent, elliptical vegetation is seated within the cusp (*arrowhead*).

- Pectinate muscles are normal structures found within the LAA and can be mistaken for thrombi (Fig. 15-11).
- Alternative approaches: contrast-enhanced MRI and contrast-enhanced CT. However, either one may give a false filling defect if contrast does not get into the LAA due to poor LAA contraction.

Left Ventricular Thrombus
Image Acquisition
- Use TTE.
- Use standard and off-axis views to optimize visualization of the apex. Care should be undertaken to avoid foreshortening the apex.
- Increase the transducer frequency.
- Left ventricular thrombus is commonly associated with abnormal wall motion.

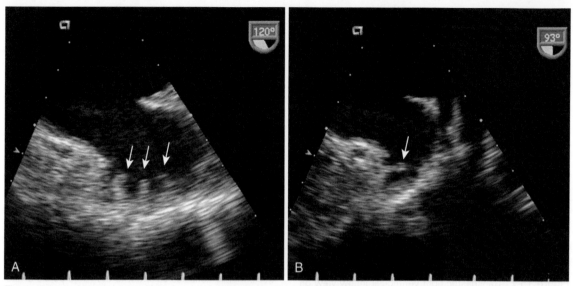

Figure 15-11. Narrow sector TEE images in different multiplane angles (**A, B**) of the LAA demonstrating normal pectinate muscles (*arrows*) that can sometimes be mistaken for abnormal masses.

Carefully examine for the presence of wall motion abnormalities.

- Mural thrombus is typically laminated against the left ventricular wall and may be more difficult to visualize than mobile thrombus.

Pitfalls

- Near-field reflection artifact is commonly encountered when imaging from the apical window. Strong reflectors are noted at the apex, which give the appearance of a mass in the apex.
- Normal variants within the ventricular apex that may be mistaken for cardiac thrombi are trabeculations or false tendons.
- Contrast agents may be useful to delineate normal structures from thrombus.

Valve Vegetations
Image Acquisition (Whether TEE or TTE)

- Narrow the imaging sector around the valve structure (Fig. 15-12).
- Examine all leaflets of the valves using multiple angles and windows.
- Examine the entire annulus closely.
- For prosthetic valves, look for valve/annular stability. The presence of annular motion may indicate valve dehiscence.
- Examine all intracardiac devices such as pacing leads and central venous catheters.

Pitfalls

- Normal variants such as Lambl excrescence (degenerative changes commonly found on

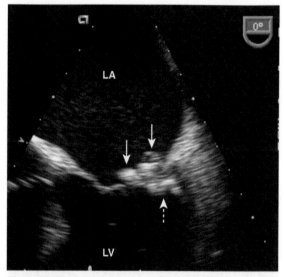

Figure 15-12. Narrow sector midesophageal TEE image of the mitral valve in a patient with streptococcal endocarditis (*solid arrows*). Note that there is associated mitral annular calcification (*dashed arrow*) that causes acoustic shadowing.

the left ventricular surface of the aortic valve usually having the appearance of linear strands [Fig. 15-13]) or nodules of Arantius (focal thickening at the coaptation point of the valve leaflets) may be mistaken for valve vegetations.

- Image artifacts such as beam width artifacts may be mistaken for valve vegetations. Identifying valve vegetations in two

ultrasound windows minimizes the likelihood of an imaging artifact.
- Mitral valve prolapse or flail chords/leaflets may be mistaken for valve vegetations.

Physiologic Data

Valve Vegetations
- Use color Doppler to identify pathologic valve regurgitation, leaflet perforation,

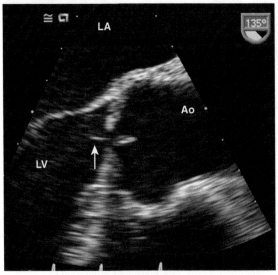

Figure 15-13. Narrow sector midesophageal TEE image of the aortic valve demonstrating a normal variant associated with aging: Lambl excrescence (*arrow*).

fistulous connections, and abnormal flow signals.
- Useful for determining the location of fistulous connections by determining the peak velocity and the timing of the flow with the cardiac cycle.

Alternate Approaches

- As with echo, MRI uses different imaging techniques to answer clinical questions. Cine MRI allows improved visualization of the cardiac apex when an ultrasound window is poor or when visualizing the cardiac apex by echo is limited by lung or rib interference. Cine MRI also allows improved endocardial delineation (Fig. 15-14). Contrast-enhanced MRI can help distinguish normal adjacent myocardium from thrombus on the basis of tissue characterization (Fig. 15-15). MRI angiography may also be helpful for distinguishing thrombus by looking for filling defects within the LAA.
- CT angiography may also be helpful to identify thrombus within the cardiac chambers by identifying filling defects.
- Invasive angiography may also be helpful to identify thrombus within the cardiac chambers.

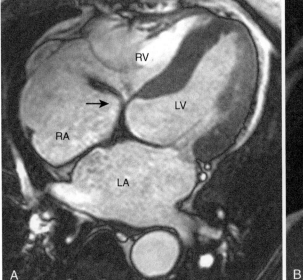
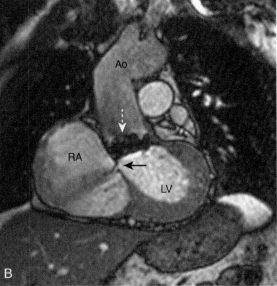

Figure 15-14. **A,** 4C SSFP cine MRI demonstrating a flow disturbance (*arrow*) from the LV into the right atrium (RA) (Gerbode-type ventricular septal defect [VSD]). **B,** In the same patient, this coronal cine demonstrates a prosthetic aortic valve (*dashed arrow*) with the Gerbode-type VSD defect (*solid arrow*) from the LV into the RA.

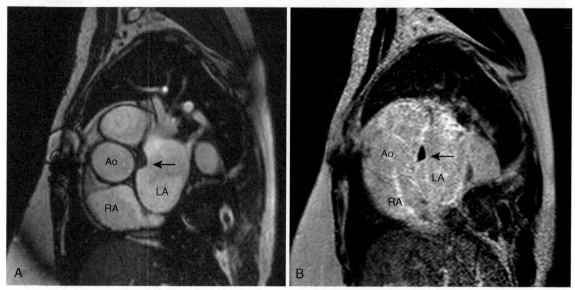

Figure 15-15. **A,** Short axis SSFP cine MRI at the level of the atria demonstrating an irregular mass (*arrow*) protruding into the lumen of the LA. **B,** Delayed-enhancement imaging with a long inversion time at the same corresponding area demonstrating laminar thrombus (*arrow*).

KEY POINTS

- The most common sources of cardiac embolization include thrombus, vegetations, and tumor.
- The location of embolization depends on the location of the source within the heart (right side versus left side) and the presence of shunts within the heart.
- Intracardiac thrombus commonly occurs in the LAA (in conjunction with mitral stenosis or atrial arrhythmias), in the LV (in the presence of regional or global dysfunction), or in the right heart (dysfunction, chamber enlargement, or trapped as the thrombus is embolizing from a deep vein).
- TTE is helpful for detecting ventricular thrombus, whereas TEE is more sensitive for the detection of atrial thrombus.
- MRI and CT are alternative modalities for the detection of intracardiac thrombus. Tissue characterization with MRI can be especially helpful in distinguishing thrombus from tumor.
- Echo remains the best modality to identify valve vegetations because of its superior temporal resolution.
- Vegetations can be visualized by 2D echo. Doppler is also helpful to suspect vegetations by identifying pathologic regurgitation, leaflet perforation, or fistulous connections.
- Prosthetic valve endocarditis is more commonly an annular disease than a leaflet disease.
- Other intracardiac devices such as pacing/defibrillator leads are increasingly common sources of thrombus and vegetations.

Suggested Reading

1. Shanewise JS, Cheung AT, Aronson S, et al. ASE/SCA guidelines for performing a comprehensive intraoperative multiplane transesophageal echocardiography examination: recommendations of the American Society of Echocardiography Council for Intraoperative Echocardiography and the Society of Cardiovascular Anesthesiologists Task Force for Certification in Perioperative Transesophageal Echocardiography. *J Am Soc Echocardiogr.* 1999;12:884-900.
2. Bonow RO, Carabello BA, Chatterjee K, et al. ACC/AHA 2006 guidelines for the management of patients with valvular heart disease: a report of the American College of Cardiology/American Heart Association Task Force on Practice Guidelines (writing Committee to Revise the 1998 guidelines for the management of patients with valvular heart disease) developed in collaboration with the Society of Cardvascular Anesthesiologists endorsed by the Society for Cardiovascular Angiography and Interventions and the Society of Thoracic Surgeons. *J Am Coll Cardiol.* 2006;48:e1-e148.
3. Zoghbi WA, Chambers JB, Dumesnil JG, et al. Recommendations for evaluation of prosthetic valves with echocardiography and Doppler ultrasound: a report from the American Society of Echocardiography's Guidelines and Standards Committee and the Task Force on Prosthetic Valves, developed in conjunction with the American College of Cardiology Cardiovascular Imaging Committee, Cardiac Imaging Committee of the American Heart Association, the European Association of Echocardiography, a registered branch of the European Society of Cardiology, the Japanese Society of Echocardiography and the Canadian Society of Echocardiography, endorsed by the American College of Cardiology Foundation, American Heart Association, European Association of Echocardiography, a registered branch of the European Society of Cardiology, the Japanese Society of Echocardiography, and Canadian Society of Echocardiography. *J Am Soc Echocardiogr.* 2009;22:975-1014.
4. Otto CM, Schwaegler RG. *Echocardiography Review Guide.* Philadelphia: Saunders, 2007.

Implications of Pediatric Renal, Endocrine, and Oncologic Disease

16

Brandy Hattendorf

Pediatric diseases of many different etiologies have cardiovascular implications. Those associated with renal, endocrine, and oncologic processes can directly or indirectly impact the cardiovascular system.

Renal

The cardiovascular complications of renal disease differ based on the etiology of the kidney disease. Cardiovascular morbidity and mortality continue to increase in association with renal disease. The most common renal diseases with cardiovascular effects include hypertension, glomerulonephritis, chronic renal failure, post-renal transplantation, and iron overload secondary to renal failure with hemodialysis.

Hypertension
- Arterial hypertension may reflect chronic kidney disease.
  - Metabolic and hormonal factors in chronic renal disease contribute to the development of both hypertension and left ventricular hypertrophy (LVH).
- Hypertension is associated with LVH.
  - Concentric hypertrophy is more common than eccentric hypertrophy.
- Volume overload contributes to hypertension in hemodialysis patients.
- LVH is an independent risk factor for coronary artery disease.
- Reduced compliance of the left ventricle (LV) secondary to LVH results in left ventricular diastolic dysfunction.

Glomerulonephritis
- Glomerulonephritis may result in:
  - LVH, right ventricular and septal hypertrophy.
  - Dilated ventricles.
  - Decreased ventricular contractility.
  - Impairment in diastolic ventricular function.

KEY POINTS
- LVH reflects pressure and volume overload on the left ventricle.
- Concentric hypertrophy occurs in the presence of pressure overload with a stiff ventricle (Fig. 16-1).
- Eccentric LVH is more likely secondary to increased volume overload (eg., in hemodialysis patients).
- Diastolic function is worse in patients with LVH.
- Regression of LVH with normalization of left ventricular mass (LVM) can occur in patients after successful treatment with antihypertensive therapy.

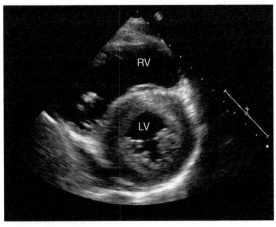

Figure 16-1. Parasternal short axis view of concentric left ventricular hypertrophy.

Chronic Renal Failure
- Adolescents are at higher risk of cardiovascular events than younger children.
- Cardiac findings: cardiomyopathy (CM), arrhythmias, and cardiac arrest of unknown origin.

215

- African American race and female sex have been reported to be risk factors for cardiovascular disease in children and adolescents on dialysis.

> **KEY POINTS**
>
> - LVH can develop even with mild to moderate chronic kidney disease.
> - Impaired diastolic dysfunction may be seen in children with chronic kidney disease, on long-term dialysis, and after transplantation.
> - Abnormalities in calcium-phosphate metabolism, particularly in dialysis patients, are associated with diastolic dysfunction.
> - Increased incidence of valvular disease in those undergoing chronic dialysis:
>   - Age older than 14 years, female African American.
>   - Aortic valve (AV) and mitral valve (MV) disease are most often involved.
>   - Annular calcification.

Post-Kidney Transplantation

- Decreased systolic function, diastolic dysfunction, and increased LVM can persist even after transplantation.

> **KEY POINTS**
>
> - The most common findings post-transplantation are:
>   - LVH.
>   - Left atrial enlargement.
>   - Left ventricular dilation.
>   - Systolic dysfunction.

Iron Overload Cardiomyopathy

- Myocardial injury due to excess iron deposition, which may occur in association with chronic renal failure/hemodialysis.

The Echo Exam: Step-by-Step Approach

Step 1: Evaluate Cardiac Size

- M-mode and two-dimensional (2D) assessment of cardiac dimensions.
  - Assess for left ventricular dilation and/or LVH using measurements indexed to body surface area (BSA).
  - Image using multiple planes including four-chamber (4C) and short axis views.
- Use indexed LVM to define LVH in pediatric patients ($g/m^{2.7}$).
  - Height should be measured (in meters).
- LVM equation is 0.8{1.04[(LVED + left ventricular posterior wall thickness + interventricular septal thickness)^3 − LVED^3]} + 0.6, where LVED is left ventricular end-diastolic dimension.

> **KEY POINTS**
>
> - Height and weight measurements should be obtained at the time of the echocardiogram to ensure accuracy rather than relying on patient history.
> - M-mode is performed from a parasternal long axis view just below the MV leaflets.
> - Leading edge to leading edge technique in end-diastole is used to measure
>   - LVED.
>   - Left posterior wall thickness.
>   - Interventricular septal thickness.
> - To evaluate LVM in patients younger than 9 years of age, percentile curves should be referenced.

- LVM is then indexed to height to the exponential power of 2.7.
  - For patients older than 9 years old: more than 40 $g/m^{2.7}$ in girls and more than 45 $g/m^{2.7}$ in boys is abnormal.

Step 2: Evaluate Systolic Cardiac Function

- Obtain end-diastolic and end-systolic measurements and calculate left ventricular fractional shortening (FS) using M-mode.
  - Parasternal short axis or long axis view at the level of the papillary muscles.
- FS greater than 38% = hyperdynamic.
- FS less than 28% = reduced systolic function.
- Use the modified Simpson's (disk summation) method for calculating ejection fraction (EF) to estimate left ventricular end-diastolic and end-systolic volumes.
  - Use the apical 4C and two-chamber (2C) views (Fig. 16-2).

Step 3: Evaluate Diastolic Cardiac Function

- Ventricular relaxation occurs during isovolumic relaxation.
  - Recorded from an apical 4C view at the MV leaflet tips.
  - Use pulsed wave (PW) Doppler with the signal aligned parallel to mitral flow.
- Normal mitral inflow Doppler pattern.
  - Isovolumic relaxation: brief interval between AV closure and the onset of ventricular filling (isovolumic relaxation time [IVRT]).
  - Blood rapidly fills the left atrium (LA) with opening of the MV (E wave).
    - E velocity of early maximum filling velocity.
    - Filling then slows (deceleration time): E peak to intersection of the slope with the zero baseline.

SIMPSON BIPLANE METHOD FOR CALCULATING LV VOLUME

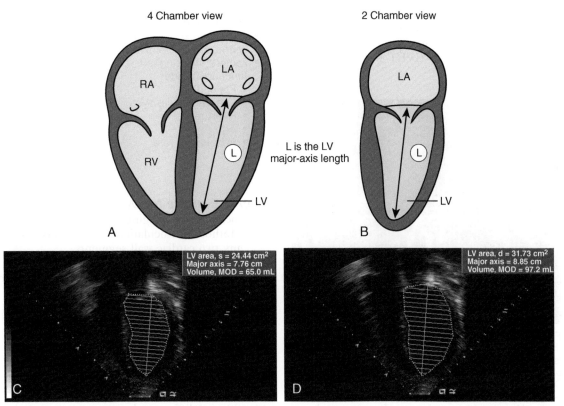

Figures 16-2. The modified Simpson method (disk summation) can be used to calculate left ventricular volumes. It involves tracing the left ventricular endocardial border in apical 4-chamber and 2-chamber views using the disk summation method for calculating ejection fraction based on estimating left ventricular volume in systole and diastole, as illustrated in **A** and **B**. Application of the modified Simpson method using an apical 4-chamber view is demonstrated estimating left ventricular end-systolic (**C**) and end-diastolic (**D**) volumes. As seen in the echo images, this technique requires adequate delineation of the left ventricular endocardium.

- Left atrial contraction causes another peak velocity (atrial velocity or A wave).
- Tissue Doppler imaging (TDI).
  - TDI is obtained at the lateral margin of the MV annulus from an apical 4C view.
  - Time interval from the end to the onset of the mitral annular velocity pattern during diastole.
  - Measurements include (Fig. 16-3).
    - Early diastolic annular velocity (E′).
    - Diastolic velocity with atrial contraction (A′).
    - Isovolumic contraction time (IVCT).
    - IVRT.
    - Ejection time (ET).
  - Used as an adjunct for evaluation of diastolic function.
  - Less dependent on preload.
    - Normal variation is less than 20%.
- In children with normal diastolic function, the E wave is larger than the A wave, reflecting that ventricular filling occurs primarily in early diastole.
- A reduced E/A ratio may be seen with diastolic dysfunction in chronic renal disease.
- Increased HR results in shorter duration of diastole with an increased A wave and lower E/A ratio.
- Impaired relaxation is associated with a prolonged IVRT.
- Decreased compliance and increased filling pressures are associated with a shortened IVRT.
- Changes seen associated with LVH secondary to hypertension include:
  - Mild left ventricular diastolic dysfunction.
    - Impaired relaxation.
    - Reduced early diastolic filling.
    - Enhanced atrial contribution:
      - Increased IVRT.
      - Reduced E velocity.

- Increased A velocity.
- E/A ratio < 1.
- The myocardial performance index (MPI) or Tei index may be calculated to assess left ventricular dysfunction.
    - MPI or Tei index = (IVRT + IVCT)/ET.

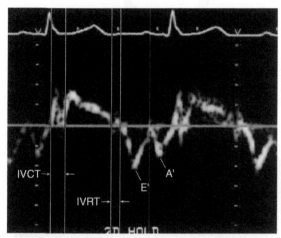

Figures 16-3. Example of tissue Doppler from the lateral mitral valve annulus samples from an apical window. Isovolumic contraction time (IVCT) is characterized by biphasic motion, first toward the apex and then away. During isovolumic relaxation time (IVRT), the IVCT motion is reversed, with motion initially away from the apex followed by motion toward the apex. There are usually two distinct apically directed peaks during diastole, one early in diastole (E′) and one following atrial contraction (A′). (*Adapted from Keane JF, Fyler DC, Lock JE. Nadas' Pediatric Cardiology, 2nd ed. Philadelphia: Elsevier/Saunders, 2006; Figure 15-18*).

KEY POINTS

- An E/A ratio can be used to evaluate left ventricular diastolic function.
- In children and adolescents with normal left ventricular diastolic function, E > A.
- Factors affecting left ventricular diastolic function include:
    - Preload.
    - Left ventricular systolic function.
    - Heart rate (HR).
    - Age.
    - Respiratory rate.

Step 4: Evaluate for Dyssynchrony

- Velocity vector imaging (VVI).
    - Method for calculation of delay between any two cardiac wall segments.
        - The endocardial border is traced in peak diastole using VVI software in the 4C and 2C views.
        - Myocardial velocity is calculated for six ventricular segments, and local velocities are tracked by the VVI algorithm.
    - Degree of dyssynchrony is quantified by comparing the regions (Fig. 16-4).
- Strain rate and strain imaging.
    - Strain rate is measured by TDI as the velocity difference between two regions in the myocardium divided by the distance between the two regions.
    - Quantifies myocardial deformation.
    - Correlates with left ventricular contractility.

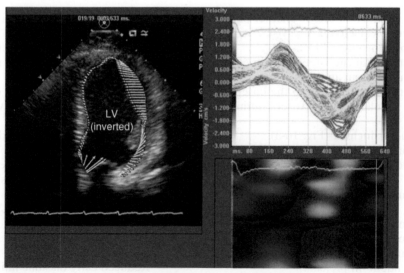

Figure 16-4. An example of velocity vector imaging (VVI) demonstrating dyssynchrony. With normal cardiac function, all vectors should be aimed toward each other in systole. The image on the left demonstrates the vectors, particularly in the basilar region, aimed in different directions. On the right of the VVI are graphic representations of standard deviation of time-to-peak velocity among different cardiac segments. These are consistent with the VVI, demonstrating that different segments of the heart reach peak velocity independently rather than simultaneously.

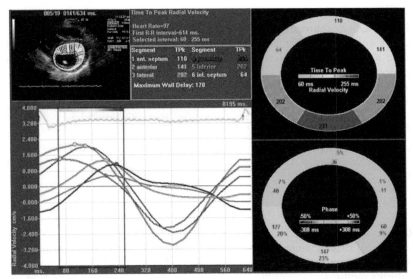

Figure 16-5. With normal cardiac function, there should be no significant difference in the time to peak strain. In this example of time to peak strain among six cardiac segments, significant dyssynchrony is noted with a maximum wall delay of 170 ms. Dyssynchrony in this patient stems from dyssynchronous motion of the lateral, posterior, and inferior segments.

- Strain is measured by integrating strain rate over time.
  - Measures the change in length corrected for the original length or fractional change from the original dimension.
  - Identifies regional diastolic asynchrony (Fig. 16-5).
  - Quantifies rate of myocardial deformation.

KEY POINTS

- Patients with CM have a greater degree of dyssynchrony.
- Strain imaging can detect myocardial dysfunction before the appearance of clinically significant global ventricular impairment.
- Useful in patients with systemic hypertension.

Step 5: Interrogate Cardiac Valves
- Use spectral and color flow Doppler for assessment of stenosis and regurgitation.

KEY POINT

- There is an increased incidence of valvular disease in patients undergoing chronic dialysis.

Endocrine

The most common endocrine diseases with cardiovascular effects include hypothyroidism, hyperthyroidism, and metabolic syndrome. A unique population in pediatrics are the infants born to diabetic mothers in whom significant congenital cardiac disease may develop, including both structural and prenatally acquired cardiac disease secondary to hyperinsulinemia.

Hypothyroidism
- Deficiency of thyroid hormone either from deficient production or a defect in the receptor, which may be congenital or acquired.
- Cardiovascular implications include
  - Bradycardia.
  - Cardiomegaly.
  - Pericardial effusion.
  - Hypertrophic cardiomyopathy (HCM).
  - Asymmetrical hypertrophy.

KEY POINT

- Amiodarone used to treat arrhythmias may cause hypothyroidism.

Hyperthyroidism
- Results from excess production of thyroid hormones triiodothyronine, thyroxine, or both.
- May be congenital in infants of mothers with untreated Graves' disease during pregnancy or acquired.
  - Cardiovascular implications include tachycardia.

KEY POINT

- Hyperthyroidism results in an increased kinetic state with hyperdynamic ventricular contractility.

Metabolic Syndrome

- Findings include obesity, atherogenic dyslipidemia, elevated blood pressure, impaired glucose tolerance, a prothrombotic state, and proinflammatory state.
- Metabolic syndrome increases the risk of atherosclerotic cardiovascular disease.

KEY POINTS

- Metabolic syndrome is present in 30% to 40% of overweight adolescents.
- Echocardiographic changes include:
  - Concentric LVH.
  - Increased LVM.

Maternal Diabetes

- Increased incidence of cardiac anomalies seen in children born to mothers with insulin-dependent diabetes mellitus.
- HCM is most commonly seen (Fig. 16-6).
  - Risk of CM is 18 times the risk among offspring of mothers not affected.
  - More commonly associated with septal hypertrophy.
  - May cause left ventricular outflow tract obstruction (LVOTO).
  - Usually regresses over time.
- Increased incidence of structural cardiac disease in children born to mothers with pregestational insulin-dependent diabetes mellitus.
  - Risk is 3.2 times higher than the risk if maternal diabetes was not present.
  - Structural lesions include ventricular septal defects (VSDs) and conotruncal lesions such as dextro transposition of the great vessels.

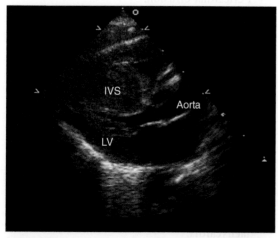

Figure 16-6. Parasternal long axis view demonstrating hypertrophic cardiomyopathy in an infant secondary to maternal diabetes exposure prenatally. Note the significant degree of septal hypertrophy that resulted in left ventricular outflow tract obstruction in this patient as well as obliteration of the left ventricular cavity in systole.

The Echo Exam: Step-by-Step Approach:

Step 1: Evaluate Cardiac Dimensions

- Use M-mode and 2D assessment of cardiac dimensions.

KEY POINTS

- Assess for left ventricular dilation and/or LVH using measurements indexed to BSA.
- Image using multiple planes including 4C and short axis views.

Step 2: Evaluate Cardiac Function

- Calculate the shortening fraction using M-mode or 2D measurements.
- Calculate the EF using a modified Simpson method or 5–6 area-length method.
- Evaluate for diastolic cardiac function including
  - Evaluation of mitral inflow (E and A wave velocities).
  - TDI.
  - VVI.
  - Strain rate and strain imaging.

KEY POINTS

- FS and EF may be increased secondary to hyperkinetic state.
- Obtain a cardiac rhythm strip during echocardiography when possible to evaluate for tachycardia.

Step 3: Evaluate Cardiac Structure

- Infants born to diabetic mothers are at increased risk of congenital heart disease.
- A full anatomic study should be performed on patients with clinical concerns.

KEY POINTS

- Fully interrogate the ventricular septum to evaluate for VSDs.
- Evaluate for structural lesions including conotruncal abnormalities and valvular lesions.
  - The aortic arch should be completely interrogated including both PW Doppler and continuous wave (CW) Doppler evaluation.
- Obtain CW Doppler measurements of both outflow tracts.
  - HCM is the most common cardiac disease seen in infants of diabetic mothers.
  - LVOTO may be present in cases of significant HCM.

Step 4: Evaluate for Pericardial Effusion

- Image from subcostal, parasternal short axis, and 4C views (Fig. 16-7).
- Measure effusion during diastole.
- Perform a spectral Doppler evaluation of the MV and tricuspid valve (TV).

KEY POINTS

- Expiratory right ventricular free wall collapse early in diastole can be a sign of tamponade.
- Expiratory right atrial collapse occurring in more than one third of the cardiac cycle indicates tamponade.
- Mitral inflow with more than 30% variation between inspiration and expiration is an indication of tamponade physiology (Fig. 16-8).

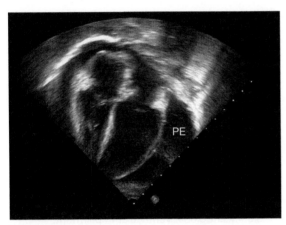

Figure 16-7. Subcostal 4C view demonstrating a large pericardial effusion (PE). Subcostal imaging is useful in identifying the location of the effusion for consideration of approach for percutaneous pericardiocentesis. In this image, the effusion is circumferential with a larger posterior pocket of fluid.

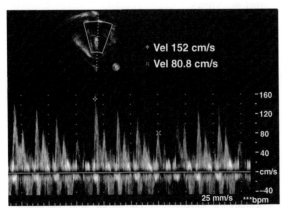

Figure 16-8. Spectral Doppler evaluation of the mitral valve inflow demonstrates more than 30% variation between inspiration and expiration, consistent with tamponade physiology.

Oncologic Disease

Chemotherapeutic agents and radiation are associated with the development of CMs.

- Dilated cardiomyopathy (DCM).
- Restrictive cardiomyopathy (RCM).
- Risk factors for CM:
  - Therapy at younger than 4 years of age.
  - Females.
  - Mediastinal irradiation.
  - Total cumulative dose; may be seen starting at a cumulative anthracycline dose of 400 to 600 mg/m^2.

KEY POINTS

- Anthracyclines.
  - Doxorubicin (Adriamycin) for oncologic processes including acute lymphocytic leukemia may cause a chronic, dose-related CM with left ventricular dysfunction.
- Can occur 3 to 8 weeks after last dose of drug.
- Incidence is related to cumulative dose, age at the time of anthracycline therapy, and duration since completion of therapy.
  - No safe dose.

Dilated Cardiomyopathy

- DCM is defined as an increased end-diastolic and/or end-systolic volume indexed to BSA in the presence of ventricular dysfunction (Fig. 16-9).
- Mitral regurgitation may be present.
- Decreased forward flow in the ascending aorta (Ao) by Doppler.
- Diastolic flow reversal can be seen in the descending aorta.

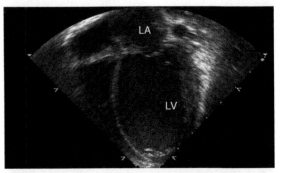

Figure 16-9. Apical 4C view demonstrating dilated cardiomyopathy with increased end-diastolic volume. The significant left ventricular dilation, which dwarfs the normal-size right ventricle, was accompanied by ventricular dysfunction in this patient.

Restrictive Cardiomyopathy

- The LA and right atrium (RA) may be markedly dilated at end-diastole and often exceed the size of the LV.
- The LV is normal in size with no appreciable LVH or dilation.
- Normal to near-normal left ventricular systolic function.
- Shortened mitral deceleration time (<150 ms) and becomes shorter with inspiration.
- May have mid-diastolic flow reversal across the MV.

The Echo Exam: Step-by-Step Approach

Step 1: Evaluate Cardiac Dimensions

- Use M-mode and 2D assessment of cardiac dimensions.
  - Measurements should be indexed to BSA to assess for left ventricular dilation and/or LVH.
  - Evaluate the RA and LA (qualitative assessment).

KEY POINTS

- Marked atrial dilation will be present with RCM (Fig. 16-10).
- Image using multiple planes including 4C and short axis views.

Step 2: Evaluate Cardiac Function

- Calculate the shortening fraction using M-mode or 2D measurements.
- Calculate the EF by a modified Simpson biplane method or 5–6 area-length method.

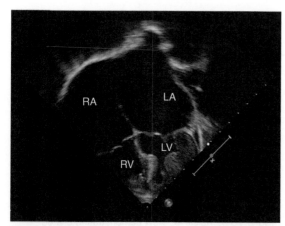

Figure 16-10. Apical 4C view demonstrating a restrictive cardiomyopathy with massive dilation of the left and right atrium (LA and RA). In this case, atrial size exceeds that of the ventricles.

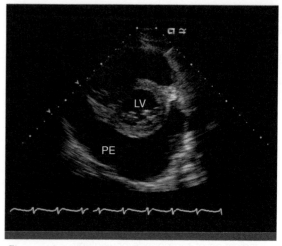

Figure 16-11. Parasternal short axis view of a large PE.

- Evaluate for diastolic cardiac function including
  - Evaluation of mitral inflow (E and A wave velocities).
  - TDI.
  - VVI.
  - Strain rate and strain imaging.

KEY POINTS

- The FS and/or EF are reduced in a cardiomyopathic state.
- Diastolic evaluation may detect myocardial dysfunction before the appearance of clinically significant global ventricular impairment.
- Patients with CM have a greater degree of dyssynchrony.

Step 3: Evaluate for Pericardial Effusion

- Image from subcostal, parasternal short axis, and 4C views.
- Measure effusion during diastole.
- Perform a spectral Doppler evaluation of the MV and TV (Fig. 16-11).

Suggested Reading

1. Lopez L, Colan S, Frommelt P, et al. Recommendations for quantification methods during the performance of a pediatric echocardiogram: a report from the Pediatric Measurements Writing Group of the American Society of Echocardiography Pediatric and Congenital Heart Disease Council. *J Am Soc Echocardiogr.* 2010;23:465-495. *This is an excellent resource for recommendations for pediatric echocardiogram measurements including left ventricular size and function.*
2. Khoury PR, Mitsnefes M, Daniels SR, et al. Age-specific reference intervals for indexed left ventricular mass in children. *J Am Soc Echocardiogr.* 2009;22:709-714. *Description of a standard method for indexing LVM in the pediatric population using height and age.*

3. Ucar T, Tutar E, Yalcinkaya F, et al. Global left ventricular function by tissue Doppler imaging in pediatric dialysis patients. *Pediatr Nephrol.* 2008;779-785. *Summary of cardiac findings and methods for echocardiographic assessment in patients with chronic renal disease including use of the MPI.*

4. Harkl AD, Cransberg K, Osch-Gevers MV, et al. Diastolic dysfunction in paediatric patients on peritoneal dialysis. *Nephrol Dial Transplant.* 2009;24:1987-1991. *This article examined the cardiovascular changes seen in pediatric renal patients on dialysis and after transplantation. Persistent changes were seen in function (both systolic and diastolic) as well as LVM even after renal transplantation.*

5. Kupferman J, Paterno K, Mahgerefeh J, et al. Improvement of left ventricular mass with antihypertensive therapy in children with hypertension. *Pediatr Nephrol.* 2010;25:1513-1518.

6. Chavers BM, Shuling L, Collins AJ, et al. Cardiovascular disease in pediatric chronic dialysis patients. *Kidney Int.* 2002;62:648-653. *Summary of cardiovascular risk factors in pediatric dialysis patients describing an increased incidence of cardiovascular morbidity and mortality in African American, female, and adolescent patients.*

7. Greenbaum LA, Warady BA, Furth SL. Current advances in chronic kidney disease in children: growth, cardiovascular, and neurocognitive risk factors. *Semin Nephrol.* 2009;29:425-434. *Comprehensive article sponsored by the National Institutes of Health reviewing the cardiovascular effects of renal disease and describing the development of LVH and diastolic dysfunction.*

8. Friedberg MK, Silverman NH, Dubin AM, et al. Mechanical dyssynchrony in children with systolic dysfunction secondary to cardiomyopathy: a Doppler tissue and vector velocity imaging study. *J Am Soc Echocardiogr.* 2007;20:756-763. *Excellent article describing how to use TDI and VVI for the assessment of dyssynchrony in pediatric patients with CM. This article specifically examines mechanical dyssynchrony in these patients rather than electrical dyssynchrony for this subset of patients.*

9. Lopez L. Advances in echocardiography. *Curr Opin Pediatr.* 2009;21:579-584. *Summary of echocardiographic assessment including strain imaging and its utility in the early assessment of cardiac dysfunction in renal and oncologic diseases in pediatric patients.*

10. DiBonito P, Moio N, Scilla C, et al. Preclinical manifestations of organ damage associated with the metabolic syndrome and its factors in outpatient children. *Atherosclerosis.* 2010;213:611-615. *A description of the cardiovascular findings associated with metabolic syndrome including LVH.*

11. Abu-Sulaiman RM, Subaih B. Congenital heart disease in infants of diabetic mothers: echocardiographic study. *Pediatr Cardiol.* 2004;25:137-140. *Summary of findings in infants of diabetic mothers including HCM and conotruncal defects.*

12. Van der Pal HJ, van Dalen EC, Hauptmann M, et al. Cardiac function in 5-year survivors of childhood cancer. *Arch Inter Med.* 2010;170:1247-1255. *Summary of the predictors for development of cardiac dysfunction in cancer patients including dose, cardiac irradiation, and younger age at diagnosis.*

Echocardiographic Assessment After Heart Transplantation

Mariska Kemna

17

Background

- Pediatric heart transplantation has been performed since the 1980s.
- Surgical technique involves left atrial anastomosis to avoid pulmonary vein (PV) stenosis as a consequence of PV anastomosis.
- Systemic venous connections are performed through a right atrial anastomosis in young children (Fig. 17-1) or a bicaval anastomosis in older children and adults (Fig. 17-2).
- Arterial connections are generally created in the ascending aorta (Ao) and main pulmonary artery (MPA).

Overview of Echocardiographic Approach

- Echocardiography (echo) serves multiple purposes after heart transplantation.[1]
- The focus of the echocardiographic exam shifts depending on the time since transplantation (Table 17-1).
- In the immediate post-transplantation period, all surgical connections should be carefully interrogated. In addition, acute graft dysfunction, pulmonary hypertension (PHTN), and pericardial effusions are major concerns.
- Surgical connections and graft function will need to be monitored indefinitely after transplantation.
- Some centers use echo for routine rejection monitoring after heart transplantation.
- Other centers monitor for rejection using cardiac biopsies, and echo can be used to guide the bioptome and screen for complications afterward.
- Dobutamine stress echo (DSE) can be used to monitor for graft coronary artery disease.

KEY POINTS

Postoperative concerns after heart transplantation that should be evaluated by echo include:
- Surgical connections.
- Pericardial effusion.
- Acute graft dysfunction: right ventricle and/or left ventricle (LV).
- PHTN.
- Rejection.
- Chronic graft dysfunction.
- Graft coronary artery disease.

Anatomic Imaging

- Focus on the surgical anastomoses between donor heart and recipient.
- All anastomoses should be interrogated in the appropriate views, either with transesophageal echo (TEE) or transthoracic echo (TTE) (Table 17-2).
- TEE should be done when the patient comes off cardiopulmonary bypass.

Venous Anastomoses

- Pulmonary side:
  - Left atrial anastomosis of the donor left atrium to recipient residual left atrial cuff is performed to avoid PV anastomosis.
  - This produces an echocardiographic image of gross atrial enlargement with an echodense suture line in the four-chamber (4C) view, which should not be mistaken for thrombus (Fig. 17-3).
  - Pulmonary venous obstruction should be excluded in the immediate post-transplantation period with echo Doppler on intraoperative TEE and subsequent TTE.
- Systemic side:
  - Right atrial anastomosis is performed in younger (smaller) children and bicaval anastomoses in older children and adults.
  - Right atrial anastomosis also creates an image of an enlarged right atrium with echodense suture line.

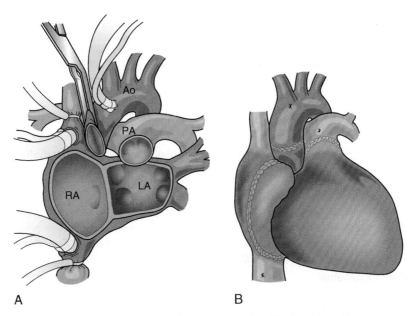

Figure 17-1. Biatrial anastomoses at the time of cardiac transplantation. The four sites of anastomoses between the donor and recipient are the left atrium, right atrium, aorta (Ao), and pulmonary artery (PA). *(From Mavroudis C, Backer CL. Pediatric Cardiac Surgery, 3rd ed. Philadelphia: Mosby; 2003.)*

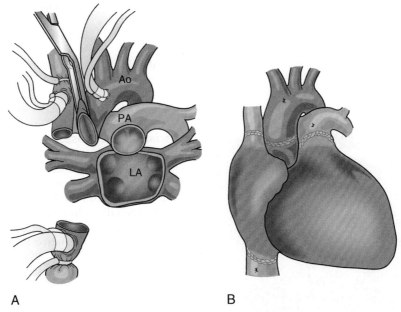

Figure 17-2. Bicaval anastomoses at the time of cardiac transplantation. The five sites of anastomoses between the donor and recipient are the left atrium, inferior vena cava, superior vena cava, Ao, and PA. *(From Mavroudis C, Backer CL. Pediatric Cardiac Surgery, 3rd ed. Philadelphia: Mosby; 2003.)*

- A bicaval connection should be interrogated for possible stenosis with Doppler imaging.
- Superior vena cava (SVC) flow velocity can be recorded from the suprasternal notch (SSN) or subcostal images. Normal SVC flow is biphasic with two distinct waves (S and D waves). A loss of this biphasic pattern or an increase in flow velocity of more than 1 m/s indicates obstruction.
- The inferior vena cava can be interrogated from the subcostal short axis (sagittal) view.
- Occasionally, abnormal congenital pulmonary and systemic connections in the native heart warrant construction of atrial

TABLE 17-1   USE OF ECHOCARDIOGRAPHIC MODALITIES AFTER TRANSPLANTATION

Immediately After Transplantation	1 Week to 1 Year After Transplantation	>1 Year After Transplantation
TEE: acute graft dysfunction (RV, LV)	TTE: RV function	DSE: graft coronary artery disease
TEE and TTE: RV pressure	TTE: RV pressure	
TEE and TTE: surgical connections	TTE: surgical connections	TTE: surgical connections
TTE: acute rejection	TTE: rejection	TTE: rejection
TTE: pericardial effusion	TTE: graft dysfunction	TTE: graft dysfunction

TABLE 17-2   TRANSESOPHAGEAL AND TRANSTHORACIC ECHOCARDIOGRAPHIC VIEWS TO ASSESS THE ANASTOMOSES BETWEEN THE DONOR HEART AND RECIPIENT

	TEE	TTE
Venous → Systemic → Right atrial	High esophageal 0 degrees (4C) or 90 degrees	Apical 4C view
→ Bicaval → SVC	High esophageal 90 degrees	SSN, subcostal coronal, and sagittal view
→ Bicaval → IVC	Gastroesophageal junction 90 degrees	Subcostal sagittal view
Venous → Pulmonary → Left atrial	High esophageal 0 degrees (4C)	Apical 4C view
→ PVs	High esophageal 0 degrees (4C) or 90 degrees	Suprasternal SAX view
Arterial → Systemic → Ascending Ao	High esophageal 120 degrees	Suprasternal LAX view
Arterial → Pulmonary → MPA	Very high esophageal 0 or 90 degrees	Parasternal SAX and LAX views

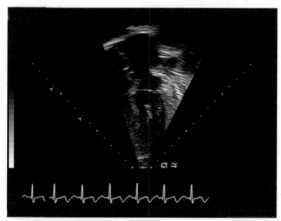

Figure 17-3. Apical four-chamber view in a heart transplant recipient showing left atrial enlargement with an echodense suture line.

baffles, which should be interrogated for obstruction.
- The presence of a left SVC in the recipient can also result in abnormal venous connections.

Arterial Anastomoses
- Pulmonary artery (PA):
  - MPA anastomosis should be interrogated for stenosis in the parasternal short axis and long axis views on TTE.
  - Occasionally, when native central PAs are abnormal, donor PAs are used, and the anastomosis with native PA tissue is made in the branch PA. These distal anastomoses will be more prone to stenosis but are sometimes poorly seen by echo, especially on TEE. When poorly seen, the presence of PA flow can be confirmed indirectly by presence of pulmonary venous flow.
- Aorta:
  - Aortic anastomosis is usually performed in the ascending Ao and can be evaluated for obstruction in the suprasternal long axis view on TTE.
  - If there is a native arch hypoplasia, an aortic arch reconstruction may be necessary, which should be evaluated for coarctation, analogous to methods described in Chapter 13, Myocardial Pathology.

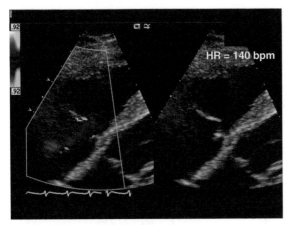

Figure 17-4. Severe tricuspid regurgitation in a heart transplant recipient secondary to a flail tricuspid valve leaflet.

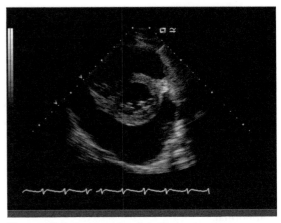

Figure 17-5. Large pericardial effusion in a heart transplant recipient with moderate cellular as well as antibody-mediated rejection.

Valve Regurgitation

- There is an increased frequency of tricuspid valve (TV) regurgitation in the transplant recipient population due to multiple factors:
  - Right atrial anastomosis.
  - Right ventricular dysfunction, especially early after transplantation.
  - PHTN, especially early after transplantation.
  - Rejection.
  - Chordal rupture as a complication of cardiac biopsy (Fig. 17-4).

Pericardial Effusion

- Pericardial effusion is relatively common after heart transplantation and has a different differential diagnosis than in the nontransplant recipient (Box 17-1).
- An effusion in the immediate postoperative period is most likely due to a surgical hematoma, but rejection is the most common cause of a new pericardial effusion at any other time after heart transplantation (Fig. 17-5).
- Pericardial effusions should be evaluated for size and signs of tamponade, according to methods described in Chapter 16.

Physiologic Data

Early Post-transplantation

- Another focus of TEE and TTE in the early post-transplantation period is acute graft dysfunction.
- TEE starts with a transgastric short axis view (probe advanced into stomach in a neutral position with anteflexion) to evaluate left ventricular systolic function (fractional shortening).

> **BOX 17-1 Differential Diagnosis of Pericardial Effusion After Heart Transplantation**
>
> Rejection
> Size discrepancy of native and donor heart
> Surgical hematoma (early post-transplantation)
> Perforation of ventricular free wall after cardiac biopsy
> Infectious pericarditis
> Inflammatory pericarditis
> Malignancy (mostly metastatic disease from lymphoma)

- Right ventricular dilation and systolic dysfunction are relatively common in the early post-transplantation period due to graft preservation injury and/or preexisting PHTN.
- Tricuspid regurgitant jet should be measured by pulsed wave (PW) Doppler for an estimation of right ventricular pressure.

Systolic Function

- Left ventricular systolic function (ejection fraction, fractional shortening, and posterior wall thickening fraction) is an important part of the TTE exam anytime after transplantation.
- A decrease in systolic function can be caused by preservation injury, rejection, transplant coronary disease, or obstruction to outflow (usually at the anastomosis site).

Diastolic Function

- LV diastolic function is often abnormal in early post-transplantation period due to perioperative ischemia, reperfusion injury, systemic hypertension, or side effects of immunosuppressive medications.

TABLE 17-3   ASSESSMENT OF DIASTOLIC FUNCTION

	Normal	Mild	Moderate	Severe
		↓ Relaxation	↓ Relaxation ↓ Compliance ↑ LVEDP	↓ Relaxation ↓↓ Compliance ↑↑ LVEDP
E/A ratio (mitral inflow)	1–2	<1 (reversed)	1–2 (pseudonormal)	>2
E′/A′ ratio (mitral annular TDI)	1–2	<1 (reversed)	<1 (reversed)	>1
IVRT (ms)	30–50 ms	↑	↓	↓

- Normalizes in the majority of patients within the first couple of months, but can remain abnormal.[2]
- Abnormal diastolic function can also be one of the first signs of rejection.
- Diastolic function can remain abnormal after rejection has been treated.

KEY POINTS

- Right ventricular dilation and decreased systolic function are relatively common in the early post-transplantation period and often normalize within days to weeks.
- Abnormal left ventricular diastolic function is often seen after transplantation.
- It will frequently recover within weeks to months but remains abnormal in a subgroup of patients.

Assessment of Diastolic Function
(Table 17-3)

- Left ventricular inflow velocity:
  - Measurement of E and A velocity performed at mitral leaflet tips in apical 4C view with PW Doppler.
  - Normal pattern of E velocity greater than A velocity is reversed with mild diastolic dysfunction.
  - More severe dysfunction can lead to a pseudonormal pattern.
  - Adult heart transplant recipients often show shortening of deceleration time of early diastolic filling.[3] However, deceleration time values have a very wide range in children[4] and therefore are not used as much as in adults.
- Tissue Doppler imaging (TDI).
  - TDI velocities of mitral annular motion (septal and lateral, obtained from the apical 4C view) are lower in transplant recipients than in normal controls.[2]
  - Can show a reversed (E′ < A′) or restrictive (E′ and A′ both <10 cm/s) pattern, especially in the first months after transplantation.

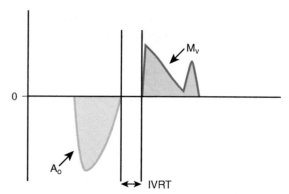

Figure 17-6. The isovolumic relaxation time (IVRT) is measured from aortic valve closure to mitral valve opening on the Doppler tracing, corresponding to the phase of the cardiac cycle where the left ventricular pressure is rapidly declining but left ventricular volume is constant. *(From Otto CM, Schwaegler RG. Echocardiography Review Guide. Philadelphia: Elsevier; 2008. Figure 7.11.)*

- Isovolumic relaxation time (IVRT).
  - IVRT is the interval between aortic valve closing and mitral valve (MV) opening at the onset of mitral forward flow.
  - It is obtained in the apical five-chamber view with the Doppler sample volume placed midway between inflow and outflow areas so that mitral inflow (above baseline) and left ventricular outflow (below baseline) are captured simultaneously (Fig. 17-6).
  - Normal values in children (30–50 ms) are lower than in adults.[4]
  - IVRT is often prolonged in pediatric heart transplant patients (55 ± 20 ms), suggesting mild diastolic dysfunction in the transplanted heart.[5]
  - Shortening of IVRT indicates more severe diastolic dysfunction with impaired ventricular compliance.

Assessment of Systolic and Diastolic Function

- Tei index or myocardial performance index (MPI).
  - A combined measure of systolic and diastolic performance.

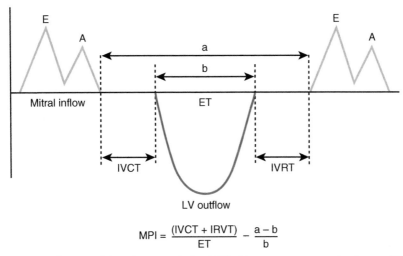

$$MPI = \frac{(IVCT + IRVT)}{ET} = \frac{a - b}{b}$$

Figure 17-7. Assessment of myocardial performance index (MPI). Measurements on pulsed wave (PW) Doppler of mitral inflow and aortic outflow. MPI = (a − b)/b; aortic ejection time (ET) = b.

- Equals isovolumic contraction time (IVCT) plus IVRT/aortic ejection time (Fig. 17-7).
- In the pediatric general population, abnormal when greater than 0.4.
- TDI is often increased in pediatric heart transplant recipients due to diastolic dysfunction.[5]
- Strain and strain rate imaging.
  - TDI technique that measures strain (shortening) and strain rate (velocity of shortening) of myocardial tissue.[6]
  - Strain is the amount of local deformation expressed as a percentage.
  - Positive strain describes thickening and negative strain describes shortening of a myocardial segment, related to its original size.
  - Able to differentiate between active and passive movement of myocardial segments, independent of overall cardiac motion.
  - Allows for early detection of myocardial dysfunction and intraventricular dyssynchrony.
  - Include myocardial viability studies and early detection of rejection and transplant coronary artery disease.
  - TDI strain rate imaging measures tissue movement compared with the transducer, in one dimension at a time, and is dependent on the angle of interrogation.
- Speckle tracking.
  - Measures regional tissue wall motion (myocardial deformation) by tracking speckles (natural acoustic markers) in a two-dimensional echo image and

determines the velocity from the changes in speckle position (with known frame rate).
  - In contrast to TDI strain rate imaging, speckle tracking can calculate strain and strain rate in multiple dimensions at a time: radial, circumferential, and longitudinal, independent of the angle of interrogation.

Rejection

KEY POINTS

- Rejection causes multiple changes in the transplanted heart.
- No single echocardiographic parameter can reliably predict rejection.
- However, an algorithm that involves multiple echocardiographic parameters increases sensitivity and can be used for rejection surveillance instead of routine cardiac biopsies.
- Echocardiographic signs of rejection:
  - Abnormal left ventricular diastolic function (early sign).
  - Decreasing left ventricular systolic function (late sign).
  - Rapidly increasing wall thicknesses (with decreased cavity size), especially in infants.
  - New pericardial effusion.
  - New-onset atrioventricular valve regurgitation (AVVR).

- Rejection causes multiple changes in the transplanted heart.
- Diastolic dysfunction occurs early in the process due to cellular infiltration and tissue edema, preceding systolic dysfunction.

- Many surveillance cardiac biopsies could be avoided with the ability to accurately diagnose subclinical rejection by echo.
- Unfortunately, no single echocardiographic parameter has sufficient negative and positive predictive power to reliably predict rejection.[7]
- Diastolic dysfunction is not specific enough because many transplant recipients have baseline abnormal diastolic function.
- Systolic dysfunction appears late in the process, and therefore systolic dysfunction alone is not sensitive enough.
- However, an algorithm that involves multiple echocardiographic parameters improves sensitivity and can reliably predict rejection.

Echocardiographic Rejection Surveillance

- Boucek et al.[8] developed an algorithm for diagnosing early rejection in pediatric heart transplant recipients that includes parameters of diastolic and systolic function (Box 17-2) as well as left ventricular mass (LVM), pericardial effusion, and AVVR.
- In the algorithm, measured patient values are compared with age-matched transplant recipients without rejection, and abnormal values provide points toward a total compiled rejection score.
- Abnormal values are dependent on patient age: younger than 6 months (Table 17-4) or older than 6 months (Table 17-5).
- A score of 5 or higher predicts significant rejection, especially if it signifies a change from the patient's own baseline values[9] (Figs. 17-8A and 17-9A).

- New-onset moderate or severe MV or TV regurgitation, newly depressed systolic function (fractional shortening <28%, with normal septal motion), or pericardial effusion predicts rejection, independent of the total rejection score.
- Echo rejection scores cannot reliably be applied until systolic and diastolic function has normalized after transplantation, although diastolic recovery is not always complete.
- In addition, there are marked variations between individuals after transplantation; hence, each patient should act as his or her own control.

TABLE 17-4   INFANT ECHO REJECTION SCORE (AGE < 6 MONTHS)

Parameter	Threshold	Score
LVEDV	<30% of predicted normal for BSA	1
LVM	>130% of predicted normal for BSA	1
LVEDV/LVM	<0.35	1
IVS thickening	<25%	1
LVPW thickening	<60%	2
Filling velocity of LV	<40 mm/s	1
Maximum velocity of LVPW thinning	<9 mm/s	1
New MR or TR	>Mild	1
E'/A'	<1.1	1

BOX 17-2 Components of the Pediatric Echo Rejection Score

Inflammatory parameters
Left ventricular end-diastolic volume (LVEDV)
LVM (increased wall thickness)
LVEDV/LVM
AVVR
Pericardial effusion

Systolic parameters
Left ventricular fractional shortening
IVS thickening fraction
LVPW thickening fraction

Diastolic parameters
Left ventricular filling velocity
Average-velocity LVPW thinning
Maximum velocity LVPW thinning
MV annulus E'/A'

TABLE 17-5   PEDIATRIC ECHO REJECTION SCORE (AGE > 6 MONTHS)

Parameter	Threshold	Score
LVEDV	<60% of predicted normal for BSA	2
LVM	>130% of predicted normal for BSA	1
LVEDV/LVM	<0.4	1
IVS thickening	<25%	1
LVPW thickening	<70%	2
Filling velocity of LV	<60 mm/s	1
Maximum velocity of LVPW thinning	<11 mm/s	2
Average velocity of LVPW thinning	<25 mm/s	1
New MR or TR	>Mild	1
E'/A'	<1.1	1

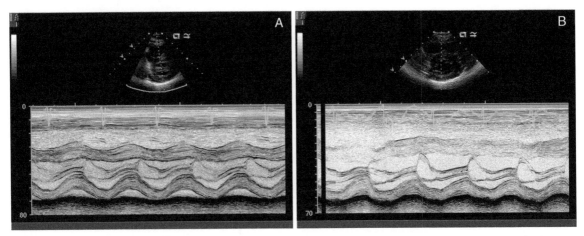

Figure 17-8. **A,** Acute cellular rejection in heart transplant recipient, diagnosed by echocardiography (echo) rejection score. The rejection score was 8 when left ventricular posterior wall (LVPW) thinning was evaluated by manual digitizer, and 6 when TDI velocities were used instead of the manual digitizer. **B,** M-mode of the LVPW of the same patient after treatment for rejection. The LVPW thinning velocity has improved, and the rejection scores are now 2 by manual digitizer and 1 by TDI velocities.

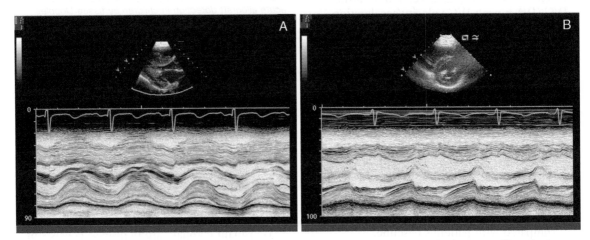

Figure 17-9. **A,** Acute cellular rejection in heart transplant recipient diagnosed by echo rejection score. The rejection score was 6 when LVPW thinning was evaluated by manual digitizer, and 9 when LV posterior wall TDI velocities were used instead of the manual digitizer. **B,** M-mode of the LVPW in the same patient after treatment for rejection. The LVPW thinning velocity has improved and the rejection scores are now 2 by manual digitizer and 1 by TDI velocities.

Requirements for Data Collection

- Echo machine with strip chart recorder at 100 mm/s.
- XY plotter to digitize endocardial tracings offline.
- Endocardial tracings are obtained from high-resolution M-mode, with gains set low for optimal definition of endocardium.
- Endocardial tracings from right ventricular septal surface, left ventricular septal surface, and left ventricular posterior wall (LVPW), as well as epicardial surface tracing of the left ventricular posterior wall from parasternal short axis view (close to the MV annulus).
- Maximum and average velocities of posterior wall thinning are determined by manual digitization of least three cardiac cycles, and results are averaged.
- This offline analysis of posterior wall thinning velocities is technically demanding, and therefore TDI velocities of the posterior wall can be used as an alternative. However, values determined by TDI are dependent on heart rate (HR) and cardiac afterload.

BOX 17-3 Criteria for Early Termination of DSE

Patient symptoms: chest pain, persistent
    headache, or discomfort
Systolic blood pressure higher than 200 mm Hg
    or more than two times the systolic blood
    pressure at rest
Diastolic blood pressure higher than 100 mm Hg
Decrease in blood pressure (>20% of resting
    value)
Arrhythmia
ST segment increase or decrease greater than
    2 mm
Definite wall motion abnormalities in two or
    more adjacent segments

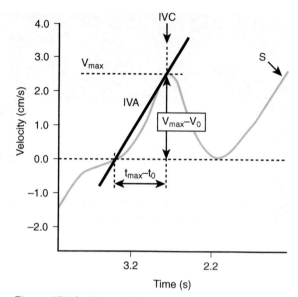

Figure 17-10. Myocardial acceleration during isovolumic
contraction was determined as the slope of the upstroke
of the isovolumic contraction wave. *(From Pauliks LB,
Pietra BA, DeGroff CG, et al. Non-invasive detection of
acute allograft detection in children by tissue Doppler
imaging: myocardial velocities and myocardial acceleration
during isovolumic contraction. J Heart Lung Transplant.
2005;24:S239–S248.)*

Other Echocardiographic Indicators of Rejection Described in Pediatric Heart Transplant Recipients

- Increase in the MPI; MPI of 0.64 or greater
  can indicate rejection.[10]
- Decrease in myocardial acceleration during
  IVC (IVA = peak IVC velocity/acceleration
  time), measured by TDI in basal left
  ventricular segments. IVA is independent of
  age or regional wall motion abnormalities and
  remains normal after heart transplantation, but
  decreases during rejection (baseline 1.1–1.4
  m/s², rejection 0.6–0.7 m/s²)[11] (Fig. 17-10).
- In the adult heart transplant recipient
  population, the following diastolic parameters
  have been associated with rejection:
  - Shortening of IVRT to less than 60 ms or
    decrease in IVRT of more than 20 ms.[12]
  - More than 10% decrease in early diastolic
    wall motion velocity of basal posterior wall
    by TDI (E′ in parasternal short axis view)
    compared with patient's baseline.
  - Longer early diastolic time (Tem = time
    from onset of second heart sound to the
    peak of the E′).[13]
- Strain and strain rate imaging might also prove
  valuable in rejection monitoring.
- A decrease in (radial) strain and strain rate has
  been associated with rejection in the adult
  transplant recipient population.[14]

Alternate Approach to Rejection Surveillance

- Although some experienced centers use echo
  to monitor for rejection, others use regular
  cardiac biopsies.
- Echo can help guide the bioptome toward the
  right ventricular side of the interventricular
  septum (IVS) for optimal tissue sampling.
- Echo is also used to monitor for complications
  after cardiac biopsy, including right ventricular

perforation with pericardial effusion or TV
regurgitation caused by rupture of TV
chordae.

Dobutamine Stress Echocardiography

- Transplant coronary artery disease consists of
  small-vessel disease with concentric intimal
  proliferation and is not easily visualized on
  coronary angiogram.
- Dobutamine increases myocardial oxygen
  demand.
- DSE provides functional assessment and can
  unmask myocardial ischemia, evidenced by
  reversible regional hypokinesis or akinesis.[15]

Protocol

- Dobutamine infusion at initial dose of 5 μg/
  kg/min, followed by 10 μg/kg/min, then
  increase every 3 minutes in increments of
  10 μg/kg/min to a maximum of 40 μg/kg/min.
- Monitor HR, blood pressure, and continuous
  12-lead electrocardiography.
- Obtain TTE images in four standard views of
  the LV (parasternal long axis, parasternal short
  axis, apical 4C, apical 2C) at baseline, each

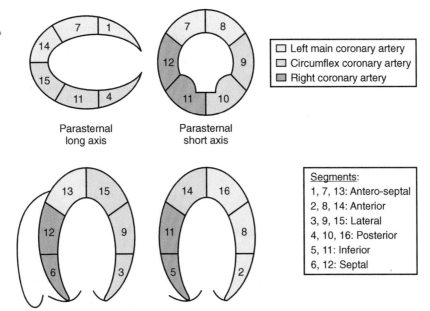

Parasternal
long axis

Parasternal
short axis

☐ Left main coronary artery
☐ Circumflex coronary artery
■ Right coronary artery

Segments:
1, 7, 13: Antero-septal
2, 8, 14: Anterior
3, 9, 15: Lateral
4, 10, 16: Posterior
5, 11: Inferior
6, 12: Septal

Figure 17-11. Echocardiographic views showing the 16-segment model of the left ventricle. *(From Di Filippi S, Semiond B, Roriz R, et al. Non-invasive detection of coronary artery disease by dobutamine-stress echocardiography in children after heart transplantation.* J Heart Lung Transplant. *2001;22:876–882.)*

stress stage (after 3 minutes of stable dose infusion), and after recovery to resting HR.

- Images are obtained in cine-loop format, with clear definition of the endocardium.
- Images are evaluated for new wall motion abnormality or worsening of baseline segmental abnormality in 16-segment model (Fig. 17-11).
- The endpoint is a target HR of 85% of the maximum HR predicted for age (220 minus age), but pediatric heart transplant recipients frequently do not reach this target, especially if general anesthesia is used during the study.
- The study is considered nondiagnostic unless the HR is at least 75% of the maximum predicted HR for age.
- DSE needs to be performed under supervision of a qualified medical professional in a procedure room with resuscitation equipment and medications readily available.
- Box 17-3 lists the criteria for early termination of DSE.

Troubleshooting
- If the target HR is not achieved, atropine (0.01–0.02 mg/kg/dose, minimum dose 0.1 mg, maximum dose 0.4 mg) may be added.
- The effects of dobutamine can be rapidly reversed with esmolol (0.1 mg/kg IV).
- Nitroglycerin sublingually or intravenously can be given for ischemia or hypertension.

Interpretation
- Integration of clinical, electrocardiographic, and echocardiographic data.
- ST segment changes indicate coronary ischemia.
- Rest and stress images are compared side by side in cine-loop format.
- Wall motion of the LV is assessed in 16 segments (see Fig. 17-11), and each segment is graded as hyperkinetic, normal, hypokinetic, akinetic, or dyskinetic.
- A normal response to dobutamine constitutes an increase in wall thickening.
- New hypokinesis, akinesis, or worsening of preexisting abnormality indicates myocardial ischemia.
- Improvement of resting wall motion abnormality with low-dose dobutamine indicates myocardial viability ("hibernating" or "stunned" myocardium).

KEY POINTS
- DSE can provide functional assessment of coronary flow and unmask myocardial ischemia.
- Myocardial ischemia is evidenced by reversible regional hypokinesis or akinesis in a 16-segment model of the LV.

References

1. Thorn EM, de Filippi CR. Echocardiography in the cardiac transplant recipient. *Heart Failure Clin.* 2007; 3:51-67.

2. Strigl S, Hardy R, Glickstein JS, et al. Tissue Doppler-derived diastolic myocardial velocities are abnormal in pediatric cardiac transplant recipients in the absence of endomyocardial rejection. *Pediatr Cardiol.* 2008;29: 749-754.

3. Burgess MI, Bhattacharyya A, Ray SG. Echocardiography after cardiac transplantation. *J Am Soc Echocardiogr.* 2002; 15:917-925.

4. Cui W, Roberson DA, Zen Z, et al. Systolic and diastolic time intervals measured from Doppler tissue imaging: normal values and Z-score tables, and effects of age, heart rate and body surface area. *J Am Soc Echocardiogr.* 2008;21:361-370.

5. Prakash A, Printz BF, Lamour JM, Addonizio LJ, Glickstein JS. Myocardial performance index in pediatric patients after cardiac transplantation. *J Am Soc Echocardiogr.* 2004 May;17(5):439-442.

6. Dandel M, Lehmkuhl H, Knosalla C, et al. Strain and strain rate imaging by echocardiography—basic concepts and clinical applicability. *Curr Cardiol Rev.* 2009;5: 133-148.

7. Mena C, Wencker D, Krumholz H, et al. Detection of heart transplant rejection in adults by echocardiographic diastolic indices: a systematic review of the literature. *J Am Soc Echocardiogr.* 2006;19:1295-1300.

8. Boucek MM, Mathis CM, Boucek RJ Jr, et al. Prospective evaluation of echocardiography for primary rejection surveillance after infant heart transplantation: comparison with endomyocardial biopsy. *J Heart Lung Transplant.* 1994;13:66-73.

9. Putzer GJ, Cooper D, Keehn C, et al. An improved echocardiographic rejection-surveillance strategy following pediatric heart transplantation. *J Heart Lung Transplant.* 2000;19:1166-1174.

10. Leonard GT Jr, Fricker FJ, Pruett D. Increased myocardial performance index correlates with biopsy-proven rejection in pediatric heart transplant recipients. *J Heart Lung Transplant.* 2006;25:61-66.

11. Pauliks LB, Pietra BA, DeGroff CG, et al. Non-invasive detection of acute allograft detection in children by tissue Doppler imaging: myocardial velocities and myocardial acceleration during isovolumetric contraction. *J Heart Lung Transplant.* 2005;24:S239-S248.

12. Dandel M, Hummel M, Meyer R, et al. Left ventricular dysfunction during cardiac allograft rejection: early diagnosis, relationship to the histological severity grade, and therapeutic implications. *Transplant Proc.* 2002;34: 2169-2173.

13. Dandel M, Hummel M, Muller J, et al. Reliability of tissue Doppler wall motion monitoring after heart transplantation for replacement of invasive routine screenings by optimally timed cardiac biopsies and catheterizations. *Circulation.* 2001;104:I184-I194.

14. Marciniak A, Eroglu E, Marciniak M, et al. The potential clinical role of ultrasonic strain and strain rate imaging in diagnosing acute rejection after heart transplantation. *Eur J Echocardiogr.* 2007;8:213-221.

15. Di Filippi S, Semiond B, Roriz R, et al. Non-invasive detection of coronary artery disease by dobutamine-stress echocardiography in children after heart transplantation. *J Heart Lung Transplant.* 2001;22:876-882.

Index

Printed and bound by CPI Group (UK) Ltd, Croydon, CR0 4YY

03/10/2024

01040303-0003